AF316733

AORTIC REGURGITATION

Collected Reprints
(1962-2019)

By

WILLIAM C. ROBERTS, MD
and
COLLEAGUES

ISBN: 979-8-88862-163-9
Printed in the United States of America on acid-free paper.

Preface

Many patients with aortic stenosis and/or mitral stenosis have some degree of regurgitation. That type of regurgitation is not the focus of this selection. The focus herein concerns patients with pure aortic regurgitation (AR), i.e., no element of valve stenosis. If a valve is stenotic, the valve cusps or leaflets are always abnormal. If a valve dysfunction is pure regurgitation, the valve structure may be entirely normal. Pure AR may result from dysfunction of the valve cusps (bicuspid aortic valve, infective endocarditis, etc.) or from abnormality of the ascending aorta (syphilis, the Marfan syndrome or its forme fruste variety, etc.). Although systemic hypertension (in 65 million Americans) can cause pure AR by dilating the ascending aorta, the degree of AR is usually mild and not life threatening and does not require aortic valve or aortic intervention. A variety of causes of pure AR are illustrated in this collection.

—*William C. Roberts, MD*

Table of Contents

*Articles are numbered based on WCR's CV.

Traumatic Aortic Regurgitation[*]

Robert J. Levine m.d., William C. Roberts, m.d. and Andrew G. Morrow, m.d.

Bethesda, Maryland

Nonpenetrating trauma to the chest often results in injury to the heart[1,2] which may vary in severity from rapidly fatal cardiac rupture to asymptomatic lesions detectable only by serial electrocardiograms or serum enzyme determinations. It is not generally appreciated that as many as 38 per cent of patients sustaining chest injuries may also show evidence of cardiac damage.[3]

A patient herein described had a variety of manifestations of trauma to the heart. These included pericardial effusion, myocardial contusion, complete heart block and rupture of the aortic valve. For several reasons the diagnosis was elusive at first. The chest trauma, which the patient considered too trivial to mention, was followed after several symptom-free days by the gradual onset of disability associated with atypical auscultatory findings. Of the several cardiac lesions in this patient, we have considered the ruptured aortic valve in greatest detail because it is potentially amenable to a definitive corrective procedure. In addition, the clinical and pathologic findings in previously reported patients with aortic regurgitation due to nonpenetrating chest trauma are summarized.

Case Report

W. R., a 35 year old prize fighter, was in excellent health until May 1960, when a box weighing over 500 pounds slid from the back of a truck and knocked him to the ground, causing sudden violent compression of his chest. He was stunned momentarily and had difficulty catching his breath but recovered spontaneously within ten minutes without residual discomfort. He regarded this trauma as trivial. Two or three days later he developed night sweats, progressively increasing fatigability and, after one week, dyspnea with exertion. Two weeks following the injury he began to have spontaneous episodes of nausea, vomiting and dizziness. After three days of such attacks he lost consciousness during a particularly severe bout of vomiting. He was brought to a hospital near his home where he was found to have a pulse rate of 30 per minute and a blood pressure of 90/50 mm. Hg. There were physical signs of complete heart block, but no murmurs or cardiomegaly were evident. The electrocardiogram (Fig. 1A) showed complete heart block with a ventricular rate of 29 but no evidence of left ventricular ischemia or hypertrophy. Laboratory studies gave normal values; these included hematocrit, white blood cell count with differential, erythrocyte sedimentation rate, urinalysis, serologic test for syphilis, serum glutamic oxalacetic transaminase, C-reactive protein, multiple blood cultures, blood urea nitrogen, fasting blood sugar, cholesterol and electrolytes. Chest roentgenogram and gastrointestinal x-ray series showed no abnormalities. On the third hospital day there was a rise in the sedimentation rate which persisted for about three weeks. The patient remained afebrile during six weeks of observation, and there was no significant alteration in the white blood count or the serum transaminase.

The heart rate responded to sympathomimetic amines, and the cardiac rhythm in the electrocardiogram gradually returned to first degree heart block within two weeks. By this time he had developed a pericardial friction rub and an apical systolic murmur. The heart sounds became quite distant, and this finding was interpreted as being due to pericardial effusion. A blowing diastolic murmur was later heard along the left sternal border. Because he was thought to have myocarditis, treatment with prednisone, 20 mg. daily, was given for about three months without apparent benefit.

In August 1960 he was readmitted to his local hospital because of persistent cough and dyspnea on exertion. At this time the pulse rate was 76 per minute and the blood pressure 110/60 mm. Hg. The heart was not clinically enlarged. A grade 2, blowing, diastolic decrescendo murmur was best heard at the left sternal border, and there was a grade 2 systolic murmur at the apex of the heart. The electrocardiogram now showed left axis deviation and persistent prolongation of the P-R interval (Fig. 1B). Again several blood cultures were negative and the sedimentation rate was elevated. Digitalis was added to his treatment because of evidence of left ventricular failure.

Physical Examination: On October 10, 1960, the

* From the Clinics of Experimental Therapeutics and Surgery, National Heart Institute and Department of Pathologic Anatomy. The Clinical Center, National Institutes of Health, Bethesda, Maryland.

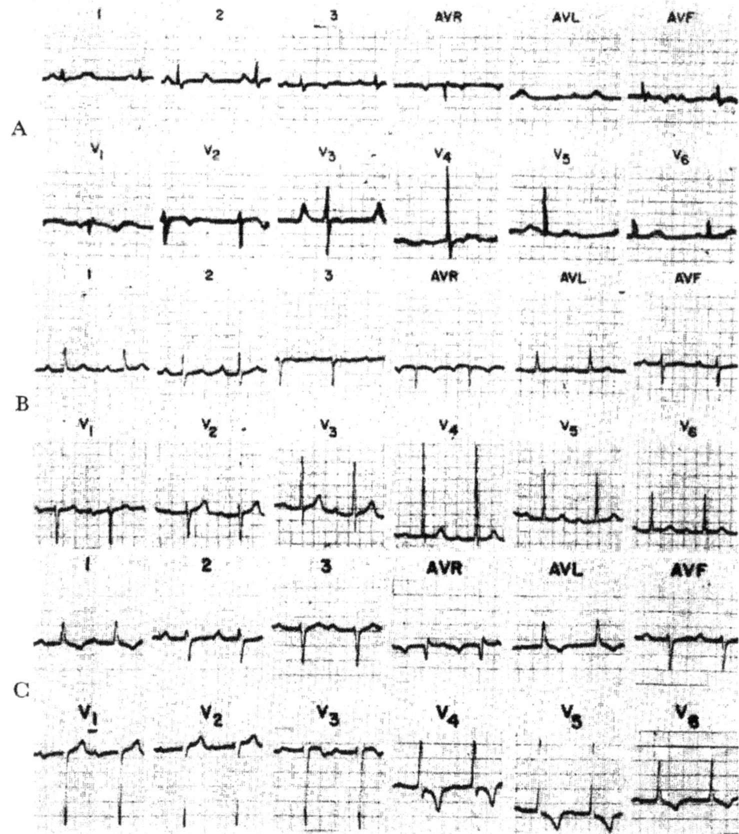

Fig. 1. Serial electrocardiograms. A, May 20, 1960, two weeks after injury. Complete heart block is present. B, July 14, 1960, seven weeks later. There is a prolonged P-R interval and a shift of the electrical axis to the left. C, October 11, 1960, five months after injury. First degree heart block persists. There is now evidence of left ventricular hypertrophy and ischemia and further shift of the electrical axis to the left.

patient was admitted to the National Heart Institute. The blood pressure was 110/60 mm. Hg, the pulse rate 100 per minute, and he was in no distress. The lungs were clear. There was a prominent left ventricular lift. The heart sounds were faint and regular. A short, rough, early systolic murmur which appeared to originate in the aortic area was heard over the entire precordium. A grade 3 early diastolic blowing murmur was heard best along the left sternal border. At the apex, in late diastole, this murmur assumed a rumbling quality (Austin Flint murmur). Near the apex was a high-pitched systolic rub heard with inspiration (pleuropericardial rub). Neither hepatomegaly nor peripheral edema was present. Numerous hematologic, bacteriologic and chemical studies were normal, with the following exceptions: The BUN was 27 mg. per 100 ml., and the sedimentation rate was 23 mm. per hour.

Roentgenographic study of the chest (Fig. 2) with barium swallow showed moderate cardiomegaly with left ventricular predominance. The ascending aorta bulged to the right, having the appearance of aneurysmal dilation. No intracardiac calcification was observed. The *electrocardiogram* showed a P-R interval of 0.34 second with evidence of left ventricular hypertrophy and ischemia and left axis deviation (Fig. 1C).

During the patient's hospital stay a marked variation in his blood pressure was recorded with systolic readings as high as 140 mm. Hg and diastolic values ranging from 0 to 60 mm. Hg. After several weeks of observation, when questioned specifically about the occurrence of chest trauma, he mentioned for the first time to a physician the injury described previously.

Cardiac catheterization was performed in November 1960. Right-sided pressures were normal with the exception of a pulmonary artery pressure of 42/25 mm. Hg (mean pressure 32). There was no evidence of an intracardiac shunt. Left heart catheterization by the transseptal technic demonstrated a mean left atrial pressure of 26 mm. Hg. The left ventricular systolic pressure was 100 mm. Hg, and the end-diastolic pressure in the ventricle was 50 mm. Hg.

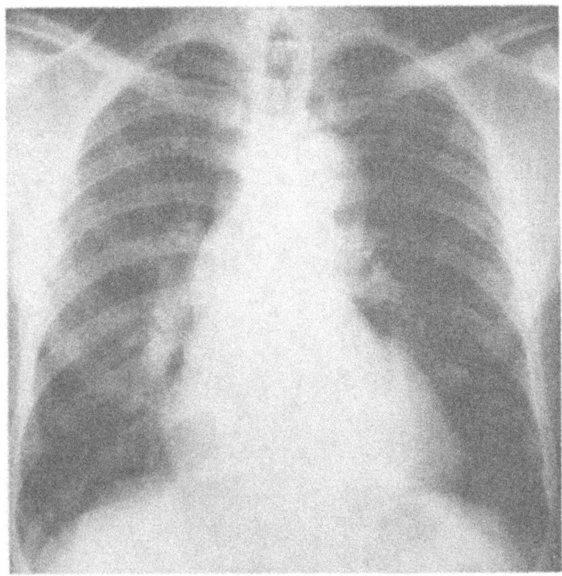

FIG. 2. Chest roentgenogram (PA projection). There is generalized cardiomegaly with left ventricular predominance and striking dilation of the ascending aorta.

The brachial artery pressure was 110/50 mm. Hg. The cardiac output, determined by dye dilution technic, was 3.1 liters per minute.

Retrograde aortography showed gross aortic regurgitation. Indicator dye injected into the aorta at the level of the eleventh thoracic vertebra was detected by sampling within the left ventricle.[4]

Surgical Findings: On the basis of the findings noted above, the diagnosis of traumatic rupture of the aortic valve seemed established, and an operation for its correction was undertaken. Through a longitudinal incision in the ascending aorta, the valve was exposed during complete cardiopulmonary bypass and hypothermic cardiac arrest. It appeared that the left anterior leaflet had been avulsed from its attachment at the commissure between it and the posterior leaflet (Fig. 3). The leaflet was re-attached and the commissure plicated with two mattress sutures reinforced with Teflon[®] felt, as shown in Figure 4. Following the repair, however, efforts to restore ventricular action were unsuccessful.

The intact, fresh heart was placed in the Davila pulse duplicator[5] in order to study the function of the aortic valve. At a rate of 70 to 80 per minute, the

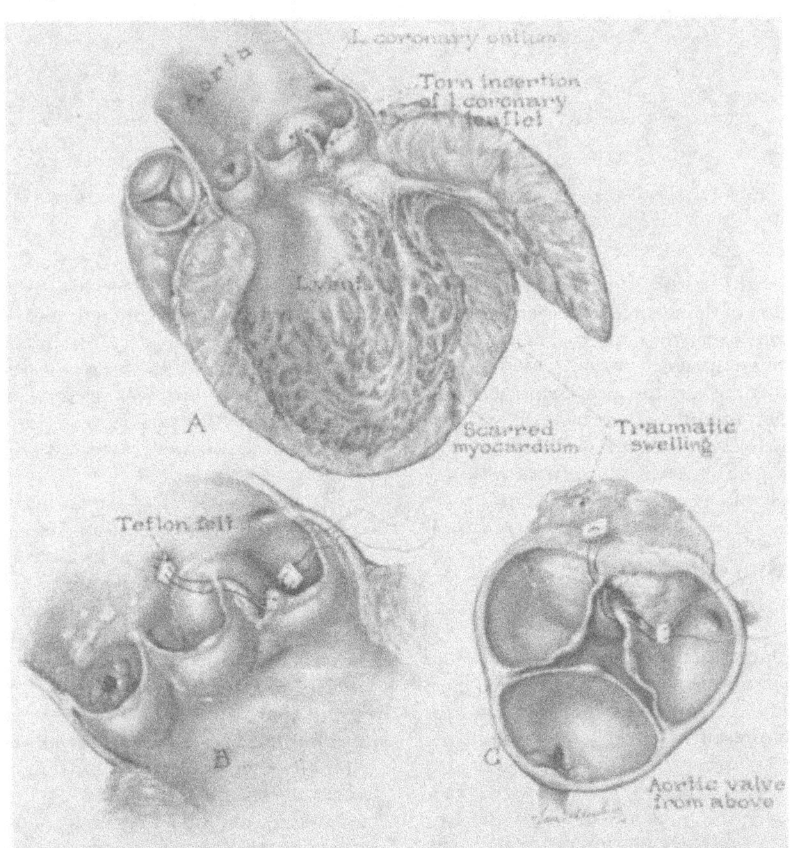

FIG. 3. Appearance of the aortic valve lesion and method of surgical repair employed.

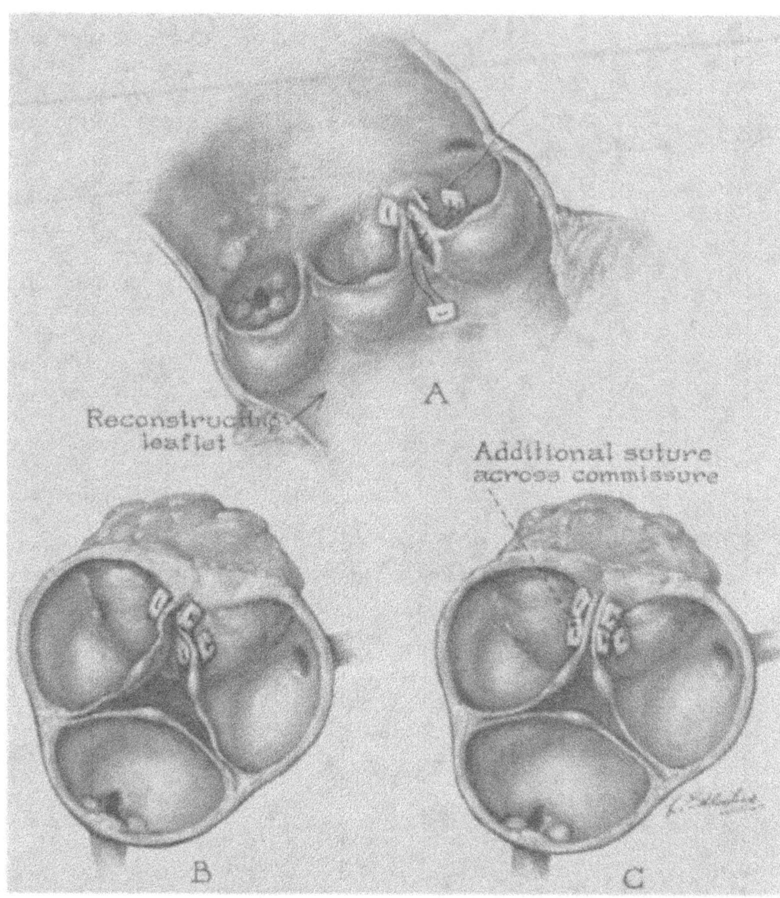

FIG. 4. Following re-attachment of the valve leaflet, another similar suture was placed across the newly reconstructed commissure.

aortic valve, both with the surgical repair intact and following the removal of the sutures, was incompetent. It was observed, however, that the more rapid the heart rate, the more competent was the reconstructed aortic valve. Indeed, when the heart rate was approximately 130 per minute, the orifice of the surgically repaired aortic valve closed well during ventricular diastole (Fig. 5). After the sutures were removed, the valve was grossly incompetent at all rates (Fig. 6).

PATHOLOGIC FINDINGS

GROSS FINDINGS

The heart was enlarged and weighed 600 gm. The right atrium and ventricle were hypertrophied and moderately dilated. A valvular-competent patent foramen ovale was present. The tricuspid and pulmonic valves were normal. The left atrium was also moderately dilated and hypertrophied, and its endocardium, particularly that portion between the anterior mitral leaflet and the foraman ovale, was thickened. The anterior leaflet of the mitral valve was thickened, but the posterior leaflet and the mitral chordae tendineae were normal. The left ventricle was hypertrophied and dilated. Its wall measured 1.7 cm. in greatest thickness, and 0.8 cm. at its thinnest point, the apex. A fibrous scar, measuring 3 by 1 by 1 cm., was present in the anterolateral wall of the left ventricle (Fig. 7). Several smaller fibrous scars also were noted in the adjacent anterolateral papillary muscle.

The aortic valve "ring" measured 8 cm. in circumference; the pulmonic valve ring, 7 cm. Within the aortic valve there was a localized, smooth-surfaced, firm "bulge," measuring 2.5 by 2.5 by 1.5 cm., which was located directly behind the commissural attachments of the posterior and left anterior aortic cusps and which protruded equally into the dilated left anterior and posterior sinuses of Valsalva (Fig. 8). In the space produced by the separation of the left anterior and posterior (noncoronary) cusps, and overlying the mid-portion of the bulge, there was a depressed area, measuring 0.2 by 0.3 cm., which was covered by necrotic material. The commissural attachment of the left anterior aortic cusp was torn free and displaced downward toward the left ventricle. The portions of the aortic leaflets adjacent to the

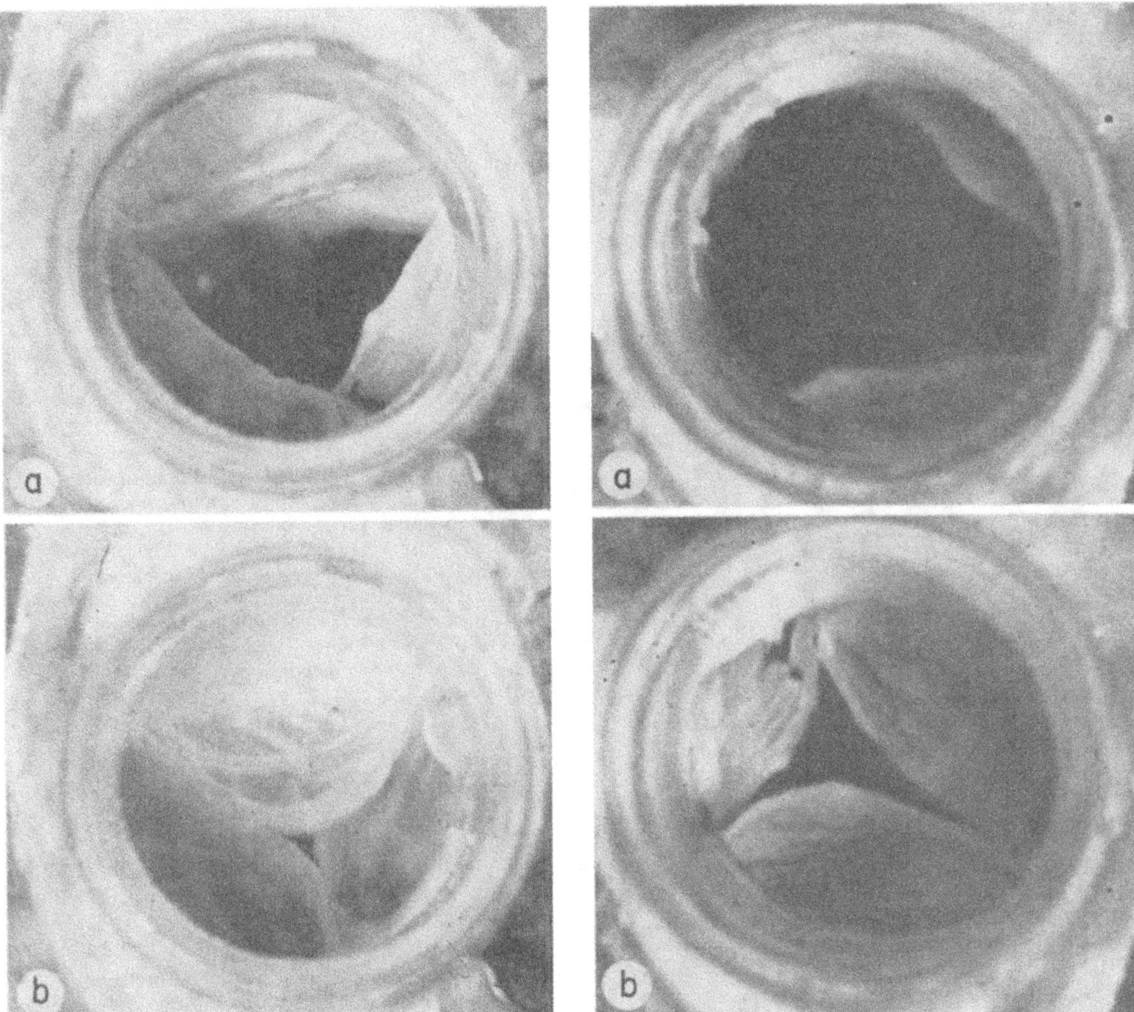

FIG. 5. Views of the aortic valve as it functioned on the Davila pulse duplicator. The surgical repair is intact. The heart rate was approximately 130 per minute. a, maximal opening of aortic valve during ventricular systole. b, maximal closure of aortic valve during ventricular diastole.

FIG. 6. Views of aortic valve functioning on the Davila pulse duplicator following the removal of the sutures re-attaching the leaflet. The heart rate was 70 to 80/min. a, maximal opening of the aortic valve during ventricular systole. b, maximal closure of the aortic valve during ventricular diastole.

protruding nodule were thickened, particularly in their margins; otherwise, these leaflets were delicate and pliable. On section through the nodule or bulge, it was found to lie between the intimal surface of the aortic sinus and the epicardial surface of the left atrium (Fig. 9A). The ostium of the left coronary artery was displaced upward, arising above the commissural attachments (Fig. 8). The ostium of the right coronary artery was normally located. The distribution of each coronary artery was normal. The right one showed a mild degree of atherosclerosis. A few atheromata were present in the ascending aorta, particularly about the ostium of the right coronary artery. Approximately one centimeter distal to the aortic valve, the ascending aorta became ex-

tremely thin and fragile, but at no point was its wall interrupted or broken.

MICROSCOPIC FINDINGS

Aorta and Aortic Valve: Histologically the nodule consisted predominantly of fibrocollagenous tissue (Fig. 9B). Within the extremely thick fibrous wall of the sinus of Valsalva an area of necrosis was present, and just proximal to the base of the aortic cusp a large abscess was noted (Fig. 10). The central portion of the abscess contained many necrotic cells surrounded by a thin irregular band of epithelioid cells. Around this was a large collection of plasma cells, lymphocytes, fibroblasts and a striking number of eosinophils. Fibrocollagenous tissue, which con-

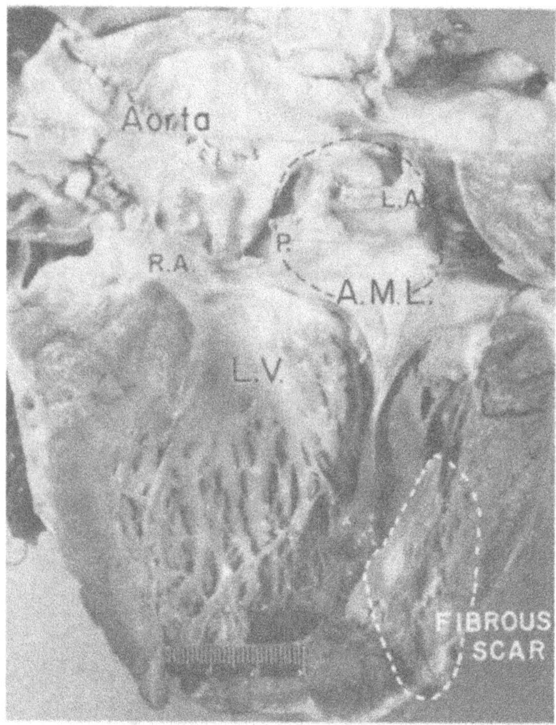

Fig. 7. The left ventricle, aortic valve and aorta are opened. The "bulge" at the aortic valve is enclosed in the black-lined circle. A fibrous scar, which probably represents an old contusion, is enclosed in the white-lined circle. L.V. = left ventricle; A.M.L. = anterior mitral leaflet; R.A. = right anterior cusp; P = posterior cusp; L.A. = left anterior cusp of the aortic valve. Both the left ventricle and aortic valve are dilated. The surgical incision is apparent in the ascending aorta.

tained dilated veins, thick-walled arteries, extravasated red blood cells, and occasional foci of plasma cells and lymphocytes surrounded these latter cells.

The area of necrosis within the sinus of Valsalva, in contrast to the abscess, was open to blood traversing the aortic valve (Fig. 10). The necrotic material was surrounded by numerous lymphocytes, plasma cells and fibroblasts, but not by eosinophils. The adventitia of the entire ascending aorta consisted of thick fibrous tissue which also contained focal collections of lymphocytes and plasma cells, and many thick-walled arteries, the lumina of some being almost completely occluded. The inflammatory cells in the adventitia were irregularly distributed and not located in the regions of the vasa vasorum. There was virtual absence of elastic fibers in the media of the aorta behind the torn aortic cusp extending approximately one centimeter distal to the sinus of Valsalva. The configuration of the elastic fibers distal to the aortic valve, however, was normal. No mucopolysaccharride material (Rinehart stain) was present in the media of the ascending aorta. Special stains of the sections of the aortic bulge for bacteria (Brown and Brenn), spirochetes (Steiner) and fungi (periodic

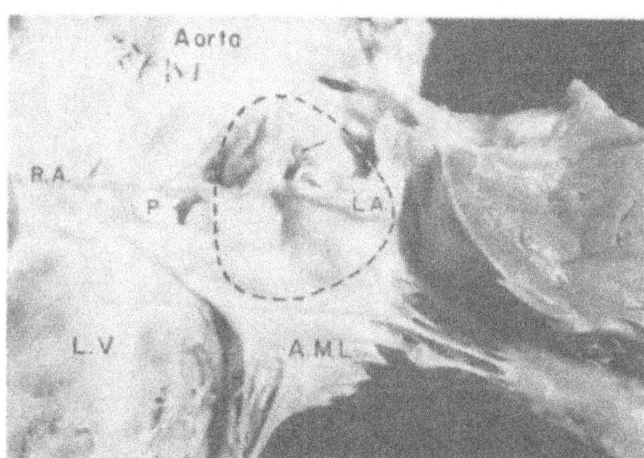

Fig. 8. A close-up view of the aortic valve "bulge." It is continuous with the anterior mitral leaflet (A.M.L.) and lies behind the left anterior (L.A.) and posterior (P) cusps of the aortic valve. The commissural attachment of the left anterior cusp has been torn. The area of necrosis in the bulge is identified by the arrow. The ostium of the left coronary artery is displaced upward. The ostium of the right coronary artery, which is normally located, is hidden behind the right anterior (R.A.) cusp of the aortic valve. The tear in the posterior (P) aortic cusp was produced by the prosector and is an artifact.

acid-Schiff and methenamine silver) showed no organisms, and no hemosiderin deposits were seen with the iron stain.

Left Ventricle: Histologic study of the left ventricular fibrous scar (Fig. 11) revealed a marked diffuse replacement of myocardial fibers by thick fibrous tissue which was free of inflammatory cells and of hemosiderin deposits (iron stain). The right and left coronary arteries were widely patent, although each showed a mild amount of intimal thickening. The myocardial fibers throughout the left ventricle were hypertrophied. The endocardium of the left atrium was thickened by fibrous proliferation.

There was acute congestion of the lungs, liver, spleen and kidneys. Sections from the vertebrae, hip and knee joints showed no evidence of arthritis. Sections from the bowel, endocrine glands and central nervous system were not remarkable.

DISCUSSION

Gore[6] suggests that many instances of heart disease are incorrectly attributed to trauma or strain, particularly when compensation or disability insurance is involved. He emphasizes the difficulty of being certain of a diagnosis of traumatic heart disease, sometimes even at autopsy. There is, however, no cause for doubt that the cardiac problem in this patient resulted from the traumatic event he described. He was in superb condition, running five miles daily, until his accident. No abnormalities had been detected at the physical examinations

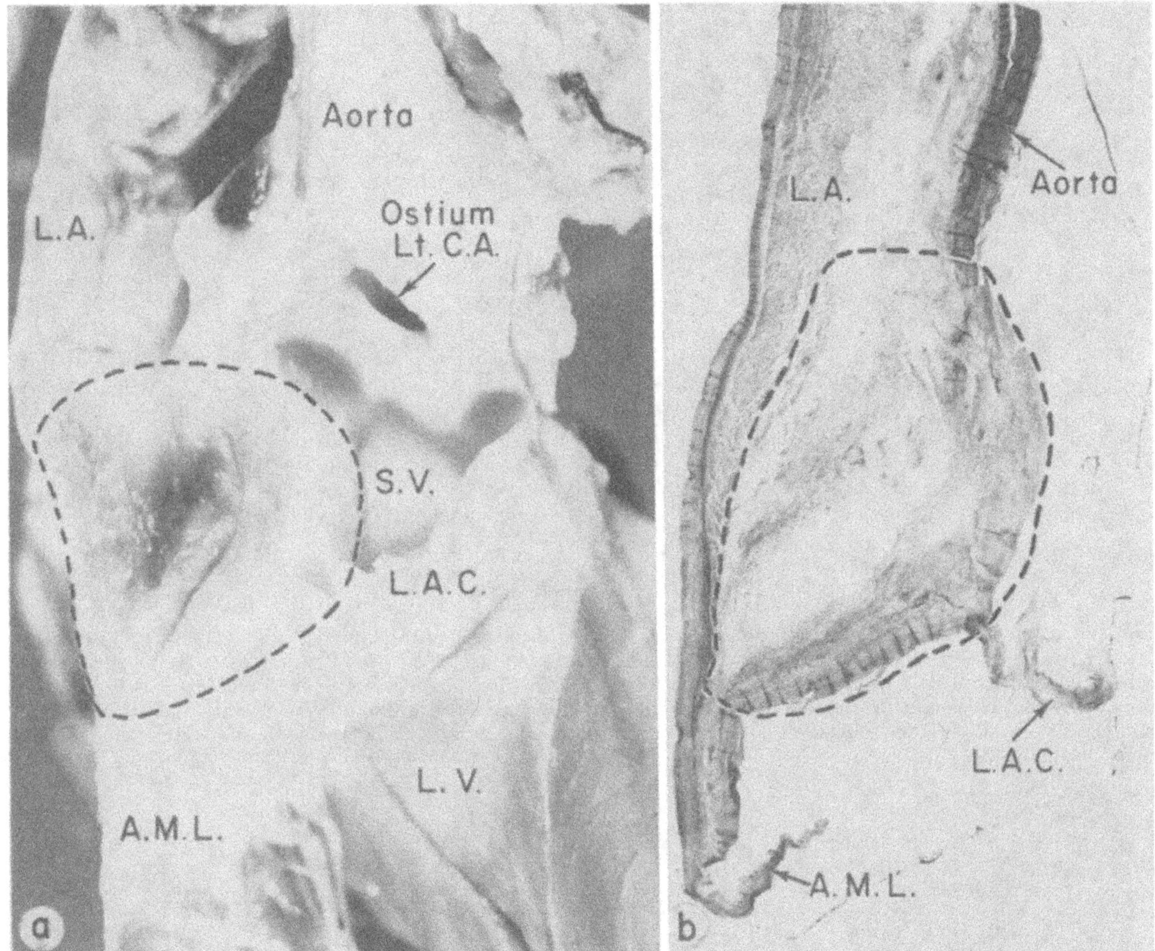

Fig. 9.   a, view following longitudinal section of the "bulge," anterior mitral leaflet (A.M.L.) left atrium (L.A.) and ascending aorta. The bulge is outlined by the black-dashed circle. The dark portion within the bulge is hemorrhagic material. The anterior portion of the bulge consists of the wall of the aorta behind the left anterior cusp (L.A.C.) of the aortic valve. The sinus of Valsalva (S.V.) is indicated.   b, photomicrograph of the cut-surface illustrated in a. The bulge again is circled. There is extreme thickening of the wall of the aorta, particularly its most proximal part. Elastic tissue stain, original magnification ×4.5.

which had preceded each of his boxing matches. Shortly following the injury his health began to deteriorate rapidly. It did not occur to him that his injury could have contributed to his illness. The clinical and postmortem studies described above disclosed no other cause of heart disease.

This patient had a pericardial effusion and extensive contusion of the myocardium. These are the most common cardiac lesions following blunt chest trauma.[2,7,8] Myocardial contusion may be so mild that it is without symptoms and can be detected only by special studies,[3] or it may be sufficiently severe to result in immediate or delayed cardiac rupture. Myocardial infarction due to coronary arterial occlusion may be closely imitated by contusion.[9] Contusion commonly involves the anterior wall of the left ventricle and the interventricular septum. Involvement of the septum and the conductive tissue may result in atrioventricular conduction defects. Complete heart block is usually transient, as in the patient described herein, but may be permanent.[10]

Rupture of the aortic valve, though unusual, is the valvular lesion most frequently observed in patients surviving nonpenetrating cardiac injury.[2] Howard[11] cities experimental evidence that tears in the cusps of the aortic valve may be produced in dogs and in human cadavers by blunt trauma to the chest or by suddenly increasing the pressure in the aorta.

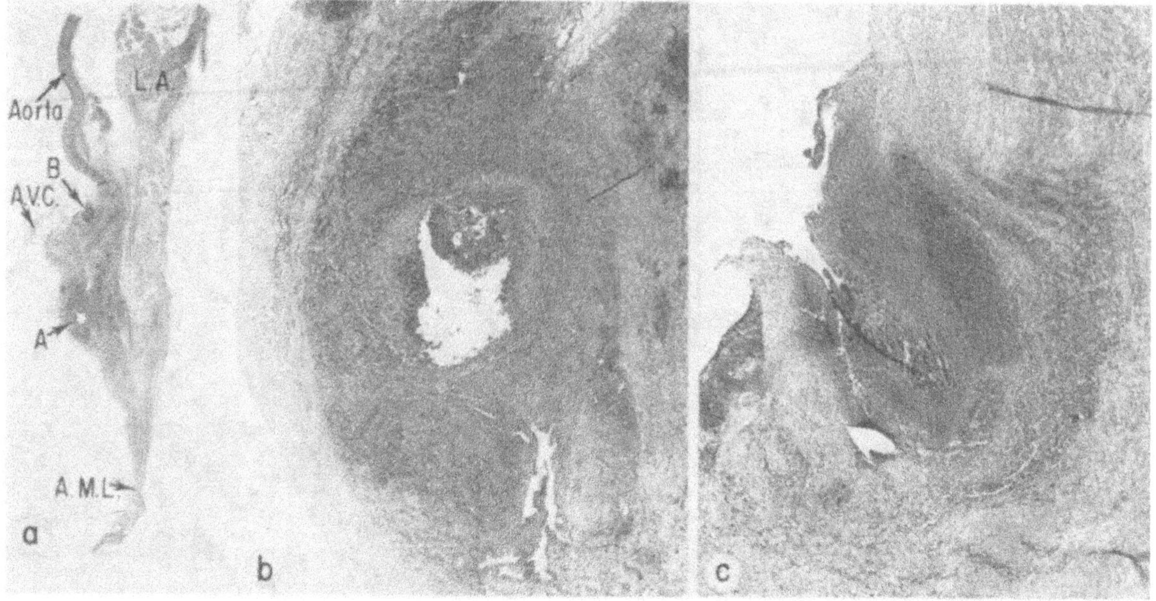

Fig. 10. *a*, photomicrograph of longitudinal section through the center of the "bulge." The anterior mitral leaflet (A.M.L.), aortic valve cusp (A.V.C.), aorta, and left atrium (L.A.) are illustrated. A designates the subendocardial abscess which is illustrated in *b*. B represents the focus of necrosis illustrated in *c*. The bulge extends from arrow A to arrow B. Hematoxylin and eosin stain, original magnification × 1.8. *b*, abscess shown in *a*. Hematoxylin and eosin stain, original magnification ×18. *c*, area of necrosis shown in *a*. Hematoxylin and eosin stain, original magnification ×28.

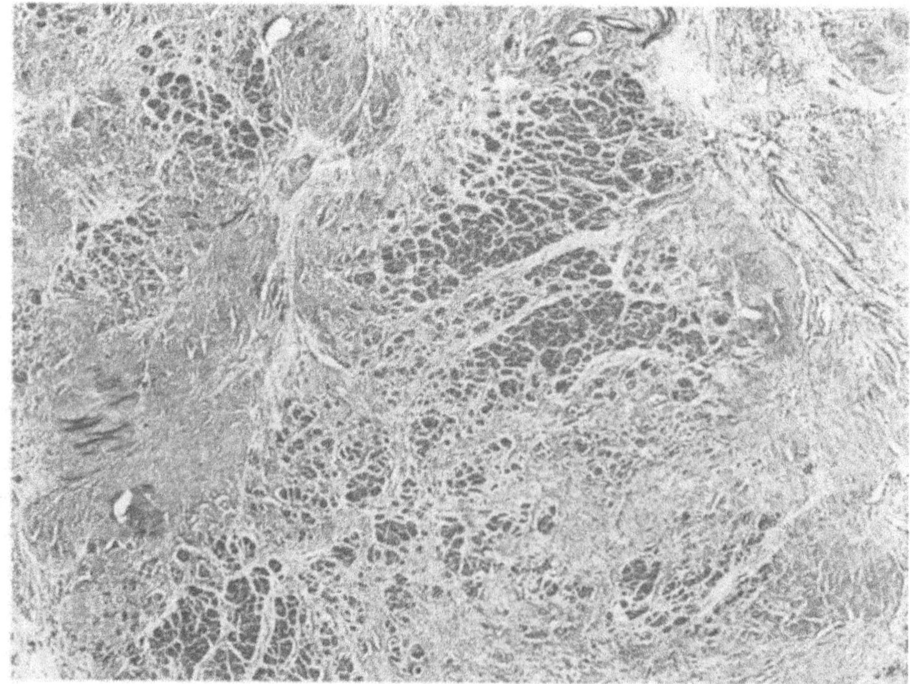

Fig. 11. Photomicrograph of section taken from the fibrous scar illustrated in Figure 5 showing severe fibrosis without inflammatory reaction. The darker portions represent myocardial fibers stranded in the fibrous tissue. The coronary artery proximal to this area of fibrosis was widely patent.

	Author & Year	Age at Accident Sex	Length of Illness from Accident to Death	Associated Cardiovascular Disease	Immediate Sign and/or Symptom(s)	Later Signs and Symptoms	Associated Injuries
1.	Kissane Koons Fidler[12] (1936)	22 M	14 mo.	0	Crushing chest pain Dyspnea	CHF* syncope	Multiple fractures, lacerations, contusions
2.	Beneke[13] (1942)	21 F	9 days	0	0	Fever CHF	0
3.	Bushong[14] (Case 1) (1947)	50 M	$2^1/_3$ mo.	0	Chest pain Dyspnea	CHF	0
4.	Kissane Koons Clark[15] (Case 2) (1948)	58 M	27 mo.	Syphilis	Purring noise in chest Sternal soreness Palpitations Dyspnea	Chest pain CHF	0
5.	Proudfit McCormack[16] (1956)	56 M	? 39 mo.	Hypertension Cerebral infarct	0	CHF Gradual lowering of blood pressure	0
6.	Dimond Larsen Johnson Kittle[17] (1957)	32 M	? 5 years†	Marfan's syndrome	Chest pain	CHF	Multiple fractures, brain concussion
7.	Ramage Morgan[18] (1957)	34 M	7 years	0	Cooing noise in chest	CHF	Sprained wrist
8.	Present authors (1961)	35 M	7 mo.‡	0	0	Night sweats Fatigability Syncope Arrhythmia CHF	0

* CHF = congestive heart failure.   † Hufnagel valve inserted 4 months before death.   ‡ Died during surgical

Previously Reported Cases: Including the patient described herein, the autopsy findings in 52 patients with aortic valvular regurgitation resulting from trauma or muscular strain have been recorded. Of these, 44 were reviewed by Howard[11] in 1928. The clinical and anatomic features in the 8 patients [12–18] described since that date are listed in Table 1. In Howard's 44 proved cases, 14 developed aortic regurgitation as a result of chest trauma and 30 as a result of muscular strain. Ninety-eight per cent were men. The age range in the traumatic group was from 19 to 85, with a mean of 45.6 years; in the strain group, from 20 to 60 with a mean of 37.2 years. Symptoms suggestive of pre-existing valvular disease were mentioned in 2 patients in his strain group, and in 5 in the traumatic group. A history of syphilis was recorded

Due to Trauma or Muscular Strain
Autopsies Performed Since 1928

Blood Pressure (mm. Hg)	Site of Tear	Aortic Valve Cusps Affected	State of Aortic Valve Cusps	State of Aorta	Heart Size (gm.)	Coronary Arteries
110/20	Cusps	All 3	"Torn, fragmented"		? normal	Normal
	Cusps Ventricular septum	Posterior R anterior	Normal	Normal	Normal	
175/55	Point of attachment of 2 cusp commissures	R anterior Posterior	Normal		650	"Slight" atherosclerosis
220/0	Point of attachment of 2 cusp commissures	L anterior Posterior	Separation of commissures Two posterior cusps, fibrous; anterior, normal	Occasional atheromata	"Enormously enlarged"	
150/50	Point of attachment of one cusp Fenestrations in 2 cusps	R anterior L anterior	Normal	Normal except for occasional atheromata	930	Moderate atherosclerosis
160/0	Ascending aorta Fenestrations in 2 cusps	L anterior Posterior	Sagging of the commissures with downward displacement of the cusps	Aneurysmal dilatation and medial cystic necrosis, asc. aorta	810	
160/30	Cusp itself	R anterior	Calcareous, fibrotic, thickened, deformed	Small aneurysm, ascending aorta	630	"Stenosis" of ostia by calcareous deposits in aorta
140–110/60–0	Point of attachment of one cusp	L anterior	Normal	Thin, fragile occasional atheromata Localized bulge in sinus of Valsalva	600	Minimal atherosclerosis

repair of the aortic valve. R = right, L = left.

only once and "rheumatism, chorea and tonsillitis" 5 times in the strain group. Neither syphilis nor rheumatic fever was mentioned in any of the 14 traumatic cases. The time interval between the accident and death varied widely, averaging 18 months in the strain group and 40 months in the traumatic group. The most common site of rupture in Howard's series was the aorta, near the base of the aortic valve (22 patients), followed by the rupture of the cusp itself (11 patients), and lastly by the detachment of the cusp from the aortic wall (10 patients). When the rupture affected the cusp itself, most commonly only one cusp was involved. There were only two instances in which all three cusps were torn. The aortic valve cusps were normal in 13 (30%) and fibrous, atheromatous or calcareous in 23 instances. None of the cusps were congenitally deformed.

The aortic regurgitation in the present patient resulted, at least initially, from a partial detachment of one aortic valve cusp from the wall of the aorta. At the time of the detachment there also was probably a tearing of the aorta immediately beneath the commissural attachment. The sequence of events thereafter was probably the following: Erythrocytes, inflammatory cells and fibroblasts entered the wall of the aorta and the adjacent adventitial tissues in the area bounded by the external surfaces of the proximal anterior mitral leaflet and the ascending aorta on one side, and left atrium on the other (Fig. 9). The tear in the aorta healed by scarring, and this fibrous proliferation produced severe thickening of the part of the aorta that bordered the sinus of Valsalva. Loose fibrous tissue clumps of chronic inflammatory cells, and scattered erythrocytes remained in the potential space thus created. The bulge thus came into being and further increased the amount of aortic regurgitation. The pathogenesis of the sterile abscess and of the focus of necrosis (Fig. 10) must remain a matter of speculation. The epithelioid cells which surrounded the focus of necrosis have not been noted previously in patients with aortic regurgitation due to trauma or muscular strain, although they have been described in patients with rheumatoid arthritis.[19] The present patient had no clinical signs nor symptoms of arthritis, and sections of two joints at autopsy were normal.

A bulge has been described in one other patient with aortic regurgitation due to muscular strain. This patient, reported by Beneke,[13] was a 21 year old woman who became febrile and in whom a basal diastolic murmur appeared nine days following the spontaneous delivery of a premature fetus. She died shortly after, and at autopsy there was a "walnut-sized nodule" in the subendocardium of the ventricular septum immediately beneath the aortic valve. Two of the aortic valve cusps were torn away at their bases from the wall of the aorta, and this tear was continuous with the nodule, which proved to be a hematoma. The hematoma had dissected through the ventricular septum, and, indeed, was apparent from the right ventricular aspect. Except for the tears, the aortic valve and aorta were normal. There was no evidence of infection at autopsy. This patient is the only recorded one in whom aortic regurgitation presumably resulted from the muscular strain exerted during parturition.

Clinical Features of Traumatic Aortic Regurgitation: The onset of symptoms of traumatic aortic valvular rupture usually follows the causative injury immediately. The most common symptom is agonizing pain in the chest often followed by faintness or syncope. There have been cases, however, in which the onset of symptoms was delayed, sometimes as long as several years. After a variable interval the usual symptoms of aortic regurgitation ensue. About half of the patients complain of a chest sound which is audible, not only to themselves, but to others.

At physical examination there are the usual signs of aortic regurgitation. Although the pulse pressure is usually wide, elevated systolic pressure is not common early in the course of the disease. A rough systolic murmur is often heard and is attributable to vibrations caused by rapid blood flow over the torn cusp. The diastolic murmur commonly has a musical quality and has been compared to such sounds as that of a sea gull, the cooing of a dove, the croaking of a frog, the spinning of a top, or whistling, whining or humming sounds.

Several clinical features that were atypical of traumatic aortic regurgitation were noted in the present patient. The onset of symptoms was delayed by several days, and then the syncope appeared to be caused by the complete heart block rather than by valvular disease. At no time was chest pain prominent, nor was the patient aware of any sound in his chest. The diastolic murmur sounded much like most murmurs of aortic regurgitation and had no musical quality.

Surgical treatment for traumatic aortic regurgitation was apparently first attempted in 1954 by Hufnagel,[20] who successfully inserted a plastic valve in the descending aorta. Fourteen months later the patient continued to do well. A similar operation in a patient with Marfan's syndrome was reported by Dimond et al.[17] This patient had no apparent relief from the operation and died a short time later. Spurny and Hara[21] attempted to repair a torn aortic cusp by direct suture but were unable to resuscitate the heart at the end of the procedure. The present patient, had he survived surgery, probably would have derived limited benefit from the operation because of the residual deformity produced by the large aortic valve nodule. It is not possible, however, to determine preoperatively the exact anatomic derangement that will be encountered at operation. Since it represents the only therapeutic approach that potentially offers lasting benefit, operative intervention would seem to be indicated in most patients with traumatic aortic regurgitation.

SUMMARY

A patient is reported who sustained myocardial contusion with complete heart block, pericardial effusion and rupture of the aortic valve following blunt chest trauma. An attempt at direct surgical repair of the valvular lesion was unsuccessful. The diagnostic difficulties presented by traumatic heart disease are discussed, and the previous reports of patients with traumatic aortic regurgitation are summarized.

ACKNOWLEDGMENT

The authors are grateful to Dr. Walter Hasbrouck, who referred this patient to the National Heart Institute.

REFERENCES

1. FRIEDBERG, C. K. Diseases of the Heart, ed. 2, p. 1057. Philadelphia, 1956. W. B. Saunders Co.
2. PARMLEY, L. F., MANION, W. C. and MATTINGLY, T. W. Nonpenetrating traumatic injury of the heart. *Circulation*, 28: 371, 1958.
3. WATSON, J. H. and BARTHOLOMAE, W. M. Cardiac injury due to nonpenetrating chest trauma. *Ann. Int. Med.*, 57: 871, 1960.
4. BRAUNWALD, E. and MORROW, A. G. A method for the detection and estimation of aortic regurgitant flow in man. *Circulation*, 17: 505, 1958.
5. DAVILA, J. C., TROUT, R. G., SUNNER, J. E. and GLOVER, R. P. A simple mechanical pulse duplicator for cinematography of cardiac valves in action. *Ann. Surg.*, 143: 544, 1956.
6. GORE, I. The question of traumatic heart disease. *Ann. Int. Med.*, 33: 865, 1950.
7. BRIGHT, E. F. and BECK, C. S. Nonpenetrating wounds of the heart. *Am. Heart J.*, 10: 293, 1935.
8. BECK, C. S. Contusions of the heart. *J.A.M.A.*, 109: 104, 1935.
9. BORODKIN, H. D. and MASSEY, F. C. Myocardial trauma produced by nonpenetrating chest injury. *Am. Heart J.*, 53: 795, 1957.
10. COFFEN, T. H., RUSH, H. P. and MILLER, R. F. Traumatic complete heart block of eighteen years' duration. *Northwest Med.*, 40: 195, 1941.
11. HOWARD, C. P. Aortic insufficiency due to rupture by strain of a normal aortic valve. *Canad. M.A.J.* 19: 12, 1928.
12. KISSANE, R. W., KOONS, R. A. and FIDLER, R. S. Traumatic rupture of a normal aortic valve. *Am. Heart J.*, 12: 231, 1936.
13. BENEKE, R. Ein Fall spontaner Aortenklappen-Ruptur mit Hämatom im Gebiet des Septum Fibrosum Ventr. als Begleiterscheinung Einer Vorzeitigen Geburt. *Ztschr. Geburtsh. u. Gynak.*, 124: 1, 1942.
14. BUSHONG, B. B. Traumatic rupture of the aortic valve: report of two cases, one a proved and the other a probable example of this condition. *Ann. Int. Med.*, 26: 125, 1947.
15. KISSANE, R. W., KOONS, R. A. and CLARK, T. E. Traumatic rupture of the aortic valve. *Am. J. Med.*, 4: 606, 1948.
16. PROUDFIT, W. L. and MCCORMACK, L. J. Rupture of the aortic valve. *Circulation*, 13: 750, 1956.
17. DIMOND, E. G., LARSEN, W. E., JOHNSON, W. B. and KITTLE, C. F. Posttraumatic aortic insufficiency occurring in Marfan's syndrome with attempted repair with a plastic valve. *New England J. Med.*, 256: 8, 1957.
18. RAMAGE, J. H. and MORGAN, J. B. Traumatic aortic incompetence. *Scottish M. J.*, 2: 299, 1957.
19. BAGGENSTOSS, A. H. and ROSENBERG, E. F. Cardiac lesions associated with chronic infectious arthritis. *Arch. Int. Med.*, 67: 241, 1941.
20. LEONARD, J. J., HARVEY, W. P. and HUFNAGEL, C. A. Rupture of the aortic valve. *New England J. Med.*, 252: 208, 1955.
21. SPURNY, O. M. and HARA, M. Rupture of the aortic valve due to strain. *Am. J. Cardiol.*, 8: 125, 1961.

Aortico-Left Ventricular Tunnel[*]

A Cause of Massive Aortic Regurgitation and of Intracardiac Aneurysm

WILLIAM C. ROBERTS, M.D. *and* ANDREW G. MORROW, M.D.

Bethesda, Maryland

AMONG the unusual causes of aortic regurgitation is an accessory vascular channel which originates in the ascending aorta, bypasses the aortic valve and communicates with the left ventricle through the upper ventricular septum. Although isolated reports of clinical and necropsy findings in patients with this lesion had appeared previously [1–4], Levy and his associates [5], in 1963, presented the first definitive characterization of the entity, and termed it "aortico-left ventricular tunnel."

This report describes the clinical, roentgenographic, hemodynamic and pathologic findings in an additional patient in whom an aortico-left ventricular tunnel not only caused aortic regurgitation, but also gave rise to an intracardiac aneurysm which was responsible for severe right ventricular outflow obstruction.

CASE REPORT

W. M. (01-21-10), a fourteen year old school boy, was found to have a precordial murmur at three months of age. He grew slowly, and at the age of five years, after cardiac catheterization and angiocardiography were performed at another hospital, his parents were told that he had aortic regurgitation. He was first seen at the National Heart Institute at the age of eight years. He was asymptomatic and played football, baseball, and swam without experiencing discomfort. On examination he was poorly developed and appeared undernourished. The heart was grossly enlarged to palpation, and there was a prominent left ventricular lift. Both systolic and diastolic thrills were present. At the base of the heart a grade 5/6 systolic ejection-type murmur was audible, and was immediately followed by a grade 5/6 high-pitched, blowing diastolic murmur which was transmitted along the left sternal border. The peripheral pulses were bounding, both systolic and diastolic murmurs were audible over the femoral arteries, and the blood pressure in the arm was 120/0 mm. Hg.

Chest roentgenograms disclosed marked enlarge-

ment of the left ventricle and ascending aorta; the electrocardiogram demonstrated normal sinus rhythm, biventricular hypertrophy and ventricular premature contractions. Retrograde arterial catheterization was performed and simultaneous measurements of left ventricular and femoral arterial pressures were 117/10 and 189/37 mm. Hg, respectively.

In the ensuing two years the patient remained asymptomatic; he was readmitted at the age of ten years for further study. At right heart catheterization the pulmonary arterial and pulmonary capillary wedge pressures were normal, but a large systolic pressure gradient was demonstrated within the right ventricle; high in the outflow tract the pressure was 22/1 mm. Hg while near the tricuspid valve it was 120/4 mm. Hg. No intracardiac shunts were demonstrated by the inhaled nitrous oxide test. A retrograde aortogram (Fig. 1) showed marked dilatation of the ascending aorta and regurgitation of dye, initially into a smooth-walled subaortic chamber and subsequently into the left ventricular cavity. The aortic sinuses of Valsalva also were dilated. It was considered that the patient had either an aneurysm of the sinus of Valsalva with rupture into the left ventricle, or cystic medial necrosis of the aorta; because of the latter possibility, and because he was asymptomatic, operative treatment was not undertaken.

The patient remained well, continued to participate in sports, despite advice to the contrary, and never experienced syncope, precordial pain, troublesome dyspnea or other symptoms of cardiac failure. His heart increased in size only in proportion to his growth (Fig. 2), but electrocardiograms (Fig. 3) showed progressive deepening of the T waves in the precordial leads. When the boy was fourteen years old a corrective operation was scheduled, but he died suddenly at home before it was performed.

Necropsy (A63-139) disclosed that the aortic regurgitation was due to a large accessory communication, an aortico-left ventricular tunnel, between the markedly dilated ascending aorta and the left ventricle. The pathologic aspects of this communication are illustrated in detail in Figures 4 through 6. Immediately below its origin from the aorta the tunnel was

* From the Clinic of Surgery, National Heart Institute, National Institutes of Health, Bethesda, Maryland. Manuscript received February 2, 1965.

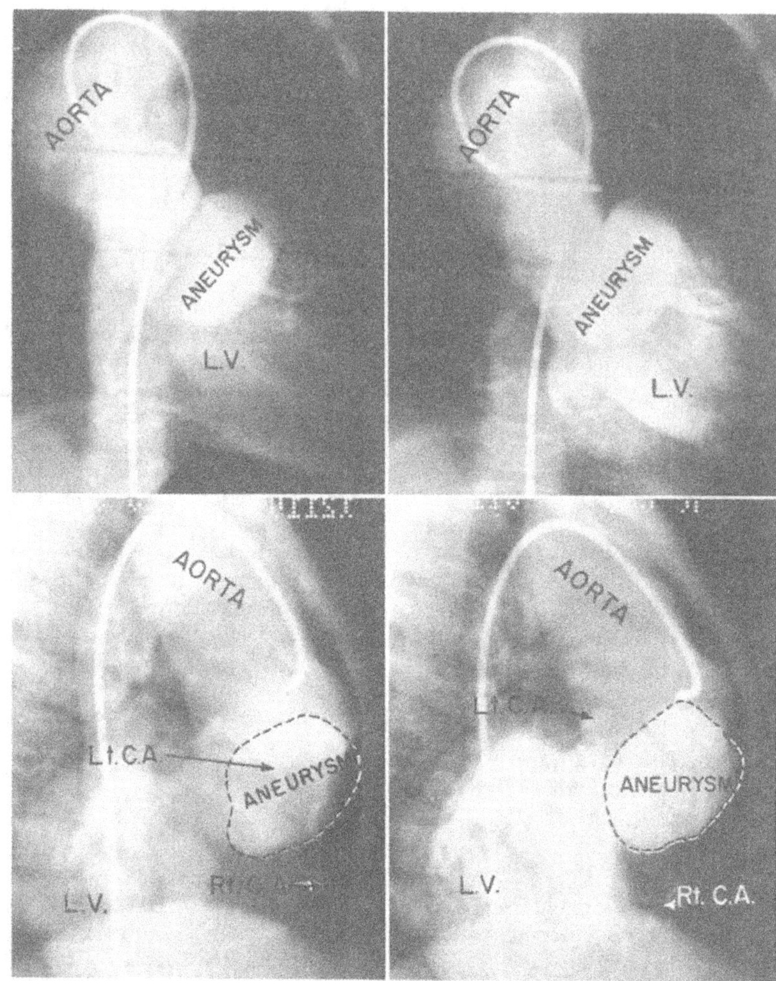

Fig. 1. Anteroposterior views (*upper*) and lateral views (*lower*) of the thoracic aortogram. Following injection of contrast material into the ascending aorta, the aneurysmal intracardiac portion of the aortico-left ventricular tunnel opacifies immediately, and is well outlined before radiopaque material enters the left ventricular cavity. The ascending aorta and sinuses of Valsalva are dilated. L.V. = left ventricle. Rt. C.A. = right coronary artery. Lt. C.A. = left coronary artery.

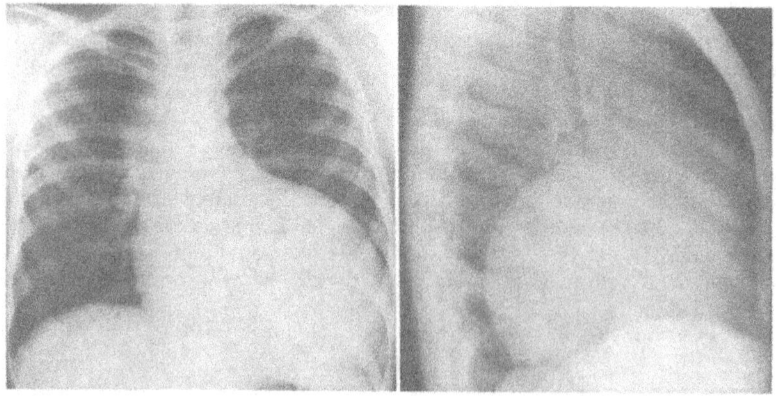

Fig. 2. Posteroanterior and lateral chest roentgenograms of the patient described. There is striking enlargement of the left ventricle and the ascending aorta is dilated.

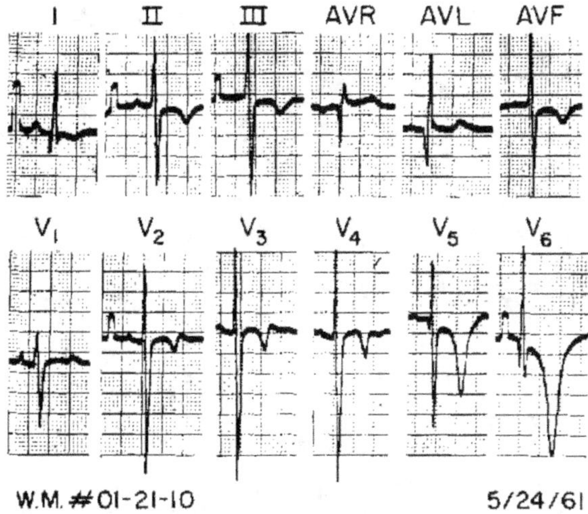

Fig. 3. Electrocardiogram. Leads ii, iii and V₂ through V₆ are at half-standardization. The T wave deflection in lead V₆ exceeds 50 mm.

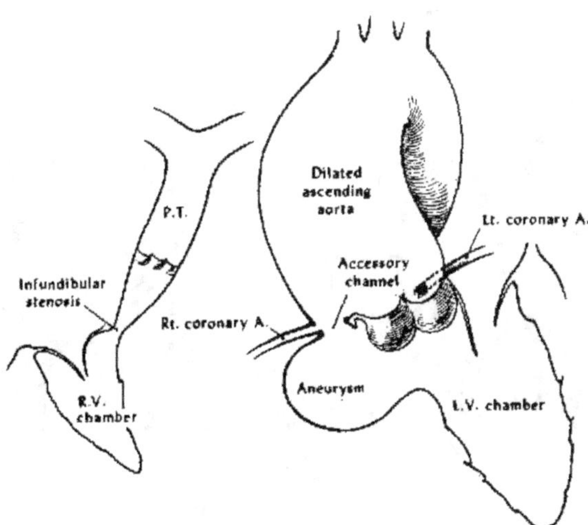

Fig. 4. Diagram illustrating the essential anatomic features of the aortico-left ventricular tunnel in the patient described. The right and left sides of the heart are shown separately for simplicity, but the comparative size of each is correct. The right ventricular (R.V.) chamber is much smaller than the left ventricular (L.V.) one. A localized area of stenosis is present at the beginning of the right ventricular outflow tract. The remainder of the infundibular chamber is of normal size as is the pulmonary trunk (P.T.). The ascending aorta is diffusely dilated. A wide open accessory channel lies between the aorta and the subaortic aneurysm and left ventricular chamber. The aneurysm is actually the tunnel located immediately behind the right ventricular infundibulum. The aortic valve is bicuspid. The ostium of the right coronary artery is located immediately above the aortic ostium of the accessory channel.

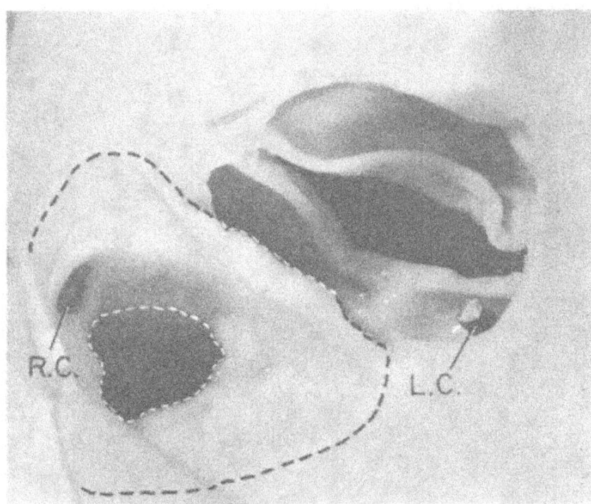

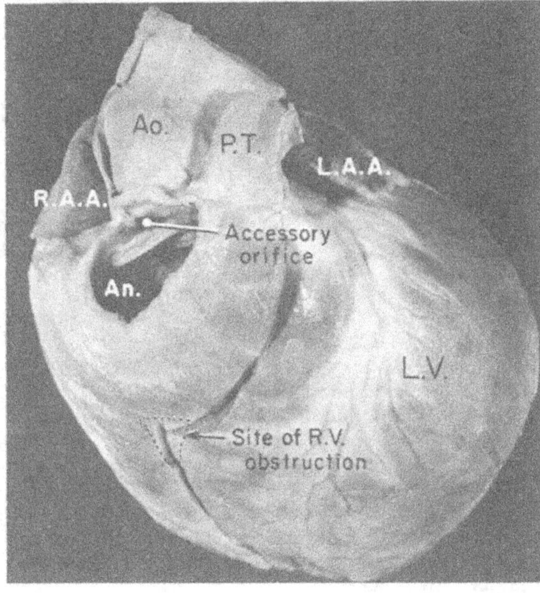

Fig. 5. Photographs of the aortic root area from above and below. *Top*, the aortic valve and ostium of the accessory channel as viewed from the aorta. The aortic valve contains only two cusps. A thick band separates the aortic valve orifice from the orifice of the accessory channel. If the top of this ridge and the surrounding aorta at this level (large black-dashed area) are considered the origin of the tunnel, then the right (R.C.) and left (L.C.) coronary arteries arise below this level. If on the other hand the actual opening into the heart (small white-dashed circle) is considered the origin of the tunnel, then the coronary arteries arise above it. *Bottom*, the heart as it appears from the anterior view. The anterior wall of the intracardiac aneurysm (An.), which is a thin fibrous membrane, has been removed allowing visualization of the accessory orifice from below. Ao. = ascending aorta. P.T. = pulmonary trunk. R.A.A. = right atrial appendage. L.A.A. = left atrial appendage. R.V. = right ventricle. L.V. = left ventricle.

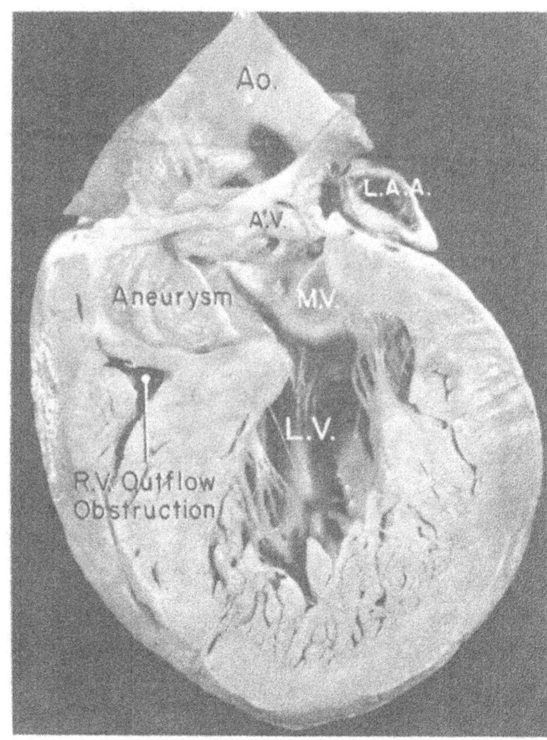

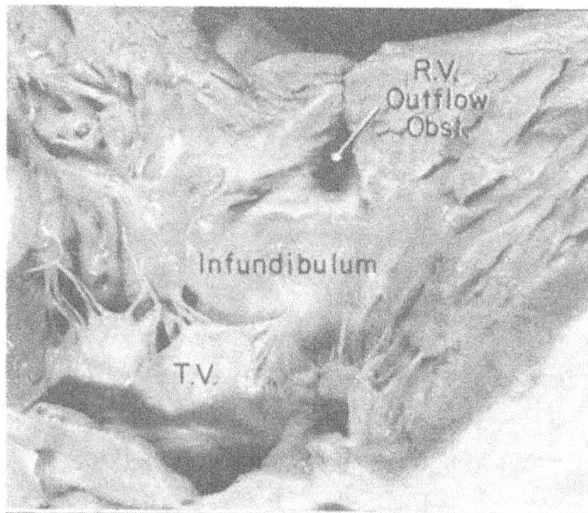

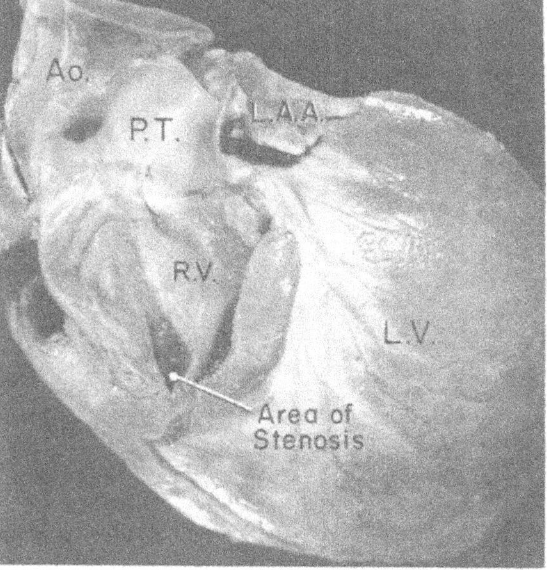

Fig. 6. Sagittal section of heart transecting the accessory aortic orifice. The intracardiac aneurysm is located between the aorta and left ventricular cavity. The tunnel penetrates the portion of the muscular ventricular septum which also forms the posterior wall of the right ventricular infundibulum. The aneurysmal dilatation of the tunnel caused the posterior wall of the infundibulum to bulge into the right ventricular cavity with resulting obstruction to right ventricular outflow. The left ventricular wall is massively hypertrophied. The ostium into the left atrial appendage (L.A.A.) is congenitally atretic. A.V. = aortic valve cusps. M.V. = anterior mitral leaflet.

Fig. 7. The area of right ventricular obstruction from below and above. *Top*, the obstruction (Obst.) is located at the beginning of the right ventricular outflow tract and is due to the infundibulum bulging anteriorly and inferiorly. There is endocardial thickening at the site of narrowing. *Bottom*, the right ventricular (R.V.) outflow tract is opened and the area of stenosis is again seen. The wall of the right ventricular outflow tract is thin, but the wall of the inflow portion (upper) is thick. Ao. = ascending aorta. P.T. = pulmonary trunk. L.A.A. = left atrial appendage. L.V. = left ventricle.

aneurysmally dilated, and the mass of the aneurysm displaced the upper portion of the ventricular septum into right ventricular outflow tract. (Fig. 7.) The coronary arteries were normal on both gross and microscopic examinations and neither was compressed by the aneurysm. Multiple sections of the left ventricular wall revealed hypertrophy of the myocardial fibers and rare foci of interstitial and replacement fibrosis. In sections of the ascending aorta, the configuration of the elastic fibers was normal and no excessive amount of mucopolysaccharide material was evident.

COMMENTS

The basic anatomic malformation in aortico-left ventricular tunnel is an abnormal vascular channel which begins in the aortic root, passes through the upper portion of the ventricular septum and enters the outflow tract of the ventricle. Aortico-left ventricular tunnel must be distinguished from an aneurysm of the sinus of Valsalva which has ruptured into the left ventricle, and Levy et al. [5] made this distinction by pointing out that in ruptured sinus aneurysm the orifice of the aneurysm is *below* the level of the ostia of the coronary arteries. In contrast, in each of the three patients with aortico-left ventricular tunnel which he described, and in the one reported by Edwards [4], the tunnel was considered to originate *above* the level of the aortic sinuses and coronary ostia. To some extent, however, the above-or-below relationship of the tunnel to the origins of the coronary arteries is a matter of semantics. In the present patient, those cited and in the patient described by Morgan and Mazur [6], the orifice of the tunnel was separated from the aortic valve by a thick ridge, the upper margin of which was on the same horizontal plane as the upper margins of the aortic valve leaflets and commissures. If the top of the ridge and the surrounding aorta at this level are designated as the origin of the tunnel, then the coronary arteries arise below it. If, on the other hand, the orifice of the tunnel is considered to be the actual opening into the heart, then the coronary arteries arise above it. (Fig. 5.)

Between the aorta and the heart, the tunnel may be tubular in shape or, more frequently, it may be dilated and appear as a discrete enlargement of the anterior portion of the aortic root [5]. In this case the angiographic appearance of the tunnel is that of a supracardiac saccular aneurysm and permits a precise diagnosis. In the present patient, however, although the tunnel was aneurysmal, the aneurysm was entirely within the heart and the dilated ascending aorta was of uniform configuration.

The tunnel enters the heart through the muscular portion of the ventricular septum, directly below the aortic root, and terminates in the left ventricle immediately below the aortic valve. The area of the ventricular septum traversed by the tunnel constitutes the posterior wall of the right ventricular outflow tract. In this patient the aneurysmal intracardiac portion of the tunnel was so large that it displaced the posterior wall of the infundibulum into the right ventricular cavity and caused obstruction to right ventricular outflow. Right ventricular outflow obstruction by this mechanism has not been documented previously, although Levy and associates postulated that such might occur.

The available evidence indicates that aortico-left ventricular tunnel is a congenital rather than an acquired malformation, and signs of cardiac disease are usually present from an early age. The patient described by Morgan and Mazur [6], for example, had aortic regurgitation from birth and died at fifteen days of age.

At autopsy there was dilatation of the ascending aorta and the appearance of the aortic root was quite similar to that shown in Figure 5. The association of aortico-left ventricular tunnel with other congenital cardiovascular anomalies also lends support to a congenital basis for this lesion. The aortic valve was bicuspid in each of the autopsy cases reported by Edwards [4] and by Levy et al., and also in the present case. In the case of Morgan and Mazur [6] the aortic valve as illustrated, although described as being tricuspid, appears malformed. In the present case there was also absence of an ostium into the left atrial appendage. Levy and associates demonstrated histologically in one of their patients that the aortic media was continuous with the wall of the tunnel, and suggested that the tunnel represented an anomalous vessel rather than an acquired tract. In the present patient, microscopic sections of the ridge separating the aortic valve from the ostium of the tunnel disclosed that this structure had the same appearance as the media of the ascending aorta, consisting predominantly of elastic fibers. The anterior wall of the intracardiac portion of the tunnel, however, was composed of dense collagenous tissue containing only an occasional elastic fibril. Thus, in this patient, if the intracardiac portion of the tunnel originally had the structure of a blood vessel, it was not apparent at the time of necropsy. It is possible, of course, that the structure of the tunnel may have been altered by the trauma of systolic and diastolic blood flow through it during the fourteen years of the patient's life.

Patients with aortico-left ventricular tunnel present physical findings indistinguishable from those observed in patients with aortic regurgitation resulting from valvular abnormalities. A congenital malformation may be suggested by an early history of a precordial murmur, but the results of conventional roentgenographic examinations, electrocardiography and cardiac catheterization are not specific. It would appear that the correct diagnosis can be established only when the origin of the tunnel from the ascending aorta, as well as regurgitant flow into the left ventricle, can be demonstrated at thoracic aortography. Even this study may not be conclusive if, as in the present patient, the tunnel is dilated only within the roentgenographic silhouette of the heart, and resembles a ruptured aneurysm of the sinus of Valsalva.

Aortic regurgitation resulting from an aortico-left ventricular tunnel may be abolished by closure of the aortic ostium, and successful surgical treatment of this type has been reported in several patients [5,7,8]. This form of aortic regurgitation would thus appear to be a relatively favorable one, particularly in a child, since the insertion of a prosthetic aortic valve, virtually always necessary in valvular aortic regurgitation, is not required.

SUMMARY

The clinical, roentgenographic, hemodynamic and pathologic findings in a fourteen year old boy with aortico-left ventricular tunnel are presented. The accessory channel between the aorta and left ventricle resulted in massive aortic regurgitation, and the portion of the tunnel which traversed the ventricular septum was aneurysmal, displaced the posterior wall of the right ventricle and caused severe obstruction to right ventricular outflow. The presence of associated cardiovascular anomalies, in this and previously reported cases, suggests that the malformation is congenital rather than acquired.

The clinical and hemodynamic manifestations of aortico-left ventricular tunnel are indistinguishable from those observed with the more common forms of aortic regurgitation, and the correct diagnosis can be established only by thoracic aortography. The malformation is usually recognized in childhood; since aortic regurgitant flow can be abolished by simple closure of the aortic ostium, and without aortic valve replacement, the indications for operative treatment differ from those which apply in aortic regurgitation due to a valvular anomaly.

ADDENDUM

Since this manuscript was submitted for publication, Cooley et al. [10] described another patient with aortico-left ventricular tunnel. The unusual features in the sixteen month old boy were the presence of associated valvular aortic stenosis and deposits of mucopolysaccharide material in the ascending aorta. The latter suggested to these workers the possibility of a relationship between aortico-left ventricular tunnel and the Marfan syndrome.

REFERENCES

1. HART, K. Uber das Aneurysma des rechten Sinus Valsalvae der Aorta und seine Beziehungen zum oberen Ventrikelseptum. *Virchow's Arch. path. Anat.*, 182: 167, 1905.
2. WARTHEN, R. O. Congenital aneurysm of the right anterior sinus of Valsalva (interventricular aneurysm) with spontaneous rupture into the left ventricle. *Am. Heart J.*, 37: 975, 1949.
3. TASAKA, S., YOSHITOSHI, Y., SEKI, K., KOIDE, K., OGATA, E. and NAKAMURA, K. Congenital aneurysm of the right coronary sinus of Valsalva with rupture into the left ventricle. *Jap. Heart J.*, 1: 106, 1960.
4. EDWARDS, J. E. Atlas of acquired diseases of the heart and great vessels. 3rd vol, p. 1142, Philadelphia, 1961, W. B. Saunders Co.
5. LEVY, M. J., LILLEHEI, C. W., ANDERSON, R. C., AMPLATZ, K. and EDWARDS, J. E. Aortico-left ventricular tunnel. *Circulation*, 27: 841, 1963.
6. MORGAN, R. I. and MAZUR, J. H. Congenital aneurysm of aortic root with fistula to left ventricle. A case report with autopsy findings. *Circulation*, 28: 589, 1963.
7. SHUMACKER, H. B., JR. and JUDSON, W. E. Rupture of aneurysm of sinus of Valsalva into left ventricle and its operative repair. *J. Thoracic & Cardiovasc. Surg.*, 45: 650, 1963.
8. SCOTT, H. W., JR., COLLINS, H. A. and SINCLAIR-SMITH, B. Surgical repair of congenital aneurysm of the right coronary sinus of Valsalva with rupture into the left ventricle. *J. Cardiovasc. Surg.*, 5: 231, 1964.
9. PALACIO, J., PERRETTA, A., SANCHEZ, B. and ALPEROVICH, M. Intrapericardial congenital supravalvular aortic aneurysm communicating with the outflow tract of the left ventricle. Hypoplasia of the aortic orifice and ascending aorta. *J. Cardiovasc. Surg.*, 5: 401, 1964.
10. COOLEY, R. N., HARRIS, L. C. and RODIN, A. E. Abnormal communication between the aorta and left ventricle. Aortico-left ventricular tunnel. *Circulation*, 31: 564, 1965.

Ankylosing Spondylitis and Aortic Regurgitation

Description of the Characteristic Cardiovascular Lesion
From Study of Eight Necropsy Patients

By BERNADINE H. BULKLEY, M.D., AND WILLIAM C. ROBERTS, M.D.

SUMMARY

Clinical and cardiovascular necropsy findings are described in eight patients with combined ankylosing spondylitis and aortic regurgitation. All were men (aged 34-55 years), each had peripheral arthritis in addition to spondylitis, all had severe congestive failure, and six had conduction disturbances. In three patients aortic regurgitation was present before distinctive radiologic changes of ankylosing spondylitis were apparent and only two patients had advanced arthritic changes of ankylosing spondylitis. Thus, cardiac dysfunction may be present before signs of spondylitis are apparent, and aortic regurgitation may be severe when signs of spondylitis are minimal. A characteristic cardiovascular morphologic abnormality was present in each patient. The aortic valve cusps and the aorta behind and immediately above the sinuses of Valsalva were thickened, the latter by dense adventitial scar tissue and by intimal fibrous proliferation. In each patient the scar tissue in the root of aorta extended below the base of aortic valve to produce a subaortic fibrous ridge. The subaortic bump involves the base of anterior mitral leaflet and may cause mitral regurgitation. Extension of the fibrous scar into ventricular septum may cause heart block. The distinctive cardiovascular morphologic findings in patients with ankylosing spondylitis clearly separate this condition from syphilis and other entities associated with aortic regurgitation.

Additional Indexing Words:

Valvular heart disease   Syphilis   Rheumatoid arthritis

ANKYLOSING SPONDYLITIS and rheumatoid arthritis were recognized as distinct entities about 15 years ago.[1-5] Subsequently, aortic regurgitation was recognized as a fairly frequent accompaniment of ankylosing spondylitis, but as an extremely rare accompaniment of rheumatoid arthritis. Despite several reports on lesions of aortic valve and aorta in ankylosing spondylitis, the distinctive features of the cardiovascular lesions have not been defined. Study of eight necropsy patients with combined ankylosing spondylitis and aortic regurgitation disclosed distinctive cardiovascular abnormalities in each. This report describes the cardiovascular findings in these eight patients, and calls attention to the unique features of the cardiovascular lesions.

From the Section of Pathology, National Heart and Lung Institute, National Institutes of Health, Bethesda, Maryland.

Address for reprints: William C. Roberts, M.D., Section of Pathology, National Heart and Lung Institute, National Institutes of Health, Bethesda, Maryland 20014.

Received May 21, 1973; revision accepted for publication June 28, 1973.

Methods

The clinical records, heart specimens and histologic sections were reexamined in all eight patients. At least two sections of ascending aorta, two of left ventricle, one of aortic valve, and two of mitral valve were examined in each patient. Radiographs, gross specimens and histologic sections of involved joints were examined in seven of eight patients. The morphologic cardiovascular findings in these eight patients were compared with the necropsy findings associated with aortic regurgitation in 20 patients with cardiovascular syphilis, three with rheumatoid arthritis, and 11 with the Marfan syndrome.

Results

Clinical Findings

Pertinent findings in the eight patients are summarized in tables 1 and 2. The patients ranged in age from 34–57 years (average 46) and all were men. In addition to spondylitis, all eight patients had peripheral arthritis. One patient also had Reiter's syndrome. Symptoms of arthritis developed at an average age of 26 years, precordial murmurs at 32 and congestive cardiac failure at 41. The duration of arthritic symptoms averaged 21 years, valvular dysfunction 16 years, and congestive

Table 1

Clinical and Necropsy Observations in Eight Patients

Patient	Age at death (yrs.)	Age at onset arthritis (yrs.)	Clinical — Age onset in years — Murmur	Clinical — Age onset in years — CHF	Clinical — Duration in years — Arthritis	Clinical — Duration in years — Murmur	Clinical — Duration in years — CHF	ECG Conduction disturbances	Hemodynamics Pressures (mm Hg) LV	Hemodynamics Pressures (mm Hg) SA	Heart weight (gms)	Cardiovascular pathology — Thick AV cusps	Cardiovascular pathology — Sub-AV fibrosis	Cardiovascular pathology — Thickening of aorta limited to sinuses
1 A61-99	52*	24	37	43	28*	15*	9	1° HB RBBB	160/18	168/30	850	+	+	+
2 A61-262	55	45	45	53	15	15	2	1° HB	114/40	124/40	680	+	+	+
3 A61-274	34*	18	31	31	16*	3*	3	1° HB	100/22	120/25	700	+	+	+
4 A64-17	35*	6	6	29	29*	29*	6	0	170/12	170/50	840	+	+	+
5 A66-127	57	42	41	55	16	17	2	0	—	180/40	520	+	+	+
6 A68-142	38*	13	14	32	25*	24*	6	1° HB	170/16	190/20	1100	+	+	+
7 A68-300	54	40	40	48	14	14	6	CHB	170/50	170/50	620	+	+	+
8 A68-350	46*	18	38	38	28*	8y*	8	LBBB	128/32	128/32	610	+	+	+
Average	46	26	32	41	21	16	6				740			

*Each underwent aortic valve replacement: 3 died within a month of operation and the other 2 at 18 and 19 months, respectively, after operation.

Abbreviations: AR = aortic regurgitation; AV = aortic valve; CHB = complete heart block; CHF = congestive cardiac failure; 1° HB = first degree heart block (P-R interval > 0.20 sec); LBBB = left bundle branch block; LV = left ventricle; RBBB = right bundle branch block; SA = systemic artery.

failure six years. Conduction disturbances were present in six patients: prolonged (> 0.20 sec) P-R intervals in four, complete left bundle branch block in one, complete right bundle branch block in one, and complete heart block in one. In four patients precordial murmurs were noted at the same time or within one year of onset of joint symptoms. In three patients aortic regurgitation was diagnosed before distinctive radiologic changes of ankylosing spondylitis were present, and a clinical explanation for valvular dysfunction was initially uncertain. All patients had severe congestive cardiac failure and each was in functional class III or IV (New York Heart Association classification). One patient had mild mitral regurgitation documented by left ventricular angiogram. Aortic valve replacement was carried out in five patients; four died within two months, the fifth 12 months later. Each of the three non-operated patients died of congestive cardiac failure.

Necropsy Findings

Cardiovascular necropsy findings in several patients are illustrated in figures 1–7. The hearts weighed 520 to 1100 gms (avg. 740). The ascending aortas including the sinuses of Valsalva were mildly dilated in all eight patients. The aortic walls behind and immediately above the sinuses of Valsalva, especially that portion behind the comissures, were thickened, up to five times normal. The thickening of aorta resulted primarily from adventitial scarring and intimal proliferation. Although focally scarred, the media was not thickened. Many vasa vasora were surrounded by collections of plasma cells and lymphocytes and their lumens often were narrowed. In all eight patients the adventitial scarring was present in the groove between aortic valve cusps and anterior mitral leaflet producing a ridge beneath aortic valve, especially the basal portion of anterior mitral leaflet. The adventitial scarring in each patient also was continuous with similar scarring in membranous ventricular septum. The aortic valves in all eight patients appeared incompetent. Both basal and distal portions of the cusps were shortened and thickened by fibrous tissue. The fibrous thickening of aortic wall behind the commissures caused the cusps to sag toward left ventricle. The commissures, however, were neither widened nor fused. The coronary ostia were widely patent. The parietal and viseral pericardia were diffusely adherent to one another in the five patients with previous thoracotomies but the pericardium was normal in the

Table 2

Arthritic Features of Eight Patients with Ankylosing Spondylitis and Aortic Regurgitation

		No. patients
I.	*Clinical abnormalities*	8/8
	Back pain	8
	Restricted spinal movement	8
	Dorsal kyphosis	4
	Peripheral arthritis	8
	Urethritis alone	2
	Urethritis + iritis (Reiter's)	1
	Negative rheumatoid factor	8
	Negative STS	8
II.	*Radiologic abnormalities*	7/7
	Sacroiliac joints	7
	Blurred (7)	
	Fused (3)	
	Vertebral bodies	6
	Squared (6)	
	Narrowing IV space (6)	
	Calcification, discs (4)	
	Calcification, ligaments (2)	
	Peripheral joints	1
	Ankylosis (1)	
III.	*Morphologic abnormalities*	7/7
	Sacroiliac joints	7
	Vertebral bodies	7
	Peripheral joints	4

three nonoperated patients. Amyloid deposits were not observed in any patient.

Discussion

Although described briefly in previous reports, the cardiovascular lesions of ankylosing spondylitis have been poorly defined and their distinctive nature not appreciated. In 1936, Mallory[6] described cardiovascular necropsy findings in two young men with combined aortic regurgitation and arthritis of both peripheral joints and spine. He described a "pannus-like overgrowth" or a "queer fibrous growth over the intima and the first portion of ascending aorta [which] . . . extended only a centimeter up the aorta but balanced this by extending about the same distance down below the aortic valve." The aortic wall lesion histologically was identical to syphilis. Twenty years later, Clark, Kulka and Bauer[7] reviewed these two patients along with eight other necropsy patients with combined aortic regurgitation and "rheumatoid arthritis with spinal involvement." These authors did not distinguish between ankylosing spondylitis and rheumatoid arthritis and, therefore, considered the aortic regurgitation to be an unusual manifestation of rheumatoid arthritis. The cardiac findings

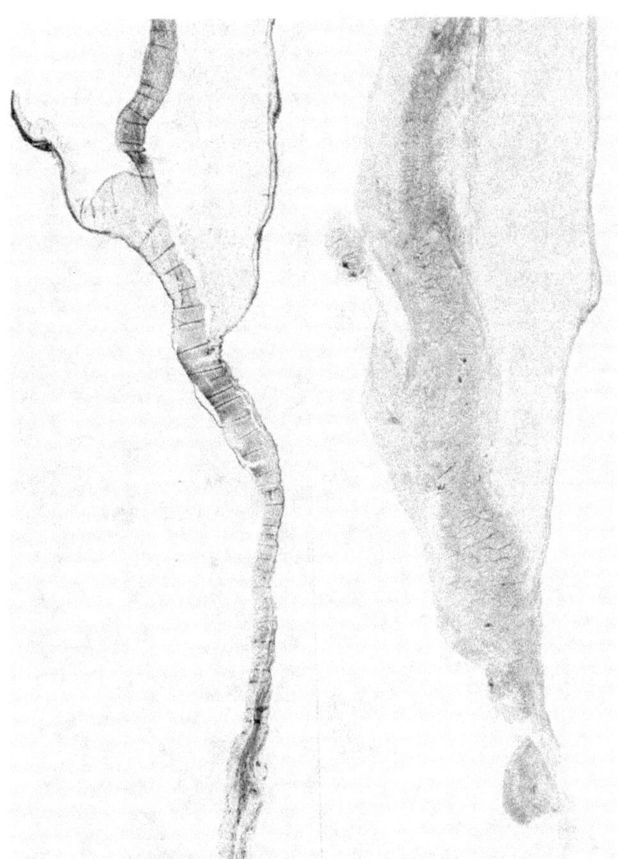

Figure 1

Heart of patient with ankylosing spondylitis compared to the normal. (left) Histologic section through aorta, aortic valve and anterior mitral leaflet from a normal heart and (right) a section from the same area from the heart of a patient (A68-300) with ankylosing spondylitis and severe aortic regurgitation. In ankylosing spondylitis the aortic wall is thickened by dense adventitial scar and less dense intimal scar. Inflammatory tissue also thickens the base of the aortic valve cusp and anterior mitral leaflet. (Elastic van Gieson stain: (left) ×4, (right) ×2.5.)

at necropsy were "strikingly similar to those of luetic heart disease." Although the subvalvular region was not described, the involvement of aorta was limited to the root area: "intimal plaques, centered about each valve commissure . . . , blended with the valvular lesion. These plaques reached into the sinuses of Valsalva and extended . . . up to 2.5 cm distally into ascending aorta." In retrospect, it appears that their patients had ankylosing spondylitis rather than rheumatoid arthritis, and that the cardiac necropsy findings were those of ankylosing spondylitis. Descriptions of the cardiovascular lesion in at least eight more necropsy patients with ankylosing spondylitis appeared subsequently,[8-13] and findings in the 16 previously reported patients

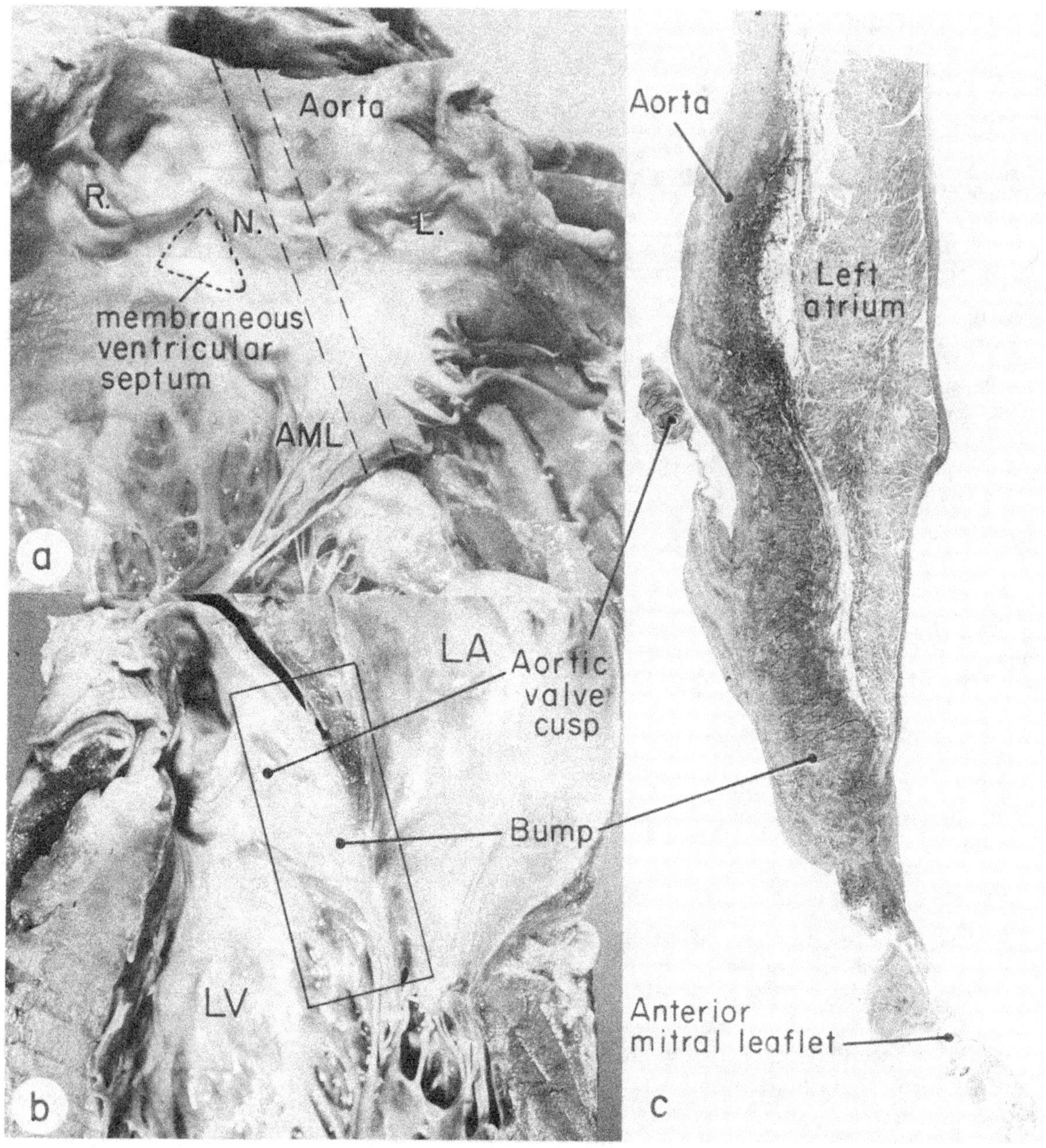

Figure 2

The heart of a 54-year-old man (A68-300) who presented with aortic regurgitation and left bundle branch block six years before death. Four years later the diagnosis of ankylosing spondylitis was made by retrospective examination of serial "spinal" roentgenograms and by a story of longstanding low back pain. The characteristic features of the cardiovascular lesion are shown. (a) Opened left ventricle, aorta, aortic valve right coronary cusp (R), non-coronary cusp (N) and left coronary cusp, and anterior mitral leaflet. The aortic wall thickening is limited to wall immediately behind and above the sinuses of Valsalva, especially behind the commissures. The basal portion of anterior mitral leaflet (AML) and the membranous septum are thickened by fibrous tissue. The dotted lines indicate the longitudinal cut through non-coronary (N) cusp of aortic valve, left atrium (LA) and ventricle (LV) which is shown in b and c. The subvalvular fibrous bump beneath aortic valve is best shown in histologic section (c). (Phosphotungstic acid-hematoxylin stain; ×3.)

are summarized in table 3. The occurrence of fibrous scarring below the aortic valve was com- mented upon in four of the 16 patients. Necropsy cardiovascular observations consistent with ankylos-

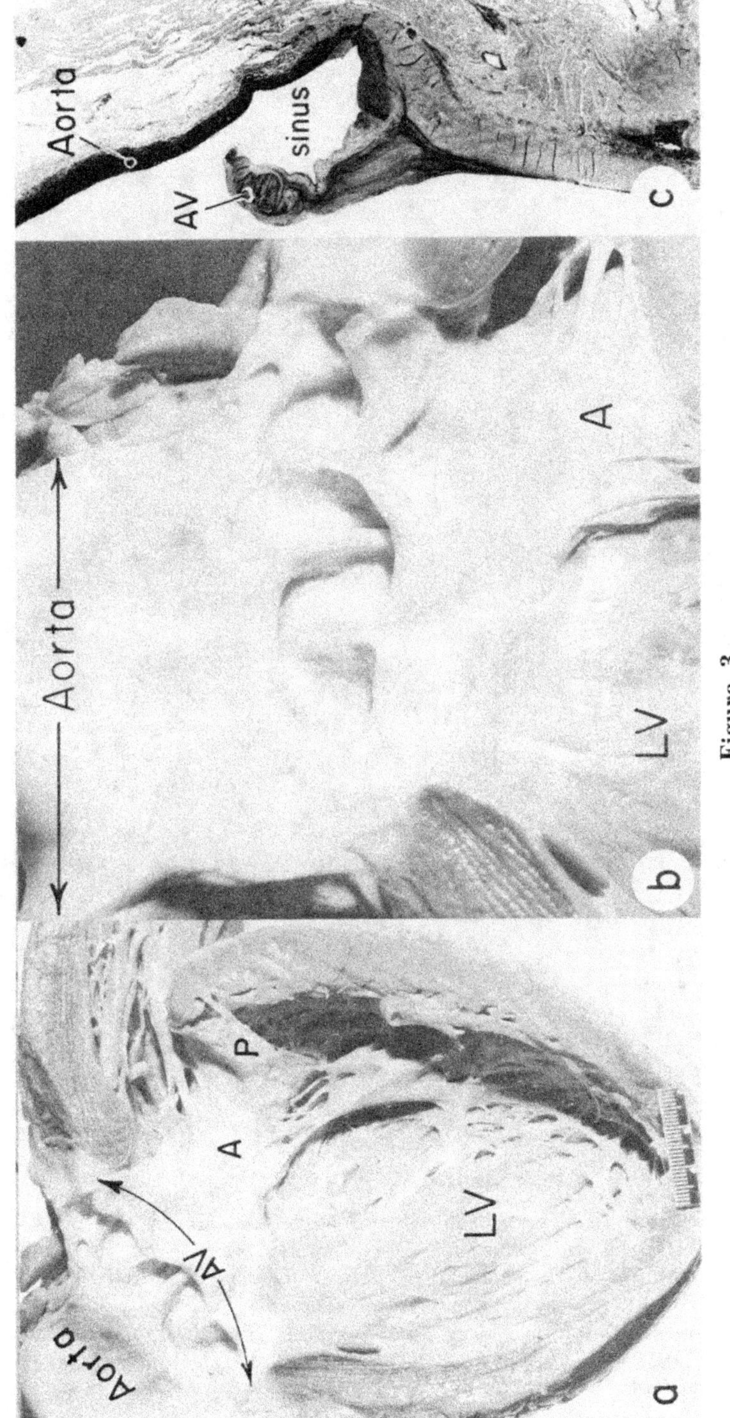

Figure 3

The heart of a 55-year-old man (A61-262) with ankylosing spondylitis who died of intractable congestive cardiac failure due to aortic valvular regurgitation. Left ventricle (LV) is opened in a and b showing aorta, aortic valve (AV) and anterior (A) and posterior (P) mitral leaflets. The scarring process of aortic wall is limited to the region of the sinuses, which are dilated. Fibrous tissue extends below the aortic valve (AV) cusps, which are thickened (b and c). (Elastic-van Gieson stain; ×3 (c).)

ing spondylitis have been described in ten other patients[1, 14] with ankylosing spondylitis, but specific information about individual cases was lacking. The mitral valve was abnormal, however, in four of these ten patients, one of whom had mitral regurgitation.

The cardiovascular lesion of ankylosing spondylitis is morphologically unique. The aortic inflammatory process is limited to aortic wall behind and immediately above the sinuses of Valsalva, particularly behind and adjacent to the commissures. The dense adventitial scar extends *below* the base of aortic valve to form a characteristic subvalvular ridge. The fibrous tissue

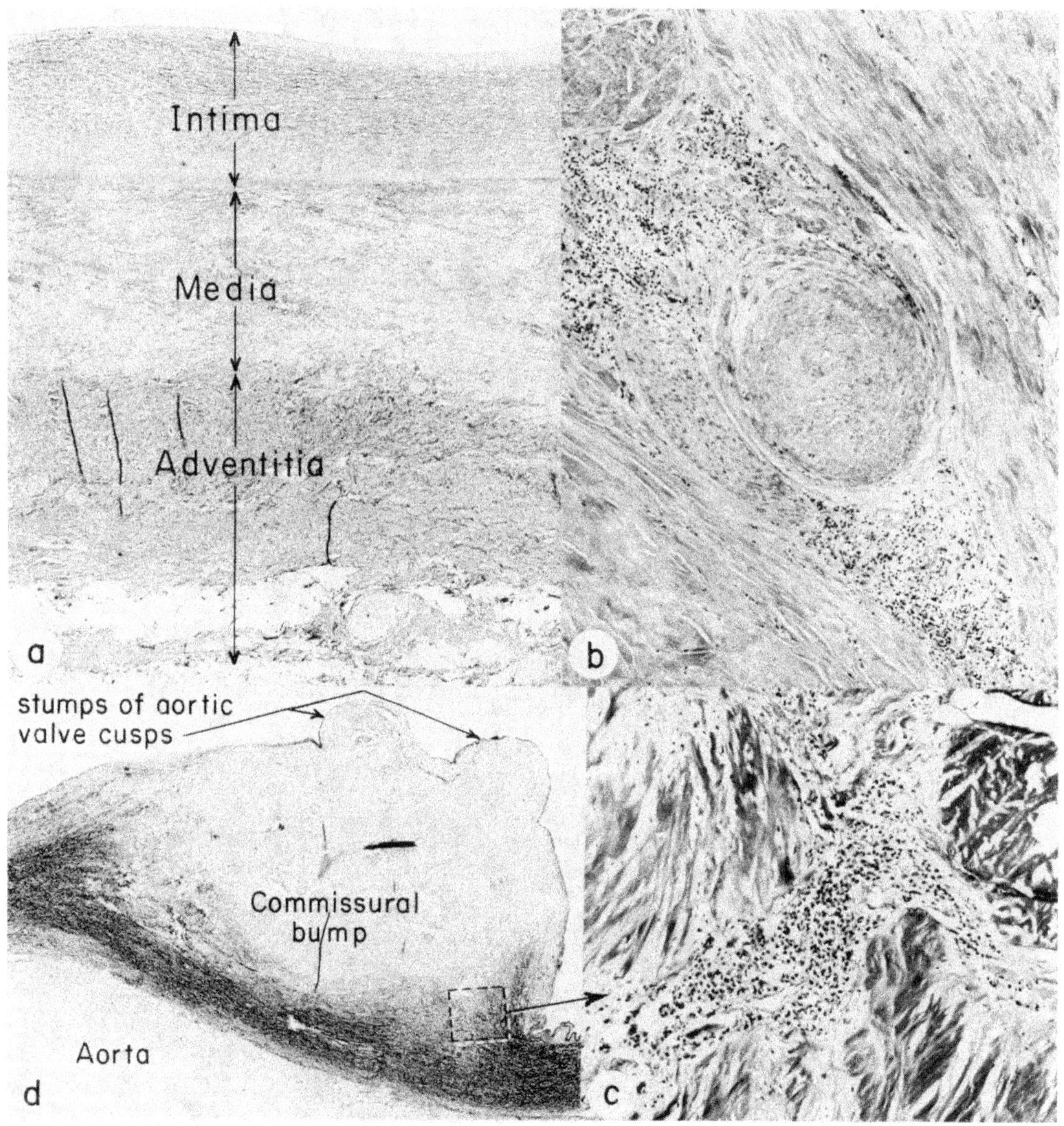

Figure 4

Aorta in ankylosing spondylitis. Aortic wall in ankylosing spondylitis is histologically similar to that in syphilis. (a) The aorta is thickened by adventitial scarring, and intimal proliferation. The media is scarred and the vasa vasora (b) are narrowed and surrounded by plasma cells and lymphocytes. The adventitial scarring (c) extends into and below the base of aortic valve. The aortic wall thickening is particularly prominent behind the commisures of aortic valve cusp (d) forming a fibrous commissural bump which causes malalignment of the cusps and their sagging toward left ventricle. (Hematoxylin and eosin stains; ×25 (a), ×88 (b), ×100 (c); Elastic van Gieson stain, ×16 (d).)

also extends into the base of anterior mitral leaflet to form a bump which may be associated with mitral regurgitation, usually of mild degree. Extension of fibrous tissue into the most cephalad portion of muscular ventricular septum is also characteristic, and it explains the associated conduction disturbances, which are frequent. The aortic valve cusps are shortened, and usually diffusely thickened. Occasionally, however, the midportion of a cusp was not thickened.

The cardiovascular lesion of ankylosing spondylitis is readily distinguished from other conditions also associated with aortic regurgitation (table 4, fig. 8). *Rheumatic disease* spares the aorta and

Table 3

Clinical and Necropsy Observations in Previously Reported Cases

Age Sex	Clinical Peripheral arthritis	Urethritis	Iritis	Age at onset arthritis (yrs.)	Age at onset cardiac disease (yrs.)	Duration of heart disease (yrs.)	CHF	ECG Conduction disturbances	Heart weight (gms)	Thick AV cusps	Sub- AV fibrosis	Cardiovascular pathology Thickening of aorta limited to sinuses	Pericarditis	Refs.
39 M	+	−	+	9	26	13	+	0	785	+	−	+	0	(7)
40 M	+	−	+	23	39	1½	+	−	550	+	−	+	foca	(7)
27 M	+	+	0	19	27	< 1	+	LBBB	580	+	+	+	foca	(7)
36 M	+	−	0	16	20	16	+	LBBB	900	+	−	+	foca	(7)
51 M	+	−	+	30	42	9	+	−	−	+	−	+	0	(7)
43 M	+	−	0	24	−	−	+	−	−	+	−	+	0	(7)
45 M	0	−	+	26	−	−	0	0	−	+	−	+	0	(7)
35 M	+	−	0	31	35	< 1	+	LBBB	−	+	−	+	0	(7)
52 M	+	+	0	11	50	2	+	1° HB	930	+	−	−	0	(8)
48 M	0	−	0	28	42	6	+	1° HB	770	+	−	+	foca	(8)
38 M	+	−	−	27	29	9	+	1° HB	700	+	−	+	0	(8)
35 M	+	−	+	27	33	2	+	RBBB 1° HB	515	+	−	0	−	(10)
54 M	+	+	+	51	51	3	+	1° HB LBBB	650	+	−	0	diffuse	(11)
50 M	+	0	0	30	50	< 1	0	1° HB	550	+	+	+	0	(11)
57 M	+	+	0	30	54	3	+	CHB	850	+	+	+	diffuse	(12)
59 M	+	−	−	39	58	1	0	CHB	550	+	+	−	0	(13)
Average 44 M	14	4	6	27	39	5	13		700					

Abbreviations: AV = aortic valve; CHB = complete heart block; CHF = congestive heart failure; 1 HB = first degree heart block (P-R interval > 0.20 sec): LBBB = left bundle branch block; RBBB = right bundle branch block.

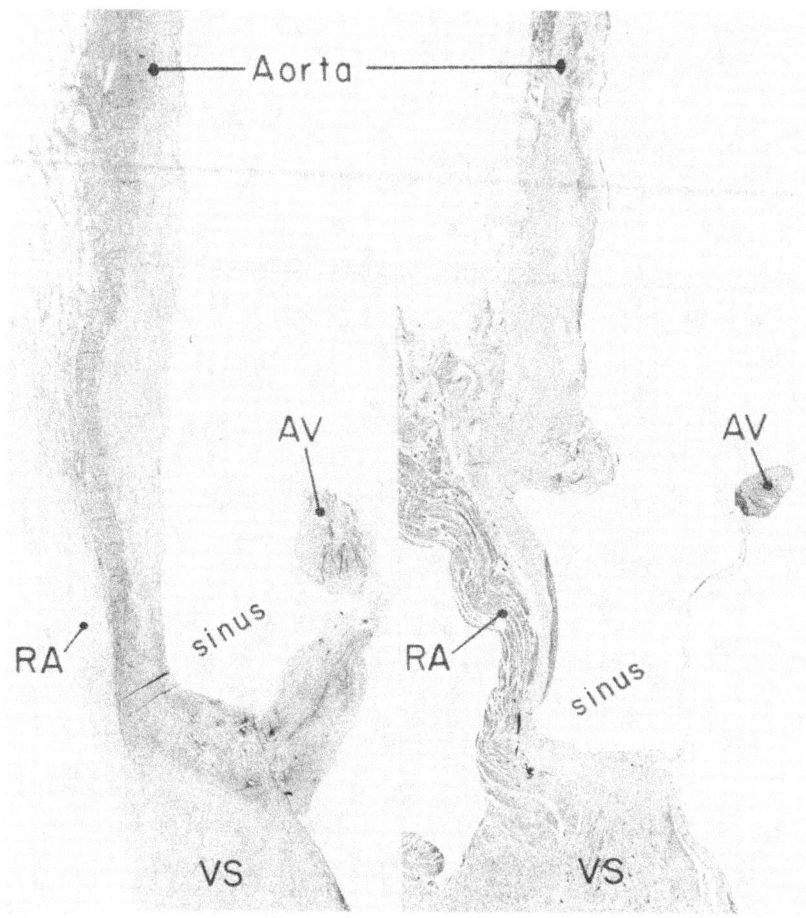

Figure 5

Longitudinal sections through wall of aorta, aortic valve (AV) cusps and ventricular septum (VS) from two patients: one (left) was a 54-year-old man (A68-300) with aortic regurgitation and ankylosing spondylitis, and the other (right), a 69-year-old man (A67-43), had aortic regurgitation from syphilis. In ankylosing spondylitis the aortic wall behind the sinuses is involved by the scarring process, whereas in syphilis a similar proces frequently begins distal to the sinus of Valsalva. Only the distal margin of aortic valve is thickened in syphilis whereas the proximal portions of valve are thickened as well in ankylosing spondylitis. RA = right atrial wall. (Elastic-van Gieson stain; ×3.5.)

always anatomically involves mitral valve.[15–16] The aortic wall lesion of cardiovascular *syphilis* is histologically identical to that of ankylosing spondylitis. The former, however, may spare the aortic wall behind the sinuses of Valsalva (fig. 6) and the adventitial scar tissue does not extend below the aortic valve or involve mitral valve or ventricular septum. Only the distal margins of the aortic valve cusps are thickened in syphilis, not the proximal portions which are always involved as well in ankylosing spondylitis. In *rheumatoid arthritis,* distinctive nodules similar to subcutaneous nodules, may infiltrate pericardium, myocardium and mural and valvular endocardium.[16–18] If valvular tissue is involved, regurgitation usually of only mild degree results. Aortic regurgitation in the *Marfan syn-*

drome is a consequence of disease of aortic wall, not of aortic valve; the aorta is thinner than normal, and usually contains medial and intimal tears. The ascending aorta is diffusely involved and dilatation of the aortic root causes the aortic regurgitation, which is usually severe. The mitral, and rarely the aortic valve, cusps may be redundant ("floppy") in patients with the Marfan syndrome.

The valular regurgitation and conduction disturbances of ankylosing spondylitis have anatomic explanations. Aortic regurgitation appears to result from a combination of three factors: 1) thickening and shortening of the cusps; 2) displacement of the cusps caudally by the fibrous tissue bump located behind the commissures; and 3) dilatation of aortic root. Mitral regurgitation, although rare, appears to

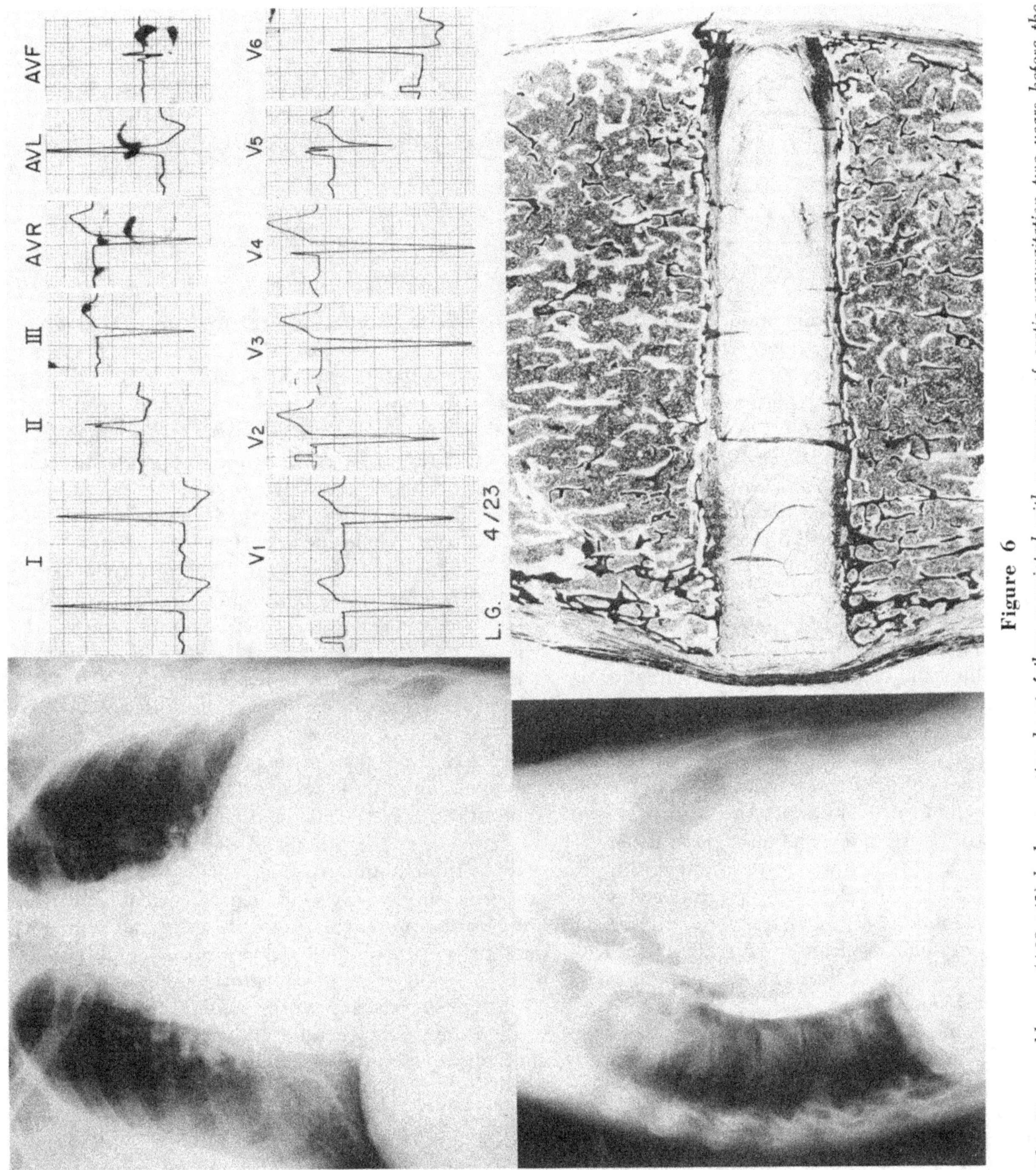

Figure 6

This 38-year-old man (A68-142) had congestive heart failure associated with a murmur of aortic regurgitation two years before the diagnosis of ankylosing spondylitis was suspected clinically. Chest roentgenograms (left), and electrocardiogram (upper right), were taken two years before death. The latter shows a prolonged P-R interval and an interventricular conduction delay. Although at necropsy early morphologic changes of ankylosing spondylitis were present in the sacroiliac joints and intervertebral spaces (lower right) the cardiac lesion had progressed to wide open lethal aortic regurgitation. (Masson stains, ×4 (d).)

Table 4

Causes of Aortic Regurgitation

	Ankylosing Spondylitis	Syphilis	Marfans	Rheumatic	Rheumatoid Arthritis
Average age	45	50	30	45	70
Usual sex	Men	Men	Men	Men	Women
Aortic regurgitation	+ + +.+	+ + + +	+ + + +	+ + +	+
Mitral regurgitation	+	0	+ + +	+ + + +	+
Conduction disturbances	+ + + +	+	0	0	+ +
Aorta:					
Adventitial scarring	+ + +	+ + +	0	0	0
Medial degeneration	+ + +	+ + +	+ + + +	0	0
Intimal proliferation	+ +	+ +	0	0	0
Limited to sinuses	+	0	0	0	0
Subaortic lump	+	0	0	0	0
Aortic cuspal thickening	Diffuse	Focal	Focal	Diffuse	Focal
Anterior mitral leaflet thickening	+ +	0	+	+ + + +	+

result from two factors: 1) dilatation of the left ventricle (from aortic regurgitation) with resulting malalignment of the papillary muscles, and 2) fibrous thickening at the basal portion of anterior mitral leaflet. Bundle branch block and complete heart block in patients with ankylosing spondylitis appear to result from extension of the fibrous process from the membranous ventricular septum into the muscular septum to interrupt or destroy the conduction fibers in the atrioventricular bundle or proximal bundle branches.

The underlying cause of pure aortic regurgitation, severe enough to be fatal, is usually readily determined. The usual etiologies include rheumatic, infective endocarditis,[19] congenitally malformed valves with and without superimposed infection,[20] "floppy" valves with and without the Marfan syndrome,[16] trauma,[16] dissecting aortic aneurysm and a few miscellaneous conditions. Among patients with pure aortic regurgitation, the etiology in a few is usually unclear. Among the latter, ankylosing spondylitis must be considered as an underlying condition. Diagnosis of ankylosing spondylitis, however, is often difficult because few patients with combined ankylosing spondylitis and aortic regurgitation have advanced and readily diagnosable skeletal deformities. Only two of our eight patients had bony ankylosis with bamboo spine, classic late arthritic changes of ankylosing spondylitis. Two others had evidence of cardiac dysfunction years before the diagnosis of ankylosing spondylitis could be made. Thus, in them and in other reported patients,[9, 11, 21, 22] aortic regurgitation clinically may exist as a forme fruste of ankylosing spondylitis. A possible reason why signs of ankylosing spondylitis may be absent or minimal in a patient with combined ankylosing spondylitis and severe aortic regurgitation is that the latter condition when severe may cause death before there has been time to develop severe arthritic signs. The average life span of patients with ankylosing spondylitis unassociated with aortic regurgitation is normal (about 70 years)[23, 24] whereas the life span of patients with ankylosing spondylitis associated with wide open and therefore fatal aortic regurgitation is much shorter (about 45 years).[7] Hence, cardiac dysfunction may appear before joint signs are definite, and the aortic regurgitation may be severe when the joint signs are minimal or absent.

The spectrum of cardiovascular disease in patients with ankylosing spontylitis is presumably wide (figure 9). Our patients represent one end of this spectrum, those with wide open fatal aortic regurgitation. Little information is available about the patients at the other end of the spectrum, i.e., those with anatomic involvement of the aortic root area but without any evidence of cardiac dysfunction. Furthermore, there is little information about patients with combined ankylosing spondylitis and minimal, mild or moderate aortic regurgitation. Of 25 necropsy patients with ankylosing spondylitis studied by Davidson et al.[14] five (20%) had anatomically abnormal aortic valves but only two of them had clinically detectable aortic regurgitation.

Although its frequency in patients with ankylosing spondylitis is unclear, aortic regurgitation does appear to increase with increasing duration of arthritis. Aortic regurgitation appears to occur in about 12% of patients with signs of ankylosing

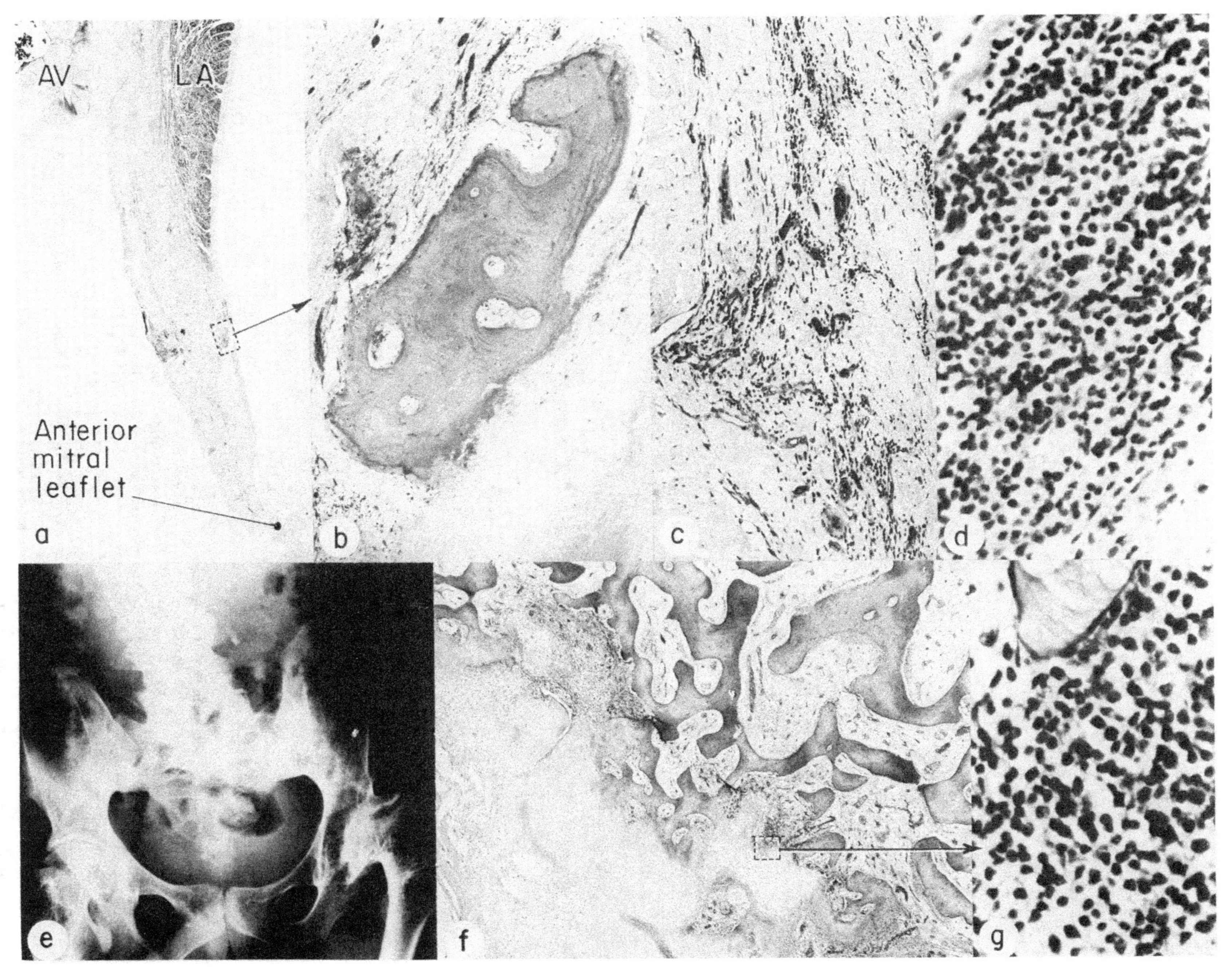

AV
LA
Anterior
mitral
leaflet
a
b
c
d
e
f
g

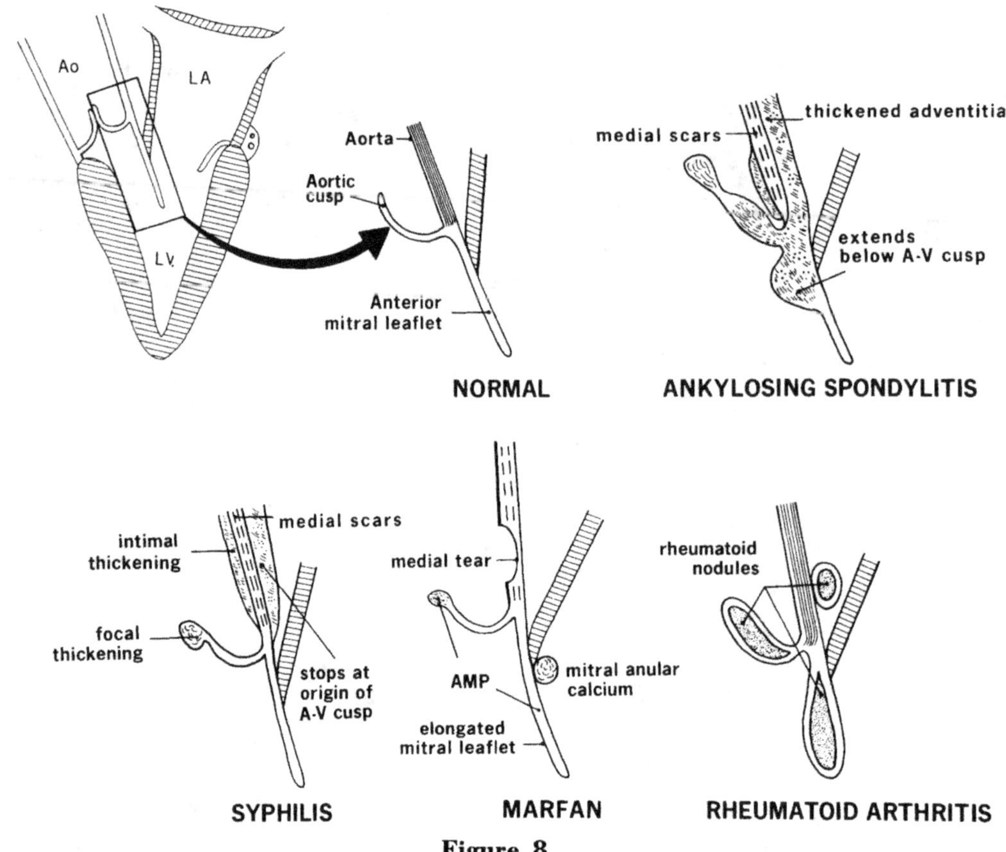

Figure 8

Cardiovascular lesion of ankylosing spondylitis compared to other conditions associated with aortic regurgitation.

spondylitis for as long as 30 years, but in only about 2% of those with signs of spondylitis for as short as 10 years.[1]

Urethritis, iritis and psoriasis occur in increased frequencies in patients with ankylosing spondylitis.[4, 25] Some patients with Reiter's syndrome (urethritis, iritis and peripheral arthritis) have aortic regurgitation, and when they do spondylitis is nearly always present as well.[25, 26] One of our eight patients had Reiter's syndrome, and all our eight patients had peripheral arthritis. The inflammatory lesion which infiltrates the central joint in ankylosing spondylitis is similar histologically to the lesion observed in the aorta in patients with

---

Figure 7

Morphologic characteristics of cardiac and skeletal involvement in ankylosing spondylitis. The inflamed fibrous tissue which infiltrates the aortic root area is histologically similar to the "pannus" which infiltrates the joints. Shown in (a) is a histologic section through aortic valve (AV), anterior mitral leaflet and left atrium (LA) from a 35-year-old man (A64-17) with ankylosing spondylitis who died almost two years after aortic valve replacement because of severe regurgitation. The subvalvular area and anterior mitral leaflet are thickened by vascularized and inflamed fibrous tissue (c) containing a few small bony spicules (b), an unusual finding in a valve not heavily calcified. Focal collections of lymphocytes and plasma cells also are present in the same area (d). This patient had severe bilateral sacroiliitis (e). A histologic section of sacroiliac joint demonstrates infiltration of the joint space with vascularized fibrous tissue (f) containing focal collections of lymphocytes and plasma cells (g) causing a "fibrous ankylosis." The latter may progress to a bony ankylosis with total obliteration of joint space.

Thus, both joint and aortic root area are involved by a similar inflammatory process. The stimulus to this process, however, remains uncertain. (Hematoxylin and eosin stain; ×3½ (a), ×90 (b), ×140 (c), ×560 (d), ×25 (f), ×560 (g).)

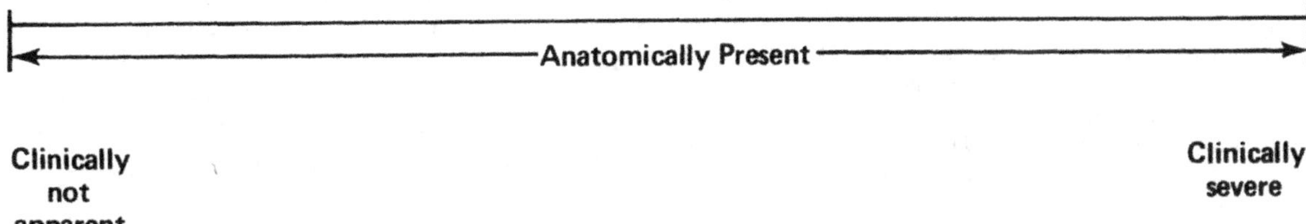

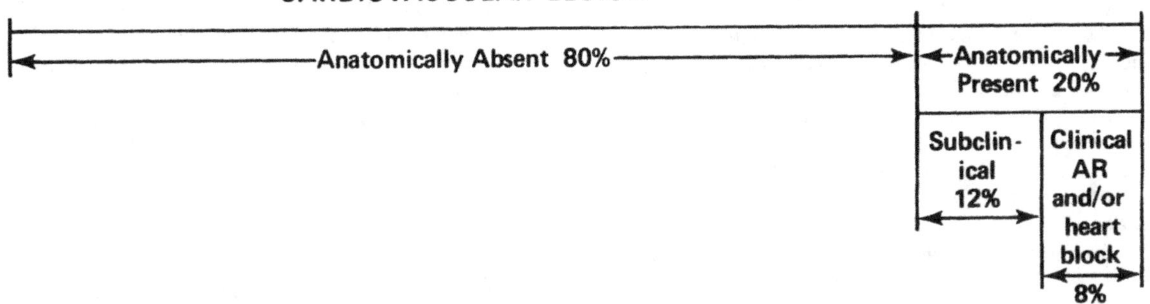

Figure 9

The spectrum of heart disease in patients with ankylosing spondylitis. Cardiovascular disease may be clinically apparent in patients with ankylosing spondylitis of any stage or severity. What proportion of patients with ankylosing spondylitis have anatomic valvular heart disease whether or not it be clinically detectable is unknown. A necropsy study by Davidson et al.,[14] however, suggests that approximately 20% of patients with ankylosing spondylitis have anatomic disease of aortic valve, but less than half of the latter group have clinically detectable valvular dysfunction.

ankylosing spondylitis and aortic regurgitation. Similar inflammatory changes occur in peripheral joints of patients with ankylosing spondylitis.[3, 27] The specificity with which certain target sites in the body are infiltrated by the inflammatory lesion suggest that a common tissue element is involved in ankylosing spondylitis and that the latter might better be termed the "spondylitis syndrome" (table 5).

Table 5

Spondylitis Syndrome

1.	Vertebral-sacroiliac joints	Spondylitis sacroiliitis
2.	Cardiovascular system	Aortic regurgitation Heart block
3.	Eye	Conjunctivitis Iritis
4.	Genitourinary system	Urethritis
5.	Skin	Psoriasis Keratodermia blennorrhagica
6.	Peripheral joints and tendons	Arthritis and tendinitis

Acknowledgment

The gross photographs were taken by Mr. Kensie L. Edwards and the histologic sections were prepared by Ms. Sandra J. Lewis.

References

1. Graham DC, Smythe HA: The carditis and aortitis of ankylosing spondylitis. Bull Rheum Dis **9**: 171, 1958

2. Graham W: Is rheumatoid spondylitis a separate entity? Arthritis Rheum **3**: 88, 1960

3. Cruickshank B: Pathology of ankylosing spondylitis. Bull Rheum Dis **10**: 211, 1960

4. Julkunen H: Rheumatoid spondylitis—clinical and laboratory study of 149 cases compared with 182 cases of rheumatoid arthritis. Acta Rhem Scand Suppl No 4, **172**: 24, 1962

5. Zvaifler NH, Weintraub AM: Aortitis and aortic insufficiency in the chronic rheumatic disorders—A reapraisal. Arthritis Rheum **6**: 241, 1963

6. Mallory TB: Case records of the Massachusetts General Hospital. N Engl J Med **214**: 690, 1936

7. Clark WS, Kulka P, Bauer W: Rheumatoid aortitis with aortic regurgitation. An unusual manifestation of rheumatoid arthritis (including spondylitis). Am J Med **22**: 580, 1957

8. SCHILDER DP, HARVEY WP, HUFNAGEL CA: Rheumatoid spondylitis and aortic insufficiency. N Engl J Med 255: 11, 1956

9. VALAITIS J, CLIFFORD GP, MONTGOMERY MM: Aortitis with aortic valve insufficiency in rheumatoid arthritis. Arch Pathol 63: 207, 1956

10. ANSELL BM, BYWATERS EGL, DONIACH I: The aortic lesions of ankylosing spondylitis. Br Heart J 20: 507, 1958

11. TOONE EC, PIERCE EL, HENNIGAR GR: Aortitis and aortic regurgitation associated with rheumatoid spondylitis. Am J Med 26: 255, 1959

12. WEED CL, KULANDER BG, MAZARELLA JA, DECKER JL: Heart block in ankylosing spondylitis. Arch Intern Med 117: 800, 1966

13. LIU SM, ALEXANDER CS: Complete heart block and aortic insufficiency in rheumatoid spondylitis. Am J Cardiol 23: 888, 1969

14. DAVIDSON P, BAGGENSTOSS AH, SLOCUMB CH, DAUGHERTY GW: Cardiac and aortic lesions in rheumatoid spondylitis. Proc Staff Meet Mayo Clinic 38: 427, 1963

15. ROBERTS WC, PERLOFF JK: Mitral valvular disease. A clinicopathologic survey of the conditions causing the mitral valve to function abnormally. Ann Intern Med 77: 939, 1972

16. ROBERTS WC, DANGEL JC, BULKLEY BH: Nonrheumatic valvular cardiac disease: A clinicopathologic survey of 27 different conditions causing valvular dysfunction. Cardiovasc Clin 1973

17. ROBERTS WC, KEHOE JA, CARPENTER DF, GOLDEN A: Cardiovascular lesions in rheumatoid arthritis. Arch Intern Med 122: 141, 1968

18. CARPENTER DF, GOLDEN A, ROBERTS WC: Quadrivalvular rheumatoid heart disease associated with left bundle branch block. Am J Med 43: 922, 1967

19. BUCHBINDER NA, ROBERTS WC: Left-sided valvular active infective endocarditis. A study of forty-five necropsy patients. Am J Med 53: 20, 1972

20. ROBERTS WC: The congenitally bicuspid aortic valve. A study of 85 autopsy cases. Am J Cardiol 26: 72, 1970

21. MALETTE WG, EISMAN B, DANIELSON GK, MAZZOLENI A, RAMS JJ: Rheumatoid spondylitis and aortic insufficiency. J Thorac Cardiovasc Surg 57: 471, 1969

22. SPANGLER RD, McCALLISTER BD, McGOON DC: Aortic valve replacement in patients with severe aortic valve incompetence associated with rheumatoid spondylitis. Am J Cardiol 26: 130, 1970

23. BLUMBERG B, RAGAN C: The natural history of rheumatoid spondylitis. Medicine 35: 1, 1956

24. WILKINSON M, BYWATERS EGL: Clinical features and course of ankylosing spondylitis as seen in follow-up of 222 hospital reference cases. Ann Rheum Dis 17: 209, 1958

25. RODMAN GP, BENEDEK TG, SHAVER JA, FENNELL RH: Reiter's syndrome and aortic insufficiency. JAMA 189: 889, 1964

26. PAULUS HE, PEARSON CM, PITTS W: Aortic insufficiency in 5 patients with Reiter's syndrome. Am J Med 53: 464, 1972

27. CRUICKSHANK B: Lesions of cartilaginous joints in ankylosing spondylitis. J Pathol 71: 73, 1956

Marfan Cardiovascular Disease without the Marfan Syndrome*

Fusiform Ascending Aortic Aneurysm with Aortic and Mitral Valve Regurgitation

*Bruce F. Waller, M.D.; Robert L. Reis, M.D., F.C.C.P.;
Charles L. McIntosh, M.D.; Stephen E. Epstein, M.D.; and
William C. Roberts, M.D., F.C.C.P.*

Dr. William C. Roberts: Herein we will discuss findings in a man with a fusiform aneurysm of the proximal ascending aorta, aortic-valve regurgitation, mitral-valve regurgitation, an anomalously arising left main coronary artery, and survival for 12 years after replacement of the aortic valve and partial replacement of the ascending aorta. Dr. Waller will describe the patient.

Dr. Bruce F. Waller: A 69-year-old Jamaican man had been asymptomatic until age 44 years. At age 17 (1927), however, a precordial murmur was heard. At age 44 (1954), he developed infective endocarditis after extraction of a tooth, and he was treated with penicillin for four weeks. Thereafter, he had exertional dyspnea which gradually progressed. At age 50 (1960), he had the sudden onset of substernal chest pain, but its etiology was never determined. Because of worsening dyspnea, he was started on a regimen of digitalis. At age 52 (1962), frequent premature ventricular beats were noted, and quinidine sulfate therapy was started. He underwent his first of four cardiac catheterizations at this time (Table 1).

Three years later, the exertional chest pain increased in frequency, the exertional dyspnea worsened, and he was admitted to the National Heart Institute (February 1956). A grade 4/6 murmur of aortic regurgitation, louder over the right than over the left sternal border, and a grade 2/6 holosystolic murmur at the apex were heard. The heart was big (Fig 1). Aortogram (Fig 1) showed a huge aortic root aneurysm and severe aortic regurgitation. An ECG (Fig 2) disclosed sinus tachycar-

dia, left ventricular hypertrophy with strain, and left atrial abnormality. On July 20, 1966, a cardiac operation was performed.

Dr. Roberts: Dr. Reis, would you describe your findings at operation?

Dr. Robert L. Reis: Each of the three aortic-valve sinuses of Valsalva and the proximal tubular portion of ascending aorta were massively dilated. The distal portion of ascending aorta was of normal or near normal size. Each of the three aortic valve cusps

Table 1—Hemodynamic and Angiographic Data (Pressures in mm Hg) at Rest*

	Age 52 (1962)	Age 56 (1966)	Age 57 (1967)	Age 69 (1978)
Right atrium (mean)	1	1	—	3
Right ventricle (s/d)	28/2	26/3	—	45/8
Pulmonary artery (s/d [mean])	28/5 [10]	26/10 [16]	—	45/20 [30]
Pulmonary wedge				
a wave	3			
v wave	10	—	—	27
mean	10	8	—	14
Left ventricle (s/d)	—	135/20	160/9	160/12
Systemic artery (s/d)	100/40	155/45	147/78	155/80
Aorta (s/d)	115/85	135/40	—	160/80
CO (CI) (L/min/sq m)	—	3.9 (2.2)	7.8 (4.4)	4.9 (2.7)
AA angiogram	—	+	+	+
AR	—	4+/4+	0	0
AA aneurysm	—	+	+	+
LV angiogram	—	—	+	+
MR	—	—	4+/4+	4+/4+

*AA indicates ascending aorta; AR, aortic regurgitation; CI, cardiac index; CO, cardiac output; LV, left ventricular; MR, mitral regurgitation; and s/d, peak systole/end-diastole.

*From the Pathology, Surgery and Cardiology Branches, National Heart, Lung and Blood Institute, National Institutes of Health, Bethesda.
Reprint requests: Dr. Roberts, NIH-NHLBI, Building 10A, Room 3E30, Bethesda, 20205

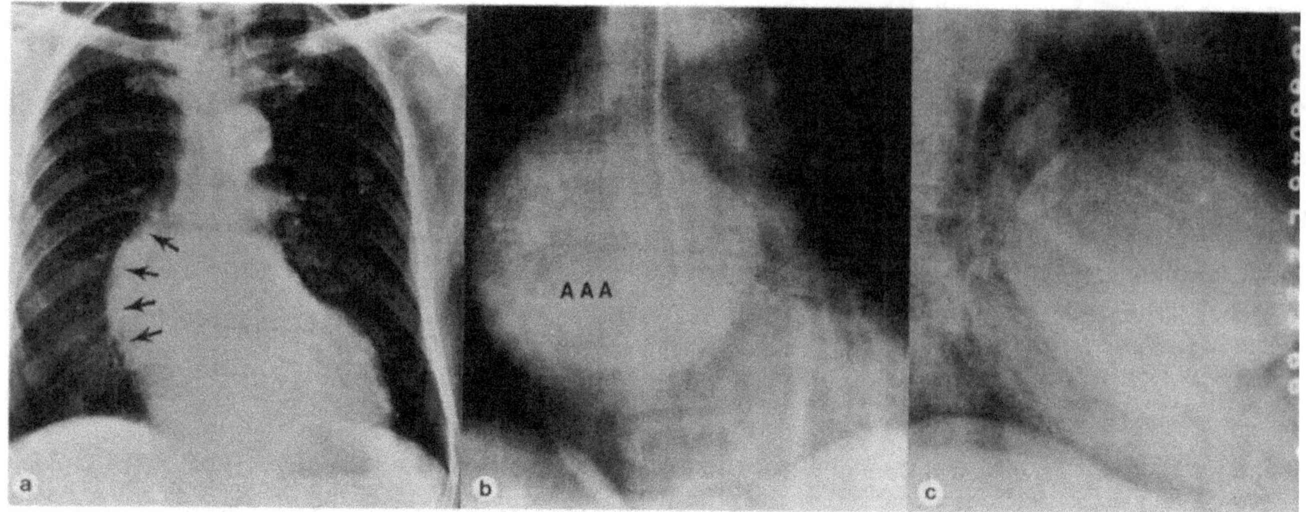

FIGURE 1. Preoperative posteroanterior chest roentgenogram showing huge ascending aortic aneurysm (*AAA*) and cardiomegaly. Anteroposterior (b) and lateral (c) aortic root angiograms demonstrate the large aneurysm.

was delicate and each appeared to prolapse toward the left ventricle. Only one coronary arterial ostium was present, and that was located in the aortic wall behind the right sinus. The aortic valve (Fig 3) was replaced with a size 9 Starr-Edwards prosthesis, and the aneurysmal wall which involved the tubular portion of ascending aorta was excised and replaced with a Teflon graft. His early postoperative period went smoothly.

Dr. Roberts: The excised portion of ascending aorta (Fig 3) had several intimal and medial tears and a thinner wall than normal. Histologically, there was massive loss of elastic fibers in the aortic media. Less than 10 percent of the expected number of elastic lamellae remained in the media, and those remaining were fragmented. The amount of acid mucopolysaccharide material in the media was focally increased. The margins of each of the three aortic valve cusps were thickened but the remaining por-

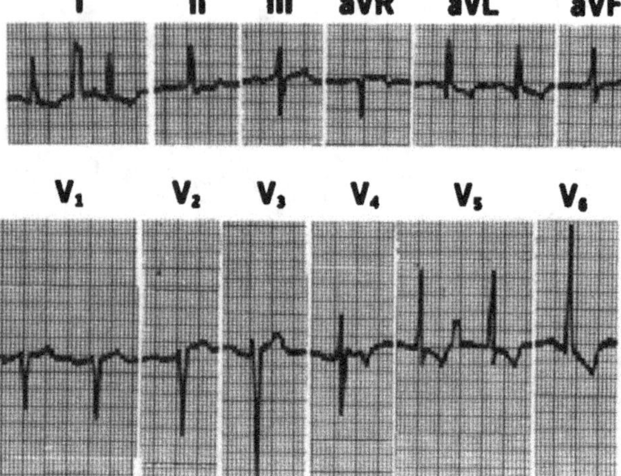

FIGURE 2. Electrocardiogram recorded immediately before first cardiovascular operation.

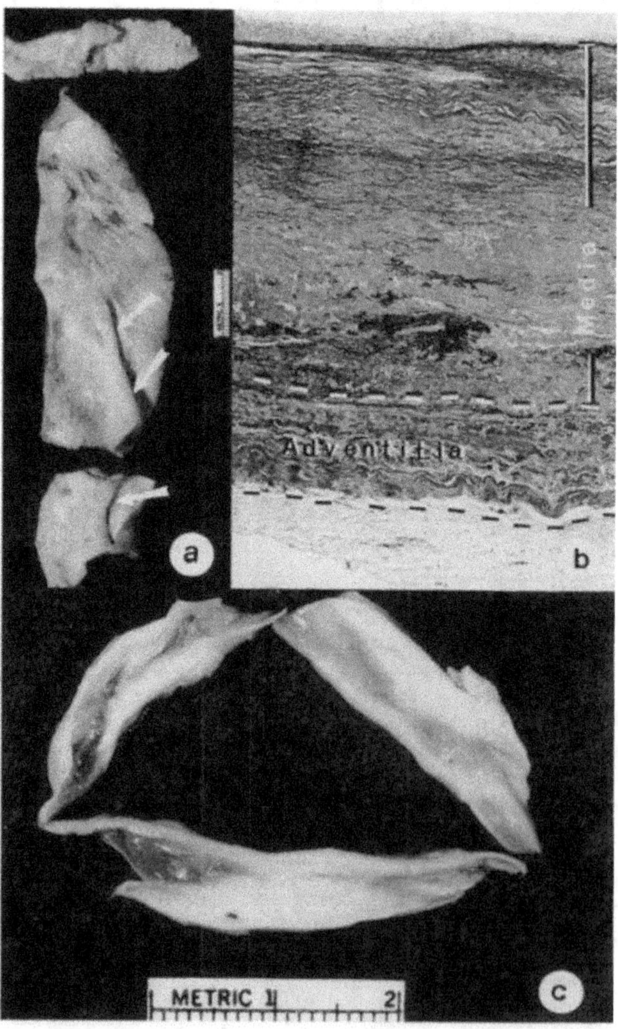

FIGURE 3. Excised portions of ascending aorta (a and b) and aortic-valve cusps (c). Intimal and medial tears (*arrows*) are present in aorta. Histologically, medial layer shows severe loss of elastic fibers (stained black). (Movat stain [b], original magnification × 40).

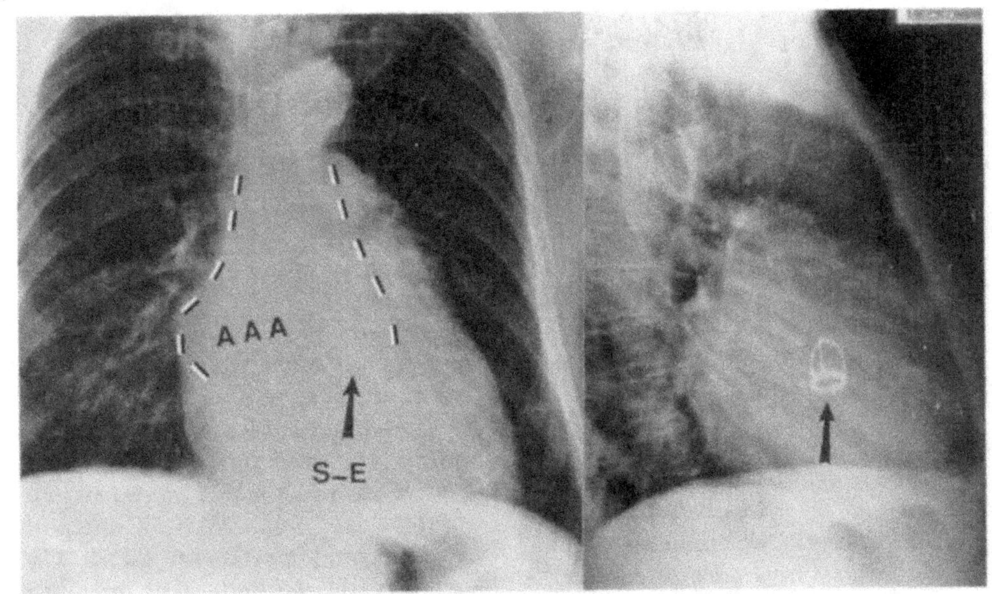

FIGURE 4. Postoperative posteroanterior and lateral chest roentgenograms showing generalized cardiomegaly, ascending aortic aneurysm (*AAA*) (outlined in dashed lines), and Starr-Edwards (*S-E*) aortic valve prosthesis.

tions were normal. The amount of acid mucopolysaccharide material was increased.

Dr. Waller, what happened to the patient after the operation?

Dr. Waller: The patient was re-evaluated nine months after the operation and was asymptomatic. The apical systolic murmur was now grade 4/6 in intensity, and it radiated into the left axilla. Aortography disclosed no aortic regurgitation but a small (13 mm Hg) peak systolic pressure gradient between left ventricle and aorta (presumably at the level of the caged-ball prosthesis) and severe

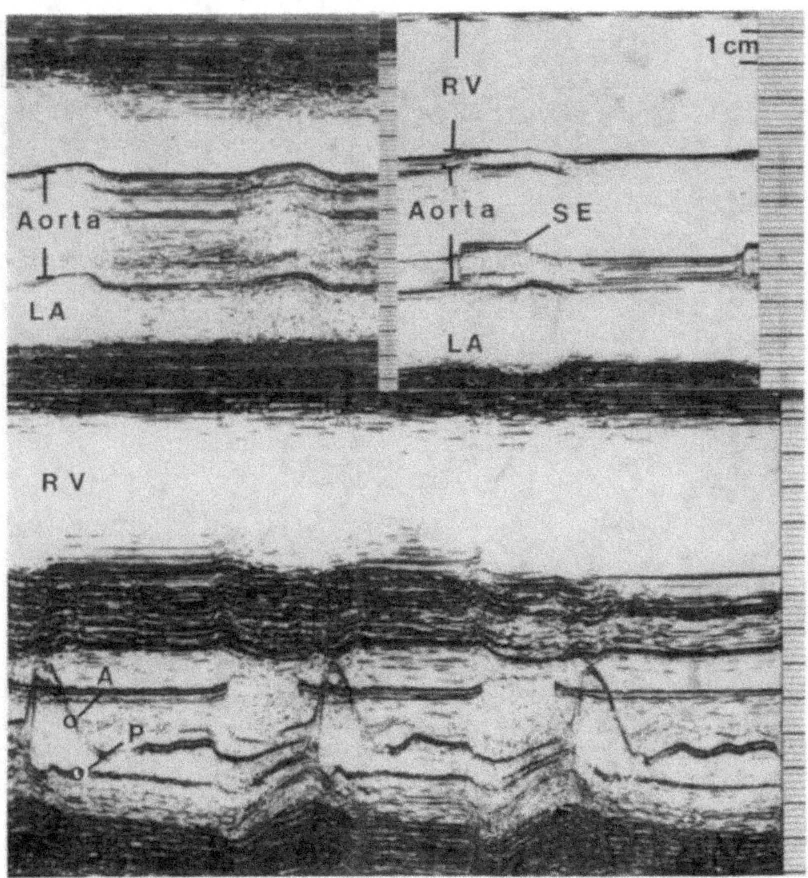

FIGURE 5. Postoperative echocardiogram. Top, view of dilated aortic root with its eccentrically healed Starr-Edwards (*S-E*) prosthesis and left atrium (*LA*). Right ventricular (*RV*) cavity is dilated and anterior (*A*) and posterior (*P*) mitral leaflets are normal.

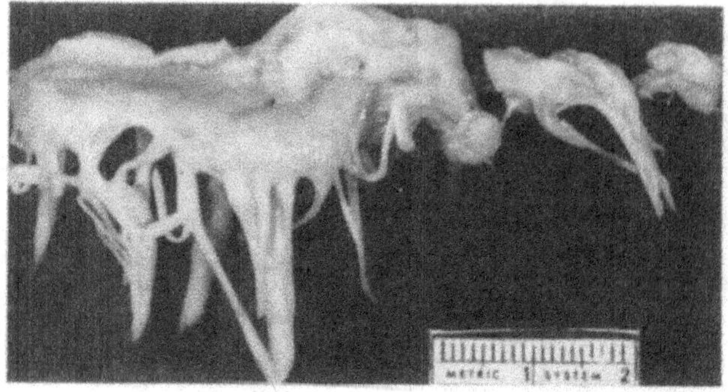

FIGURE 6. Excised mitral valve. Anterior leaflet and its chordae tendineae are thickened by fibrous tissue.

(4+/4+) mitral regurgitation (Table 1). He remained asymptomatic for another seven years, until age 64 (1974), when mild exertional dyspnea and chest pain reappeared. Because of gradual worsening of the dyspnea and the appearance of considerable fatigue, he was reevaluated in October 1978 when he was 69 years old (12 years after the aortic operation). He was unable to walk more than one flat block because of dyspnea. Precordial examination was unchanged. Repeat chest roentgenograms disclosed the cardiac silhouette to be about the same size as it was on the preoperative roentgenogram, but the left atrial cavity was larger (Fig 4). The ECG was unchanged. Echocardiogram (Fig 5) dis-

closed the aortic "root" to be much larger than the left atrial cavity, and the aortic-valve prosthesis to be eccentrically located. Repeat catheterization (Table 1) and angiography showed massive mitral regurgitation and elevation of pulmonary arterial pressures. A second cardiac operation was done.

Dr. Roberts: Dr. McIntosh, would you describe your operative findings?

Dr. Charles L. McIntosh: The second operation was to replace the severely regurgitant mitral valve via a transatrial septal approach. The anterior leaflet had protruded toward left atrium, and both leaflets were mildly thickened. The anulus was severely dilated. The mitral valve was replaced with a porcine prosthesis (size 31 mm). No calcific deposits or ruptured chordae tendineae were found. The wall of left atrium was firmly adherent to the thin aneurysmal wall of the ascending aorta, and during valve replacement, a retractor tore the atrial wall and the aortic aneurysmal wall. Repeated attempts to close the atrial and aortic wall tears were unsuccessful.

Dr. Roberts: The excised mitral valve disclosed an entirely normal posterior leaflet and chordae tendineae. The anterior leaflet, in contrast, was thickened by fibrous tissue, and its basal to distal margin was

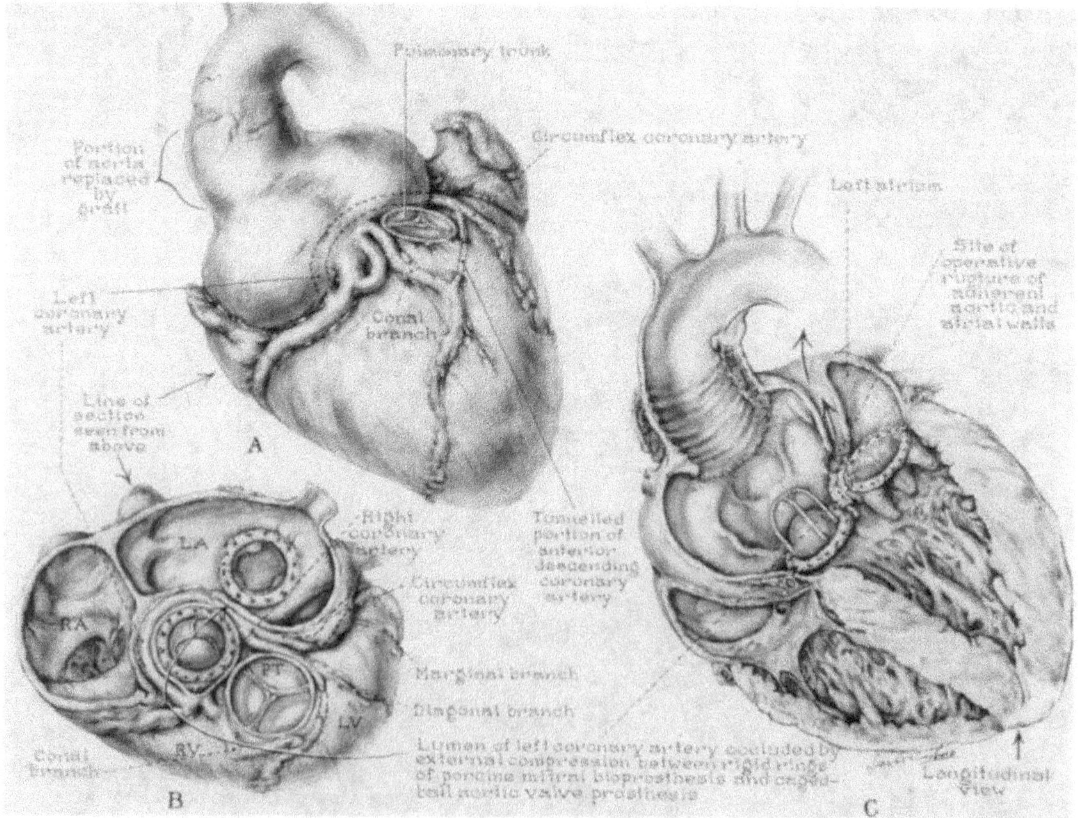

FIGURE 7. Drawing showing external anterior view of the heart (A), the anomalously arising left main coronary artery from the right coronary artery, and a longitudinal view (C) showing site of operative rupture of aorta and left atrium.

shorter than normal. (Fig 6). Several of its attached chordae also were thicker than normal. Histologically, the amount of acid mucopolysaccharide material in it was not increased.

Dr. Waller, could you summarize the cardiovascular findings at necropsy?

Dr. Waller: The tear in the wall of left atrium and aorta was readily apparent (Fig 7 and 8). The heart weighed 750 g. The aortic root aneurysm measured 9 × 7 × 5 cm (Fig 9). The poppet of the aortic valve prosthesis was yellow, but its surface was smooth and intact. The prosthesis was free of thrombus. The left main coronary artery arose as the first branch of the right coronary artery, and after coursing behind the aorta, it branched into the left anterior descending and left circumflex arteries (Fig 7). A large conus artery also connected the right and left anterior descending coronary arteries.

Dr. Roberts: The above described patient with cardiovascular features of the Marfan syndrome but without the Marfan syndrome is unusual for several reasons, as follows: (1) He lived a long life, namely 69 years and 57 of those were before a cardiovascular operation. The average age of death in patients with the Marfan syndrome is 35 years, and nearly all die from cardiovascular complications.[1,2] (2) Our patient lived 12 years after replacement of the aortic valve and a portion of ascending aorta, a very long survivor with this type operation. (3) He developed severe mitral regurgitation, severe enough to warrant mitral valve replacement. It is well known that patients with the cardiovascular disease of the Marfan syndrome often have mitral regurgitation, but usually the mitral regurgitation is not severe enough to warrant valve replacement.[2] (4) His aortic root aneurysm was extremely large, much larger than in most patients with the Marfan type cardiovascular disease. (5) He also had a congenital anomaly of the coronary arteries, namely only one aortic ostium with origin of the left main from the right coronary artery.

Dr. Epstein, you have studied clinically many patients with aortic root aneurysms of the Marfan type. What factors determine whether or not you recommend aortic valve replacement or aortic resection or both in these patients?

Dr. Stephen E. Epstein: In patients with aortic root aneurysms of the Marfan type, but without aortic regurgitation, operation is recommended under the following circumstances: (1) the patient develops, even in the absence of medical treatment, paroxysmal nocturnal dyspnea, an episode of pulmonary edema, angina pectoris, or near syncope or syncope; (2) the patient has dyspnea or fatigue that seriously interferes with his (her) normal daily living; or (3)

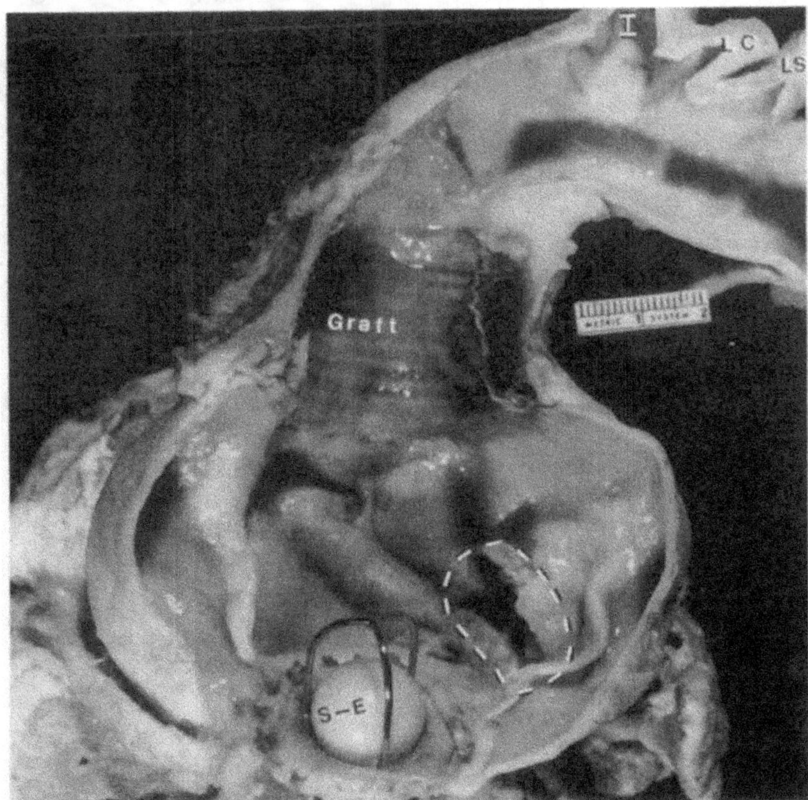

Figure 8. View of ascending aortic aneurysm and the Starr-Edwards (*S-E*) prosthetic valve. CAD (*dashed area*) designates site of operative rupture. *I* indicates innominate artery; *LC*, left common carotid artery; and *LS*, left subclavian artery.

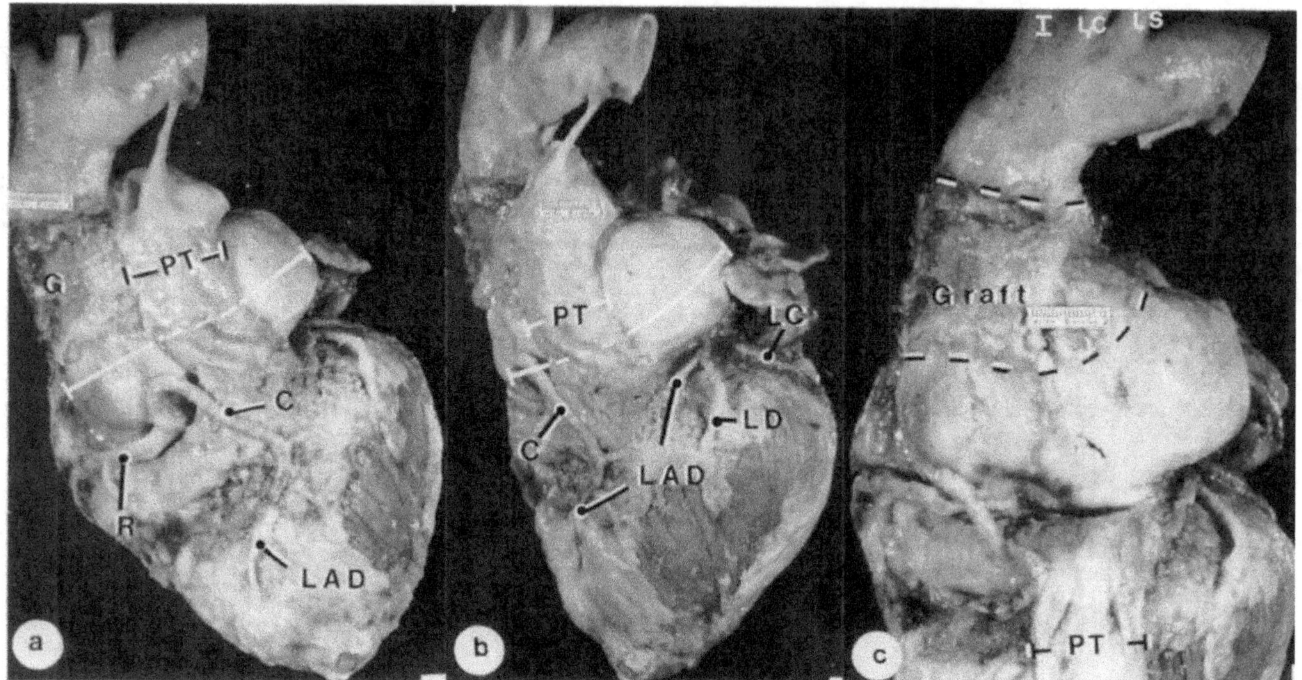

FIGURE 9. Exterior views of the heart at necropsy. a, Anterior view, b, left lateral view, and c, anterior view with pulmonary trunk (*PT*) retracted. The *white solid and dashed line* shows dimensions of aortic aneurysm. *C* indicates conal branch of right coronary artery; *R*, right coronary artery; *LAD*, left anterior descending coronary artery; *LD*, left diagonal coronary artery; *LC*, left circumflex coronary artery; *I*, innominate artery; *LC*, left common carotid artery; and *LS*, left subclavian artery.

there is evidence of left ventricular systolic dysfunction at rest, demonstrated by echocardiographic, radionuclide or catheterization studies. It is not necessary, in my view, however, that any of these three criteria of left ventricular dysfunction be present to recommend operation in a patient with an aortic root aneurysm of the Marfan type associated with aortic regurgitation. When aortic root aneurysm is suspected clinically because of an atypical location of the aortic regurgitant murmur (to the right rather than to the left of the sternal border), or an inappropriately dilated ascending aorta is observed on chest roentgenogram or echocardiogram, aortic root angiography is recommended. If a dilated aortic root with effaced sinuses is demonstrated, the patient is an operative candidate regardless of symptomatic status or degree of left ventricular dysfunction. The reason for this view is that the presenting manifestation of the Marfan-type aortic disease can be aortic dissection or rupture, both of which can cause sudden death or make subsequent operation impossible or extremely difficult.

Dr. Roberts: Possibly in the asymptomatic individual with a relatively small aortic root aneurysm of the Marfan type without or with only minimal aortic regurgitation, operatively *wrapping the ascending aorta* with a synthetic cloth (Teflon) might be considered. This procedure might prevent the develop-

ment of aortic regurgitation or possibly prevent or delay its progression. Furthermore, the wrapping might prevent additional aneurysmal dilatation of the aorta. Moreover, the wrapping procedure might stimulate the formation of considerable fibrous tissue around the aorta and this in turn might prevent aortic rupture.

Dr. Waller, the present patient had an echocardiogram which showed the ascending aorta to be much larger than the left atrium. In addition, the aortic valve prosthesis occupied a very small portion of the aortic root area, and it was very eccentrically located in the aorta. Can you summarize echocardiographic findings in patients with the Marfan type aortic root aneurysm?

Dr. Waller: Echocardiographic findings in patients with the cardiovascular disease associated with the Marfan syndrome or its form fruste varieties include the following: (1) dilatation of the aortic root; (2) mitral leaflet prolapse; (3) diastolic fluttering of the anterior mitral leaflet (if aortic regurgitation is present); and (4) dilatation of both ventricles and of the left atrium. Of 35 patients with the Marfan syndrome reported by Brown and associates,[3] 21 (60 percent) had dilated aortic roots (using at least two or three of the following criteria: absolute aortic dimensions >3.7 cm; body surface area correction for aortic diameter > 2.2 cm/sq m, and left atrial/ aortic ratio < 0.7) and 32 (91 percent) had prolapsed mitral leaflets. Payvandi and colleagues[4] found aortic root dilatation in five of nine patients with the Marfan syndrome and in seven (18 percent) of 40 relatives; mitral leaflet prolapse was present in all nine patients and in 13 (33 percent) of the 40 relatives. Neither of these studies, however, had angiographic documentation of aortic root enlargement or mitral leaflet prolapse.

The severe eccentric location of our patient's aortic valve prosthesis within the aorta on the echocardiogram deserves comment. To my knowledge, this echocardiographic eccentricity of an aortic prosthesis has not been described previously in a patient with the Marfan syndrome or its forme fruste variety. The posterior location of the prosthesis within the aorta suggests that the ascending aortic aneurysm protruded more anteriorly than posteriorly. This feature, however, could not be confirmed at necropsy. The recorded echoes of the aortic prosthesis itself appear to represent both anterior and posterior surfaces of the silicone rubber poppet, which was present in our patient, in addition to the prosthetic struts.[5-7] Most current models of the caged-ball prostheses contain hollow metal poppets, and in them only, the anterior surface of the poppet can be visualized echocardiographically.

Dr. Roberts: Dr. McIntosh, what type of operation is preferred today for the aortic disease of the Marfan or Marfan type syndromes?

Dr. McIntosh: The initial operative treatment for aortic root aneurysm of the Marfan type was replacement of most or all of the ascending aorta above the sinuses of Valsalva by a graft with or without the addition of nylon or Teflon aortic wrapping.[7-8] Later, aortic-valve replacement in addition was added.[9] These procedures, however, were associated with a high frequency of postoperative bleeding, and the diseased wall of aorta behind the sinuses of Valsalva was not excised. The next major operative advancement in treatment of aortic root aneurysm of the Marfan type with aortic regurgitation and the one preferred today is insertion of an aortic graft-aortic valve composite unit after excision of the aortic valve with or without excision of the ascending aorta.[10-13] The problem of restoring coronary flow has been handled by implanting the native coronary ostia into side holes of the composite graft or attaching saphenous vein conduits for bypass of each of the three major coronary arteries.

The later technique has lowered early mortality rates by reducing postoperative bleeding and operating times. Mayer and associates[13] recently reported a 4.5 year experience with 16 patients with the Marfan or Marfan-like aortic root disease in whom composite replacement of the aortic valve and ascending aorta with implanted native coronary ostia was accomplished. Although 11 of the 16 patients are alive and have minimal or no symptoms of cardiac dysfunction, two developed aneurysms at the site of coronary anastomoses on the aortic graft and a third developed an aneurysm at the anastomosis of the graft to the distal aorta. Despite these late complications, the composite graft method is clearly superior to the older operative procedures.

Dr. Roberts: Most students of cardiovascular diseases are aware that patients with the Marfan syndrome and form fruste varieties of it may have *floppy or prolapsing mitral leaflets.*[2] Our patient had severe mitral regurgitation and yet, at operation, the posterior mitral leaflet was normal, and the anterior leaflet did not protrude enough toward the left atrium to be considered "a prolapsed leaflet." Both grossly and histologically, the anterior leaflet was thickened by fibrous tissue and the amount of acid mucopolysaccharide material in it was not increased. Our patient indicates that there are causes of mitral regurgitation in these patients other than a prolapsing or floppy leaflet. Another major cause is *dilatation of the mitral anulus.* The anulus in the present patient, however, was 12.5 cm in circumference, which is not enough to produce severe mitral regurgitation.[14] Another cause of mitral regurgitation in these patients is *mitral anular calcific deposits,* but none occurred in the present patient.[15] A fourth cause of mitral regurgitation in these patients is *marked dilatation of the left ventricle from associated aortic regurgitation.* The present patient, however, had no aortic regurgitation during his last 12 years, and his left ventricle was not very dilated at necropsy. Thus, it appears that the mitral regurgitation in our patient resulted mainly from the fibrous contracture of the anterior mitral leaflet, possibly a process initiated by *infective endocarditis* which healed.[16] The leaflet thickening, however, could be the *anatomic equivalent of the "Austin-Flint" murmur* from the previously severe aortic regurgitation.

A final unusual finding in our patient was the *origin of the left main coronary artery as the first branch of the right coronary artery.* The left main passed behind the ascending aorta and between the wall of aorta and anterior wall of left atrium. Consequently, only one ostium of a coronary artery was present in the aorta. Dr. Waller, is there any specific danger of replacing both mitral and the aortic valves in a patient in whom either the left main or the left circumflex coronary arteries course behind the aorta in between the mitral and aortic valve "rings"?

Dr. Waller: In this laboratory, we have studied two patients who had anomalous origin of the left circumflex coronary artery as the first branch of the right coronary artery and in whom either the mitral or both the mitral and aortic valves were replaced with rigid-frame prostheses.[17] The anomalous coronary artery had not been diagnosed preoperatively or at operation in either patient. In the patient with two prostheses, the lumen of the anomalous left circumflex coronary artery was compressed between the two prosthetic-valve rings causing severe narrowing with resulting lateral wall myocardial infarction. Thus, in the present patient, the danger could have been even greater, since not only was the left circumflex potentially compressed, but the entire left system could have been compressed by the rigid frames of the porcine mitral and that of the caged-ball aortic prosthesis.

Dr. Roberts: A final word regarding nomenclature. The lesion in the aorta in patients with the Marfan syndrome or the form fruste varieties of it has been called "medial cystic necrosis." This term, however, is poor because "cysts" are relatively infrequent, and "necrosis" is extremely difficult to be sure of when examining histologic sections of ascending aorta. This term "medial cystic necrosis" was introduced by Gsell in 1928[18] and further used by Erdheim in 1929.[19] These authors had access only to hematoxylin eosin stains at that time, and these stains are simply not adequate to study the configuration of the elastic fibers in the media of aorta. Use of superb elastic tissue stains during the past 25 years has indicated that the dominant histologic finding in the ascending aorta in patients with the Marfan syndrome or in its form fruste varieties is *massive degeneration of elastic fibers* which occurred in the present patient. We estimated that less than 10 percent of the expected number of elastic fibers were present in the media of the wall of the aneurysm in the present patient. Massive elastic-fiber degeneration is the *sine qua non* of the Marfan type aorta. The strength of the aorta is due to the integrity of its elastic fibers, collagen fibrils, and smooth muscle cells. There is no evidence that the smooth muscle cells are abnormal in the aorta in these patients, but there is some ultrastructural evidence that the collagen fibers are abnormal. By simple histologic examination, however, the major and dominant histologic feature is massive degeneration of elastic fibers, and, therefore, the term "medial cystic necrosis" might best be avoided.

REFERENCES

1 Murdoch JL, Walker BA, Halpern BL: Life expectancy and causes of death in the Marfan syndrome. N Engl J Med 1972; 286:804-808

2 Roberts WC: Congenital cardiovascular abnormalities usually "silent" until adulthood: morphologic features of the floppy mitral valve, valvular aortic stenosis, hypertrophic cardiomyopathy, sinus of Valsalva aneurysm, and the Marfan syndrome. *In*: Roberts WC, ed. Congenital heart disease in adults. Philadelphia: FA Davis Co, 1979; 407-453 (Cardiovascular Clinics 10 [#1]: 1-574, 1979)

3 Brown OR, DeMots, Kloster FE, Roberts A, Menashe VD, Beals RK: Aortic root dilatation and mitral valve prolapse in Marfan's syndrome: an echocardiographic study. Circulation 1975; 52:652-802

4 Payvandi MN, Kerber RE, Phelps CD, Judisch GF, El-Khoury G, Schrott HG: Cardiac, skeletal and ophthalmologic abnormalities in relatives of patients with the Marfan syndrome. Circulation 1977; 55:797-802

5 Johnson ML, Paton BC, Holmes JH: Ultrasonic evaluation of prosthetic valve motion. Circulation 1970; 42 (suppl 2):3-15

6 Siggers DC, Srwongse SA, Deuchar D: Analysis of dynamics of mitral Starr-Edwards valve prosthesis using reflected ultrasound. Br Heart J 1971; 33:401-406

7 Bahnson HT, Nelson AR: Cystic medial necrosis as a cause of localized aortic aneurysms amenable to surgical treatment. Ann Surg 1956; 144:519-529

8 Cooley DA, DeBakey ME: Resection of entire ascending aorta in fusiform aneurysm using cardiac bypass. JAMA 1956; 162:1158

9 Wheat MW, Wilson JR, Bartley TD: Successful replacement of the entire ascending aorta and aortic valve. JAMA 1964; 188:717-719

10 Bloodwell RB, Hallman GL, Cooley DA: Aneurysm of the ascending aorta with aortic valvular insufficiency. Arch Surg 1966; 92:588-599

11 Ferlic RM, Goot B, Edwards JE, Lillehei CW: Aortic valvular insufficiency associated with cystic medial necrosis. Ann Surg 1967; 165:1-9

12 Bentall H, DeBono A: A technique for complete replacement of the entire ascending aorta. Thorax 1968; 3:338-339

13 Mayer JE, Lindsay WG, Wang Y, Jorgensen CR, Nicoloff DM: Composite replacement of the aortic valve and ascending aorta. J Thorac Cardiovasc Surg 1978; 76:816-823

14 Bulkley BH, Roberts WC: Dilatation of the mitral anulus: a rare cause of mitral regurgitation. Am J Med 1975; 59:457-463

15 Roberts WC, Perloff JC: Mitral valvular disease: a clinicopathologic survey of the conditions causing the mitral valve to function abnormally. Ann Intern Med 1972; 77:936-975

16 Roberts WC, Buchbinder NA: Healed left-sided infective endocarditis: a clinicopathologic study of 59 patients. Am J Cardiol 1977; 40:878-888

17 Roberts WC, Morrow AG: Compression of anomalous left circumflex coronary arteries by prosthetic valve fixation rings. J Thorac Cardiovasc Surg 1969; 57:834-838

18 Gsell O: Wandnekrosen der Aorta als Selbstandige Erkrankung und ihre Beziehung zur Spontanruptur. Virchows Arch Path Anat Physiol 1928; 270:1-9

19 Erdheim J: Medionecrosis aortae idiopathica. Virchow's Arch Path Anat Physiol 1929; 273:454-463

Severe Aortic Regurgitation From Systemic Hypertension (Without Aortic Dissection) Requiring Aortic Valve Replacement

Analysis of Four Patients

BRUCE F. WALLER, MD
JEREL M. ZOLTICK, MD
JEFFREY H. ROSEN, MD
NEVIN M. KATZ, MD
MARIO N. GOMES, MD, FACC
ROSS D. FLETCHER, MD, FACC
ROBERT B. WALLACE, MD
WILLIAM C. ROBERTS, MD, FACC

Washington, D.C.
Bethesda, Maryland

Clinical and morphologic observations are described in four patients who had *severe* aortic regurgitation from severe systemic hypertension unassociated with aortic dissection; each patient underwent aortic valve replacement. Although aortic regurgitation of minimal or mild degree is well recognized to occur in patients with systemic hypertension, severe degrees of aortic regurgitation are rare in such patients; aortic valve replacement in such patients has not previously been reported. Why these four patients had such severe aortic regurgitation was not determined. Although systemic hypertension is rarely a cause, it nevertheless must be added to the list of causes of severe pure aortic regurgitation.

It is well recognized that a small proportion (about 9 percent[1]) of patients with systemic hypertension have a basal diastolic blowing murmur indicative of aortic regurgitation, which is usually of minimal or mild degree. The development of *severe* aortic regurgitation purely on the basis of elevated intraaortic pressure in the absence of aortic dissection is extremely rare and, to our knowledge, aortic valve replacement for pure aortic regurgitation secondary to systemic hypertension unassociated with dissection has not been reported. However, four patients with this condition are described in this report.

Patients Studied

Blood pressure: Pertinent clinical and morphologic observations in the four cases are summarized in Tables I and II and illustrated in Figures 1 to 4. Each patient had systemic hypertension treated with combinations of antihypertensive drugs including afterload-reducing agents. Patient 3 had the shortest duration of clinically recognized systemic hypertension (1 year) and Patient 2 the longest duration (30 years). The highest indirect systolic brachial arterial pressures in the four patients ranged from 195 to 270 mm Hg (average 241) and the lowest from 140 to 170 mm Hg (average 157). The highest indirect diastolic brachial arterial pressures in the four patients ranged from 110 to 150 mm Hg (average 125) and the lowest from 35 to 70 mm Hg (average 59). Pre- and postoperative systemic arterial pressures in Patient 4 are summarized in Figure 3. The cause of the systemic hypertension in Patients 1 and 2 was renal disease (bilateral polycystic disease [each kidney weighed 4,000 g] in Patient 1 and probably congenital hypoplasia [each kidney weighed 70 g] in Patient 2); the cause was considered essential or idiopathic in Patients 3 and 4.

Cardiac findings: All four patients had a precordial diastolic blowing murmur typical of aortic regurgitation. On aortic root angiography, the degree of aortic regurgitation was either 3+ or 4+ on a 1+ to 4+ scale[2] in all four patients (Fig. 1). None of the four patients had clinical or anatomic evidence of mitral valve dysfunction. All four patients had evidence (dyspnea, pulmonary, rales and third sound gallop) of chronic congestive heart failure, in three patients for 6 months or less and in one patient for 24 months. Preoperatively, all four patients were

From the Division of Cardiology, Department of Medicine, and the Department of Surgery, Georgetown University, Washington, D.C., the Department of Cardiology, Department of Medicine, Veteran's Administration Hospital, Washington, D.C., and the Pathology Branch, National Heart, Lung, and Blood Institute, National Institutes of Health, Bethesda, Maryland. Manuscript received June 1, 1981; revised manuscript received July 21, 1981, accepted July 27, 1981.

Address for reprints: William C. Roberts, MD, Building 10A, Room 3E30, National Heart, Lung, and Blood Institute, National Institutes of Health, Bethesda, Maryland 20205.

TABLE I

Clinical and Morphologic Observations in Four Patients With Aortic Valve Replacement (AVR) for Pure Aortic Regurgitation (AR) Secondary to Systemic Hypertension (SH)

Observation	Patient			
	1 (43 m)	2 (59 m)	3 (48 m)	4 (55 m)
Duration (yr) of SH	12	30	1	7
Duration (mo) of AR	24	10	6	36
Duration (mo) of congestive heart failure	6	4	2	24
Grade 1–6 murmur of AR	3	4*	3	4
Indirect systemic pressure (mm Hg) (systolic/diastolic [s/d] [avg])	240–170 (193) / 120– 70 (110)	270–140 (176) / 150– 60 (105)	230–160 (188) / 110– 70 (116)	195–160 (182) / 85–35 (66)
Serum creatinine (mg/100 ml)	2.4†	1.8	1.1	1.2
Blood urea nitrogen (mg/100 ml)	28	38	17	23
Indirect systemic pressure (s/d) (mm Hg) 1 mo after AVR	170/90	—	120/70	110/55
Direct LV pressure (s/d) (mm Hg)	150/8	170/22	160/12	184/12
Direct aortic pressure (s/d) (mm Hg)	150/65	170/70	160/75	184/45
Status 2 mo after AVR	Dead	Dead	Alive	Alive
Heart weight (g)	595	810	—	—
Circumference (cm) of aortic sinotubular junction	11	11	—	—
LV wall fibrosis or necrosis	0	0	—‡	—‡
One or more major coronary arteries narrowed >75% in cross-sectional area	0	0	0	+§

* Diastolic thrill along left sternal border. † Mean of 3 values. ‡ By angiography, no left ventricular segmental wall motion abnormalities were present. § Right coronary artery was severely narrowed and an aortocoronary arterial bypass graft was inserted.

avg = average; LV = left ventricular; m = male.

considered to be in New York Heart Association[3] functional class III or IV. The congestive heart failure progressed rapidly in Patients 1, 2 and 3 and more slowly in Patient 4 and was not related to acute elevations in systemic arterial pressures. Patients 2 and 4 had at least one episode of acute pulmonary edema. None of the four patients ever had chest pain or syncope.

On electrocardiography, all four patients had sinus rhythm and a normal P-R interval; one (Patient 1) had left axis deviation, one (Patient 1) had complete left bundle branch block and the other three had voltage criteria for left ventricular hypertrophy. Echocardiographic findings in the four patients are summarized in Table II and illustrated in Figure 2. On both echocardiography and angiography, the ascending aorta was dilated (Fig. 1).

Surgical and autopsy findings: At operation, in each of the four patients the aortic valve was tricuspid. Each cusp was delicate, freely mobile and free of calcific deposits and none of the three commissures were fused. The wall of the ascending aorta in all four patients at operation was normal; and at necropsy the wall in Patients 1 and 2 also was grossly and histologically normal. In the two necropsy patients (Cases 1 and 2 [Fig. 4]), the left ventricular walls were free of foci of fibrosis and necrosis. Patient 1 died of aortic dissection 45 days after

TABLE II

M Mode Echocardiographic Measurements Preoperatively in Four Patients With Aortic Valve Replacement for Pure Aortic Regurgitation Secondary to Systemic Hypertension

Measurement (mm)	Normal Values Range (avg)	Patient			
		1	2	3	4
Ventricular septum					
End-systole	—	30	25	24	20
End-diastole	6–11 (9)	22	14	18	16
Left ventricle free wall					
End-systole	—	26	24	22	21
End-diastole	6–11 (9)	14	12	16	15
Left ventricular cavity					
End-systole	—	60	38	59	46
End-diastole	37–56 (47)	80	67	75	71
Left atrial cavity					
End-systole	—	38	40	37	40
End-diastole	19–40 (29)	35	35	34	32
Aorta					
End-systole	—	47	49	48	46
End-diastole	20–37 (27)	41	40	42	41

avg = average.

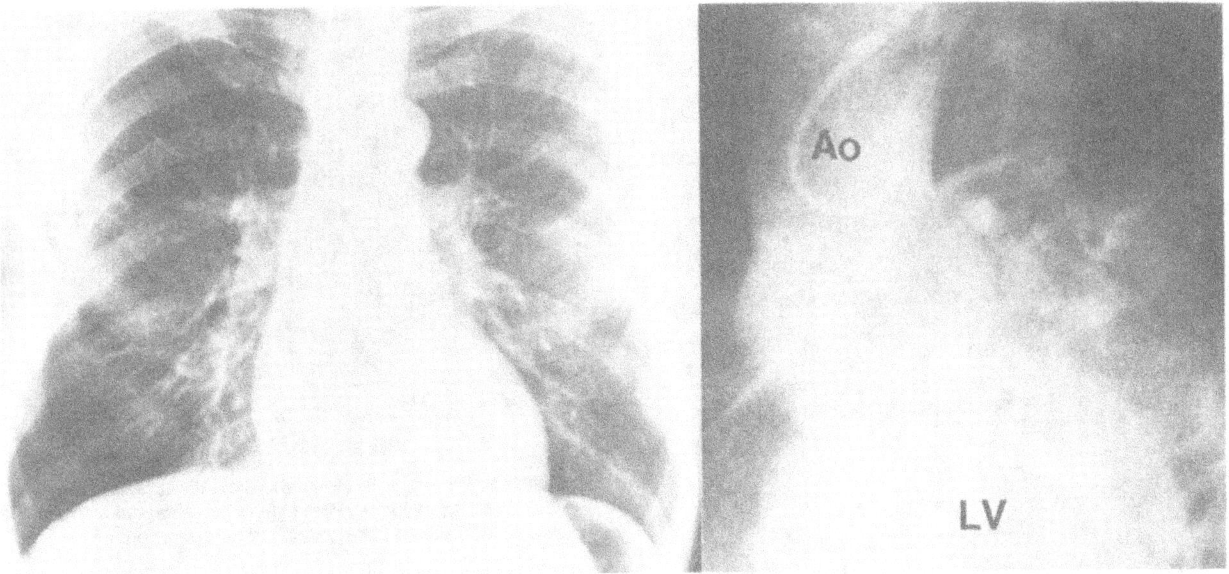

FIGURE 1. Left, chest radiograph in Patient 4. **Right,** aortogram in Patient 2. Ao = ascending aorta; LV = left ventricle.

operation; except for the acute dissection, the wall of the aorta in this patient was normal. Patient 2 died of excessive bleeding 36 hours after operation.

The major epicardial coronary arteries in Patients 1, 2 and 3 on preoperative selective angiography were free of significant narrowings; the right coronary artery in Patient 4 was narrowed greater than 75 percent in diameter and an aortocoronary bypass graft was inserted.

Comments

Each of the four patients had severe aortic regurgitation, severe systemic hypertension and chronic congestive heart failure. In no patient was there an explanation for the aortic regurgitation other than systemic hypertension, and the cause of the chronic congestive heart failure in at least three and probably all four patients appears to have been the severe aortic regurgitation. All four patients underwent aortic valve replacement. One died of excessive bleeding early postoperatively and one of an aortic dissection 45 days postoperatively; in the remaining two patients evidence of congestive failure disappeared in the early postoperative period. The systemic arterial pressures about

TABLE III

Summary of Previously Reported Patients With Systemic Hypertension and Pure Aortic Regurgitation (AR)

First Author (yr)	Garvin[4] (1940)	Gouley[5] (1943)	Hamman[6] (1944)	Fenichel[7] (1950)	Puchner[8] (1960)	Barlow[1] (1960)	Matalon[9] (1971)	Total
Patients (n)	9	8	1	16	27	9	9	79
Age (yr)	38–78 (59)	45–72 (–)	54	59–75 (67)	—(54)	—	23–71 (–)	23–78 (59)
Men:Women	5:4	8:0	0:1	10:6	—	—	8:1	31:12
Systemic arterial pressure (mm Hg): Range (avg)	160–250 (194) 50–160 (103)	150–190 35–100 (–)	220 120	150–240 (203) 60–120 (107)	180–260 (216) 110–160 (131)	>180 — (–)	—	150–260 (204) 35–160 (114)
Pulse pressure (mm Hg): Range (avg)	60–120 (85)	85–128 (105)		60–170 (115)	40–130 (85)	—		40–130 (96)
Patients (n) with severe AR	7	8	0	2	0	0	0	17
Patients (n) with chronic CHF	9	8	0	8	0	0	9	34*
Dead patients (n)	9	8	1	4	0	3	4	29*
Patients (n) with autopsy confirming anatomically normal ascending aorta and aortic valve	9	8	1	0	0	3	4	25
Heart weight (g) Range (mean)	450–700 (550)	400–700 (590)[†]		—	—	—	(418)	400–700 (570)
Circumference (cm) of aortic "ring": Range (mean)	7–10 (8.3)	8–12 (—)[‡]	9	—	—	↑	↑[§]	7–12 (8.3)

* Includes all 17 patients with severe aortic regurgitation. [†] Four patients. [‡] Six patients. [§] One patient.
avg = average; CHF = congestive heart failure; ↑ = increased.

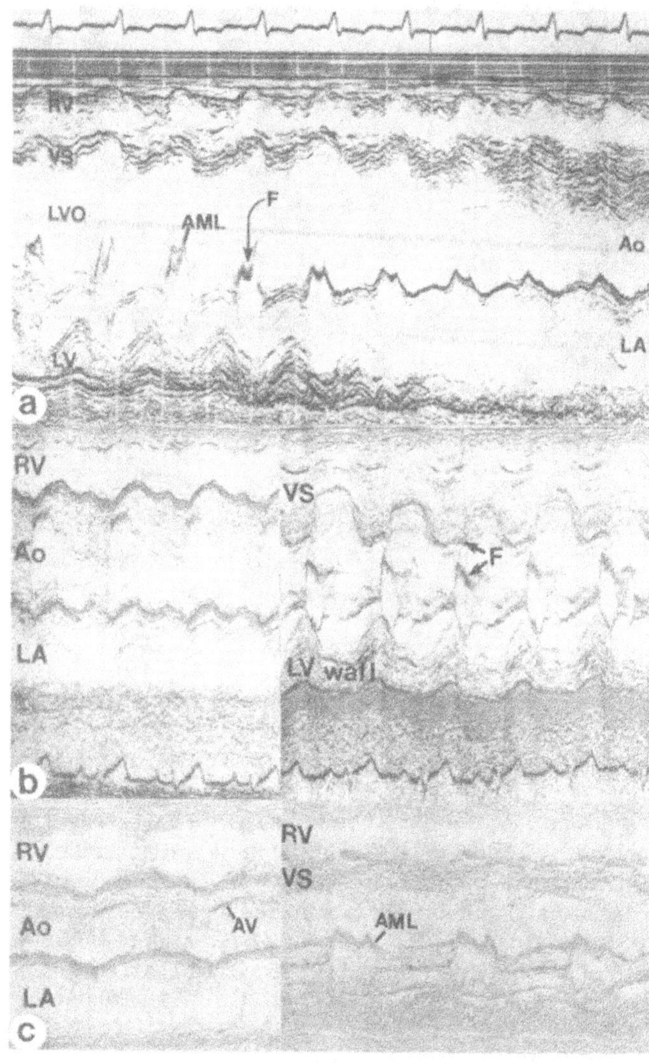

FIGURE 2. M mode echocardiograms. **a,** Patient 1. Sweep from left ventricular outflow (LVO) to aorta (Ao). The left ventricular cavity is dilated and there is fluttering (F) of the anterior mitral leaflet (AML). **b,** Patient 2. Both the aorta (Ao) and left ventricular outflow tract are dilated and there is fluttering (F) of the anterior mitral leaflet. **c,** Patient 4. The diameter of the aorta (Ao) is about the same as that of the left atrium (LA). The left ventricular cavity is dilated. LA = left atrium; LV = left ventricle; RV = right ventricle; VS = ventricular septum.

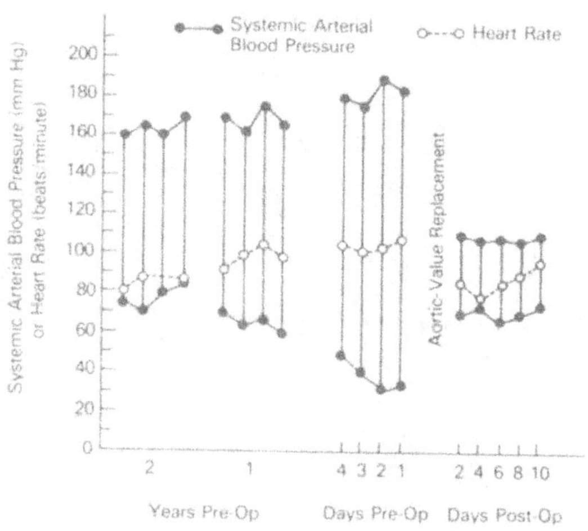

FIGURE 3. Patient 4. Systolic and diastolic arterial pressures before (Pre-Op) and shortly after (Post-Op) aortic valve replacement. The pulse pressure decreased considerably after operation.

1 month postoperatively remained elevated in two of the three survivors. Until these four patients were encountered (and all were seen in a 12 month period), we had not observed a patient with severe aortic regurgitation from systemic hypertension alone and we are not aware of any report describing aortic valve replacement in such patients.

Incidence of severe aortic regurgitation in arterial hypertension: The frequency with which severe aortic regurgitation develops in patients with systemic hypertension is unclear. In Table III, we tabulated data from previous reports describing precordial murmurs consistent with aortic regurgitation in patients with systemic hypertension. Of the 79 patients analyzed in these seven studies,[1,4–9] 17 (all from three studies reported in 1940, 1943 and 1950[4,5,7]) appear to have had severe aortic regurgitation. All 17 patients had evidence of congestive heart failure and all died. However, in 6 of the 17 another definite, probable or possible cause of the congestive heart failure other than aortic regurgitation appears to have been present. Of the remaining 11 patients, necropsy information was provided in seven

TABLE IV

Clinical and Autopsy Findings in Seven Previously Reported Patients With Severe Aortic Regurgitation and Chronic and Eventually Fatal Congestive Heart Failure Caused by Severe Systemic Hypertension

Author (yr)	Age (yr) & Sex	Duration of CHF (mo)	Indirect SAP (mm Hg) (s/d)	PP (mm Hg)	HW (g)	Normal AA & AV at Autopsy	Circ of Ao "Ring" (cm)	Dilated LV Cavity
Garvin[4] (1940)	53F	13	180/60	120	575	+	9	+
	41F	12	220/100	122	525	+	7	−
	58M	6	160/100	100	460	+	8	−
	78M	8	190/70	120	625	+	9	+
	68F	18	210/100	110	510	+	10	−
Gouley[5] (1943)	70M	"months"	160/45	115	560	+	8	+
	66M	10	225/80	145	700	+	12	0

AA = ascending aorta; Ao = aorta; AV = aortic valve; Circ = circumference; CHF = congestive heart failure; HW = heart weight; LV = left ventricular; PP = pulse pressure; s/d = systolic/diastolic; SAP = systemic arterial pressure. + = positive or present; 0 = negative or absent; − = no information available.

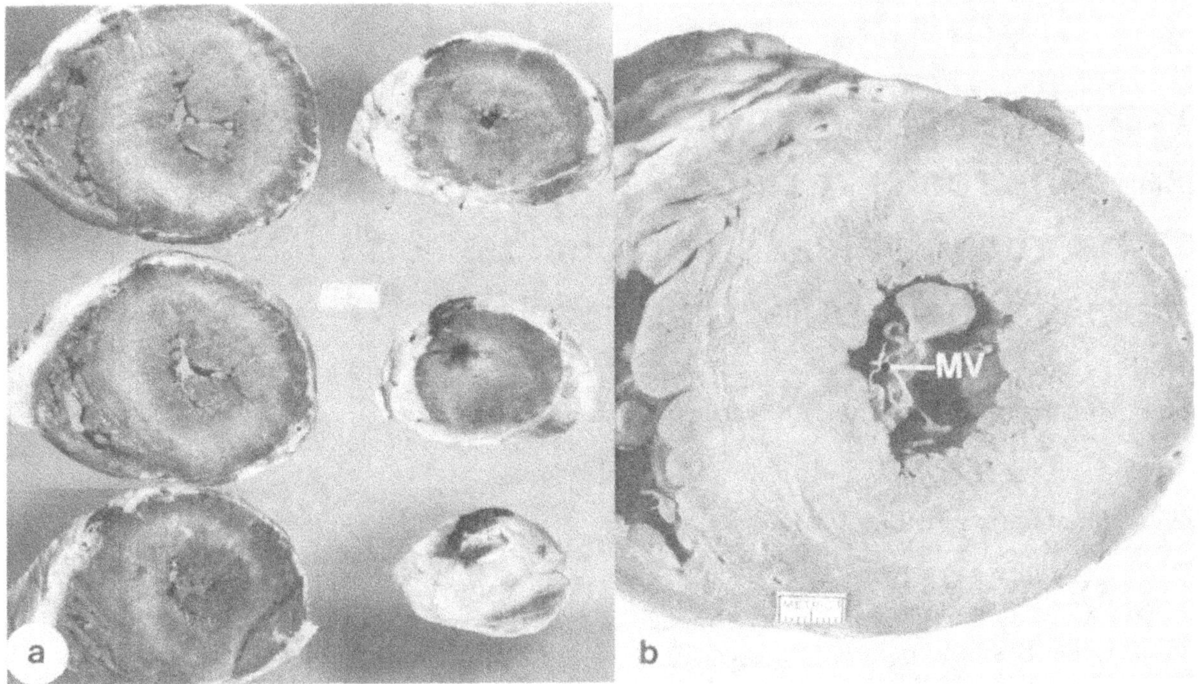

FIGURE 4. Patient 2. **a**, photographs of transverse slices of both cardiac ventricles from base to apex showing a nondilated left ventricular cavity and thickened ventricular walls. **b**, close-up of basal portion of left ventricle showing a portion of mitral valve (MV).

(Table IV). Thus, these seven patients appear to be similar to our four patients, although none of the seven had undergone aortic valve replacement or had received antihypertensive medications.

Mechanisms of aortic regurgitation in hypertension: The mechanism by which severe aortic regurgitation develops in a few patients with systemic hypertension is unclear. The aorta was dilated in all four of our patients and in six of the seven necropsy patients whose data are summarized in Table IV. We presume that dilation of the aortic root, causing stretching of the aortic valve cusps so that they fail to coapt during ventricular diastole with a resulting central leak, is the cause of the regurgitation, but it appears that the aorta dilates to a similar degree in many other patients without development of aortic regurgitation.

Although severe aortic regurgitation appears to be rare in patients with systemic hypertension, minimal and mild degrees of aortic regurgitation are common in hypertensive patients. Of 100 patients with systemic arterial systolic pressures greater than 180 mm Hg described by Barlow and Kincaid-Smith,[1] diastolic blowing murmurs consistent with aortic regurgitation were found in 9. Their report and reports of others[4,8] pointed out that among hypertensive persons, the *higher the systemic arterial pressure*, the greater the chance that aortic regurgitation will develop. Among patients with similar levels of systemic arterial pressure, *older patients* have a higher frequency of aortic regurgitation than do younger patients. Of patients of similar age and similar blood pressure, those with systemic hypertension of *longer duration* have a higher frequency of aortic regurgitation than do those with hypertension of shorter duration. Among the few patients with severe aortic regurgitation due to systemic hypertension, arterial diastolic pressure is usually greater than 60 mm Hg, but nevertheless the pulse pressure is greater than 100 mm Hg.

References

1. **Barlow J, Kincaid-Smith P.** The auscultatory findings in hypertension. Br Heart J 1960;22:505–14.
2. **Delany DJ.** Aortography. In: Grossman W, ed. Cardiac Catheterization and Angiography. Philadelphia: Lea & Febiger, 1976:150.
3. The Criteria Committee of the New York Heart Association. Nomenclature and Criteria for Diagnosis of Diseases of the Heart and Great Vessels. 8th ed. Boston: Little, Brown, 1979:290.
4. **Garvin CF.** Functional aortic insufficiency. Am J Med 1940;13:1799–804.
5. **Gouley BA, Sickel EM.** Aortic regurgitation caused by dilatation of the aortic orifice and associated with a characteristic valvular lesion. Am Heart J 1943;26:24–38.
6. **Hamman L.** Diagnostic implications of aortic insufficiency. Cincinnati J Med 1944;25:95–125.
7. **Fenichel NM.** Arteriosclerotic aortic insufficiency. Am Heart J 1950;40:117–24.
8. **Puchner TC, Huston JH, Hellmuth GA.** Aortic valve insufficiency in arterial hypertension. Am J Cardiol 1960;5:758–60.
9. **Matalon R, Moussalli ARJ, Nidus BD, Katz LA, Eisinger RP.** Functional aortic insufficiency—a feature of renal failure. N Engl J Med 1971;285:1522–3.

The spectrum of cardiovascular disease in the Marfan syndrome: A clinico-morphologic study of 18 necropsy patients and comparison to 151 previously reported necropsy patients

William C. Roberts, M.D., and Howard S. Honig, M.D. *Bethesda, Md.*

Cardiovascular abnormalities are the most common cause of death in patients with the Marfan syndrome, and a variety of lesions have been described in the aorta and heart in such patients. Although some information has been reported in at least 151 necropsy patients with the Marfan syndrome,[1-91] no studies are available describing in detail large numbers of such patients at necropsy. Indeed, of the 151 necropsy patients reported, 65 were isolated case studies[1-5, 7, 8, 10-12, 14, 15, 18, 20, 23-26, 28, 29, 31-36, 38-41, 43-51, 54, 56-62, 64-70, 72-75, 79, 80, 85, 87-89, 91]; each of 14 reports described only two patients[6, 9, 13, 16, 17, 21, 22, 30, 63, 71, 76-78, 81, 83]; each of three reports described three patients[19, 37, 53]; three reports described four patients[52, 84, 90]; and five reports described five,[86] six,[27, 55] seven,[42] and 11[82] patients, respectively. The amount of detailed information available on each necropsy patient tended to be much less in the reports describing more than two patients than in those concerned with only one or two patients. Although virtually all of the previously reported necropsy patients with the Marfan syndrome had characteristic musculoskeletal features of this syndrome,[82] not all had histories of this syndrome in other family members or the characteristic ocular features.[82] To determine more precisely the type and frequency of the cardiovascular lesions in the Marfan syndrome, this report reviews findings in 18 necropsy patients with this syndrome studied in the Pathology Branch, National Heart, Lung and Blood Institute, and compares the observations in them to those in previously reported necropsy patients.

From the Pathology Branch, National Heart, Lung and Blood Institute, National Institutes of Health.

Received for publication Dec. 1, 1981; accepted Dec. 10, 1981.

Reprint requests: William C. Roberts, M.D., Pathology Branch, NHLBI-NIH, Bldg. 10A, Room 3E-30, Bethesda, MD 20205.

METHODOLOGY

All 18 necropsy patients had typical musculoskeletal features of the Marfan syndrome[82]: of the 16 patients with adequate historical information, 14 had other family members with typical musculoskeletal features and 13 had severe eye problems typical of this syndrome (dislocated lens, iridesis, severe myopia with scleral defects, retinal detachment or glaucoma).[82] All 18 patients had either a history of this syndrome in other family members or ocular abnormalities or both.

Certain clinical and morphologic observations in the 18 patients are tabulated in Table I. All 18 patients died between 1956 and 1977: four died before 1960, eight died from 1961 to 1970, and five died since 1970. The ages at death in the 18 patients ranged from 15 to 52 years (mean 34); seven were women (mean age = 42 years) and 11 were male (mean age = 29 years). Eight were black and 10 were white. All 18 had one or more abnormalities in the aorta or atrioventricular valves or both. The 18 patients were divided into three major groups according to the status of the aorta: (1) those with fusiform ascending aortic aneurysm (patients No. 1 to 13); (2) those with aortic dissection (patients No. 14 to 16); and (3) those with isolated mitral regurgitation (patients No. 17 and 18).

GROUP I. FUSIFORM ASCENDING AORTIC ANEURYSM (FIGS. 1 to 10)

Chronic aortic regurgitation (AR) was present in all 13 patients in this group, and it was known to be of severe degree in at least 10 of them. The AR was confirmed by aortic angiogram in nine patients. The systemic arterial diastolic pressure in 11 of the 13 patients was 60 mm Hg or less, including eight in whom it was 40 mm Hg or less. Six of the 13 patients also had precordial murmurs typical of *mitral regurgitation* (MR), which was considered mild in three

Table I. Clinical and necropsy observations in 18 personally studied patients with the Marfan syndrome

| Pt | Age (yr) | Race | Sex | Marfan features | | | Ht (cm) | Wt (kg) | CHF | Murmur (0-6/6) | | Indirect SAP (mm Hg) | | Direct (mm Hg) | | AR (0-4+) |
				M-S	Ocular	FH				AR	MR	S	D	LVP (s/d)	SAP (s/d)	
Fusiform aneurysm of ascending aorta																
1	15	W	M	+	+	?	193	68	+	3	3	140	0	—	—	—
2	20	W	M	+	0	+	198	49	0	3	3	220	70	170/20	170/65	3+
3[a]	21	B	M	+	+	+	203	—	0	1	0	130	80	—	—	—
4	21	B	M	+	+	+	147	67	+	4	3	160	60	136/18	158/62	4+
5	26	W	M	+	0	+	198	—	+	5	0	110	40	—	—	3+
6	31	W	M	+	+	+	183	45	+	2	4	135	40	—	—	—
7	35	W	F	+	+	+	158	50	+	3	0	110	40	120/25	120/50	4+
8	36	B	F	+	0	+	185	49	+	3	0	100	40	—	130/38	4+
9	38	B	F	+	+	+	173	50	+	3	4	140	20	—	—	—
10	38	B	M	+	0	+	191	59	0	3	0	115	55	—	140/65	3+
11	41	B	M	+	+	−	193	82	+	5	0	150	50	110/35	110/35	3+
12	47	W	M	+	+	+	187	64	+	4	2	140	40	108/24	108/39	4+
13	48	W	F	+	0	+	179	54	+	3	0	150	40	150/12	150/40	3+
Dissection of aorta																
14	43	W	M	+	+	0	193	86	0	0[b]	0	210	100	—	—	—
15	49	B	F	+	+	+	173	47	0	0[b]	3	110	70	—	—	—
16	52	B	F	+	+	0	178	72	0[b]	0[b]	0	180	100	—	—	—
Isolated mitral regurgitation																
17	28	W	M	+	+	+	175	59	+	0	5	130	80	—	130/80	—
18	35	W	F	+	+	0	184	66	+	0	4	120	80	100/14	100/75	0
Total or mean	34	10 W 8 B	11 M 7 F	18	13	13	173	60	12	13	9	142	56	128/21	132/55	9

Abbreviations: AA = ascending aorta; AAR = ascending aortic replacement (graft); AR = aortic regurgitation; AV = aortic valve; AVR = aortic valve replacement; Ca⁺⁺ = calcium; CAD = coronary heart disease; CHF = congestive heart failure; C of A = aortic isthmic coarctation; CMN = cystic medial necrosis; C-V = cardiovascular; D = end-diastole; F = female; FH = family history of Marfan syndrome; Ht = height; IE = infective endocarditis; LVP = left ventricular pressure; M = male; MR = mitral regurgitation; M-S = musculo-skeletal; MV = mitral valve; PDA = patent ductus arteriosus; PV = pulmonic valve; RCT = ruptured chordae tendineae; S = peak systole; SAP = systemic arterial pressure; TV = tricuspid valve; yr = years; Wt = weight.

[a] = Daughter of patient No. 9.

[b] = Not present before the dissection but appeared afterwards.

[c] = The aortic dissection, which occurred 8 years before death, was operatively plicated at the time. Severe AR developed thereafter due to the dissection to the aortic root and AVR was done 3 days before death, the consequence of excessive bleeding.

[d] = Aortic dissection, 14 days before death, was plicated 13 days before death which resulted from rupture of the aorta into the pericardial sac.

and moderate or severe in three. *Periodic chest pain of a nonanginal type* occurred in 7 of the 13 patients. At necropsy, five of them had healed tears in the ascending aorta (to be described later). The heart and ascending aorta were enlarged by chest roentgenogram in all 13 patients. The aortic dilatation was confirmed in nine by aortogram. ECGs in 12 patients disclosed evidence of left ventricular (LV) hypertrophy in all but patient No. 13, but at necropsy he too had cardiomegaly (520 gm heart).

The cause of death was variable. *Chronic congestive heart failure* (CHF), present in 10 of the 13 patients, proved fatal in four. Of the three patients without chronic CHF, two (No. 3 and 10) died suddenly from rupture of the ascending aorta; the third (patient No. 2), a 20-year-old man, died of bleeding soon after resection of an aortic isthmic after a cardiovascular operation: patient No. 6 bled excessively after insertion of a Hufnagel prosthesis into the descending thoracic aorta; patient No. 4, who underwent replacement of the aortic valve and of the ascending aorta 9 months earlier, died from bleeding 3 days after mitral valve replacement; the remaining four patients died from 1 to 5 months after replacement of the aortic valve with a prosthesis (caged ball in three, porcine bioprosthesis in one) and a portion of ascending aorta with a graft.

In addition to the ascending aortic fusiform aneurysms, two patients (No. 4 and 11) also had fusiform aneurysms of the descending thoracic aorta (Fig. 10). The ascending aortic aneurysms in all 13 patients involved both the sinus and proximal tubular portions of aorta. The most distal portion of ascending aorta, i.e., that portion immediately prox-

| Operation | | | Heart weight (gm) | Aortic tears | CMN AA | Circumference valve anuli (cm) | | | | Prolapse | | RCT MV | Ca⁺⁺ MV anulus | Associated C-V lesions |
AAR	AVR	Other				TV	MV	PV	AV	TV	MV			
0	0	0	730	0	+	16	16	8	12	+	+	+	0	0
0	0	+	900	0	+	12	10	7	8	0	+	+	+	C of A
0	0	0	460	+	+	14	13	8	9	+	0	0	0	0
+	+	+	700	+	+	12	13	9	9	0	0	0	+	0
+	0	0	725	+	+	14	12	9	16	0	0	0	0	0
0	0	+	700	0	+	14	16	9	12	+	+	+	+	IE
+	+	0	375	+	+	9	9	7	9	0	0	0	0	PDA
0	0	0	750	+	+	14	13	10	10	0	0	0	0	0
+	0	0	750	+	+	14	15	9	18	0	+	+	0	IE
0	0	0	520	+	+	13	10	9	14	0	0	0	0	0
+	+	0	750	0	+	11	12	7	9	0	0	0	0	0
+	+	0	830	+	+	—	—	—	—	0	0	0	0	CAD
+	+	0	520	0	+	12	11	8	12	0	0	0	0	0
0	0	+ᵈ	500	0	0	12	9	8	8	0	0	0	0	0
0	0	0	480	0	0	12	14	8	9	0	+	0	0	0
0	+ᶜ	+	700	0	0	11	10	8	9	0	0	0	0	0
0	0	0	830	0	0	13	17	9	8	+	+	+	+	0
0	0	0	555	0	0	12	17	7	9	0	+	0	+	0
7	6	5	654	8	13	13	13	8	11	4	7	5	5	5

dilated only in the patient with an associated isthmic coarctation and congenitally bicuspid aortic valve. In eight patients, nontransmural tears, either transverse or longitudinal or both, were present in the aneurysmal portion of ascending aorta (Figs. 1, 2, 6 to 8). In two of the eight patients with aortic tears, the final tear extended through the entire thickness of aortic wall causing fatal pericardial tamponade (Figs. 1 and 8). In all eight patients with aortic tears, the wall of aorta at the site of the tears was thin. Multiple histologic sections of ascending aorta showed severe elastic fiber degeneration of the aortic media in all 13 patients (Figs. 1, 4, 8, and 9). This loss was most evident at the sites of the gross tears, but it also was present in areas of aorta which grossly appeared normal. The intima was mildly thickened by fibrous tissue in the area of the "healed" tears. The adventitia in all 13 patients was normal except in the patients who had undergone aortotomy months earlier, and in them it was considerably thickened by fibrous tissue and was adherent to adjacent tissues.

The aortic valve cusps in the 12 patients with three-cuspid valves were grossly normal except for increased size and mild marginal "rolling." The former apparently was the result of stretching of the cusps between the commissural attachments and the latter resulted from the severe AR. Histologically, the aortic valve cusps in all 13 patients had increased amounts of acid mucopolysaccharide material (Fig. 9). The mitral leaflets in 9 of the 13 patients appeared "stretched," i.e., the lengths of the leaflets from their basal attachments to their distal margins were increased. In the other four patients actual prolapse or overshooting of portions of the posterior mitral leaflet was evident, but each of them had several ruptured chordae tendineae and two of them had histories of active infective endocarditis which had healed (Fig. 3). Three of the four patients with mitral prolapse had mitral "anular" calcific deposits: grade 2+/4+ in severity in two patients and grade 3+/4+ in one (patient No. 4) (Fig. 2). The mitral anular circumferences in the 13 patients ranged from 10 to 16 cm (mean 13) (normal < 10 cm): in the four patients with mitral prolapse, the range was 10 to 16 cm (mean 12) but three were 15 cm or above; in the nine patients without prolapse, the range was 10 to 13 cm (mean 12) and none was above 13 cm. Histologic sections of the mitral leaflets in all 13 patients disclosed excessive quantities of acid mucopolysaccharide material. The tricuspid valve anuli were above 11 cm in circumfer-

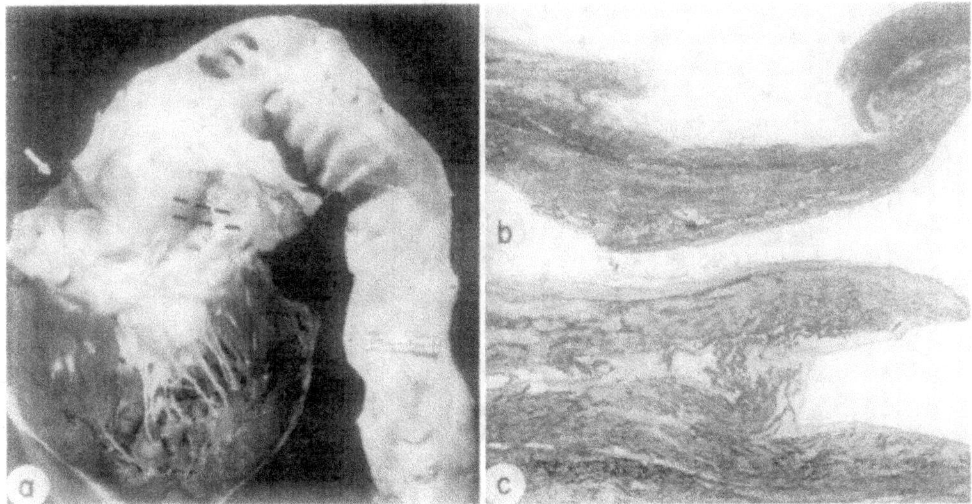

Fig. 1. Case No. 3 (Table I). *a*, Opened left ventricle, aortic valve, and aorta in a 21-year-old man (A67-120) who died suddenly while sitting in his automobile. Necropsy disclosed the pericardial sac to be filled with blood and the ascending aorta to contain a large through-and-through tear *(arrow)*. Other incomplete healed tears also are present in the aorta. *b*, Photomicrograph of a transverse cut across a tear at the site of the *parallel dashed lines* shown in *a*. The tear causes considerable thinning of the media. *c*, Close-up at edge of a healed tear showing loss of many elastic fibers. (Movat stains; original magnifications ×7 *b*, ×18 *c*.) The diagnosis of the Marfan syndrome was made at age 12 years. The patient's blood pressure at that time was 130/80 mm Hg and a precordial diastolic murmur was not heard. He was asymptomatic until his sudden death.

ence in 10 of the 12 patients in whom this measurement was done and in at least three of the 13 patients the elongated leaflets appeared to protrude abnormally toward the right atrium, i.e., to prolapse. No actual scalloping was present in the tricuspid valve leaflets, which in all patients appeared delicate.

GROUP II. AORTIC DISSECTION (FIG. 11)

Each of the three patients with aortic dissection was free of symptoms of cardiovascular dysfunction until the sudden appearance of chest pain, which was found to result from dissection extending from the tubular portion of ascending aorta to at least the common iliac arteries. *Before the aortic dissection,* none of the three patients had radiographic evidence of enlargement of either the aorta or the heart, none had a precordial murmur, and none had evidence of CHF. Patients No. 14 and 15 died soon after the occurrence of the aortic dissection (Fig. 11). Patient No. 16 had clinical evidence of aortic dissection when 44 years old, and at that time the false channel in the aorta was operatively closed and the prolapsed aortic valve (due to the dissection) was resuspended. The ascending aorta was noted to be normal in size at this operation carried out 8 years before death. Severe AR, nevertheless, resulted from the aortic dissection and progressive CHF necessitated aortic valve replacement, performed 3 days

before death. At the second operation, the ascending aorta was severely dilated. She died from severe postoperative thoracic bleeding.

Patients No. 14 and 16 had systemic hypertension for many years before the aortic dissection occurred. In patients No. 14 and 15, the aorta was not dilated and obvious tears were present in the ascending aorta just above the aortic valve (Fig. 11). The origin of the right coronary artery was completely disrupted from the true channel and an acute myocardial infarct involving the posterior wall of LV resulted in each patient. In patient No. 16, the ascending aorta was quite dilated at necropsy and the false channel was no longer visible (having been interrupted at operation 8 years earlier). No tears were present in the aorta in any of these three patients, except those associated with the sites of origin of the dissection. Histologically, the media of ascending aorta was within the range of normal (for age) in all three patients. The mitral and tricuspid valves were normal except for anular dilatation in all three patients.

GROUP III. ISOLATED MITRAL REGURGITATION (FIGS. 12 and 13)

Each of these two patients (No. 17 and 18) had *severe mitral regurgitation* without AR and normal-sized ascending aortas by chest roentgenogram. Chronic CHF, which proved fatal, occurred in

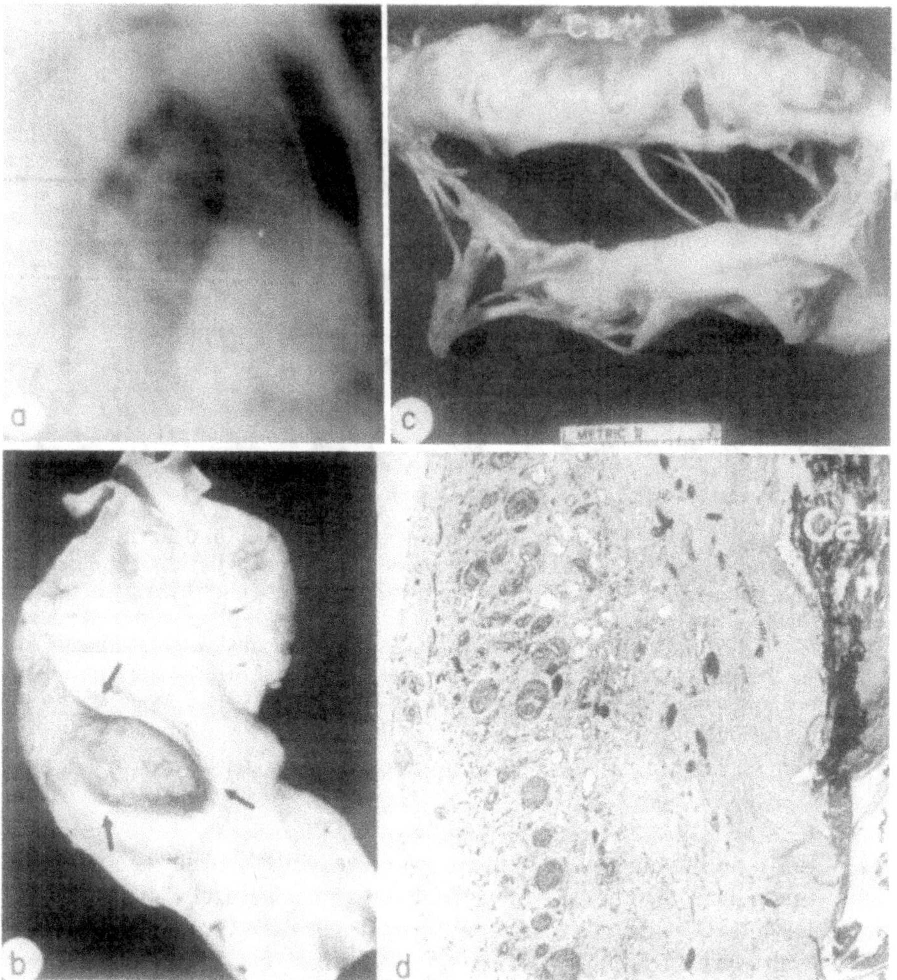

Fig. 2. Case No. 4. Heart in a 21-year-old man (A64-224) who had been asymptomatic until about 11 months before death when he had the onset of episodic retrosternal pain with exertion. Angiogram *(a)* disclosed a dilated aortic root and 9 months before death the ascending aorta *(b)* and aortic valve were replaced. A large incomplete tear *(arrows)* was present in the aorta and the aortic valve cusps were thin and stretched. He bled extensively postoperatively. Later postoperatively, severe mitral regurgiation became apparent and 15 days before death the mitral valve *(c)* was replaced. Calcific deposits (Ca^{++}) were present in the anular region and the anulus was very dilated. Histologic section *(d)* disclosed many vascular channels as well as calcific deposits (Ca^{++}) in the basal portion of the posterior mitral leaflet. (Hematoxylin-eosin stain; original magnification ×56.)

patient No. 17; patient No. 18 died suddenly. The ascending aorta and aortic valve by histologic examination were normal in each patient. Both had floppy, i.e., scalloped mitral leaflets which prolapsed toward the left atrium (Figs. 12 and 13). Both had massively dilated mitral anuli (17 cm in circumference; normal = about 9 cm) and both had heavy (3+/4+) deposits of calcium in the mitral anular region (beneath the posterior leaflet). One or more mitral chordae tendineae appeared to have been ruptured in patient No. 17.

COMMENTS

The Marfan syndrome generally involves the bones, joints, eyes, heart, and blood vessels. The extremities are long and thin (dolichostenomelia), the ligaments and joint capsules are redundant, the lenses are dislocated (ectopia lentis), the ascending aorta often is dilated, and one or both left-sided cardiac valves frequently are incompetent. Cardiovascular disease is by far the most common cause of death in patients with the Marfan syndrome. Of our 18 necropsy patients fulfilling McKusick's rigid criteria for this syndrome,[82] all died from cardiovascular disease and death in each was premature (mean age = 34 years [range 15 to 52]). Of 56 deceased patients with this syndrome studied during life by Murdoch et al.,[92] cardiovascular disease was the cause of death in 52 (93%) and the mean age at death was 32 years. Of the 151 previously reported

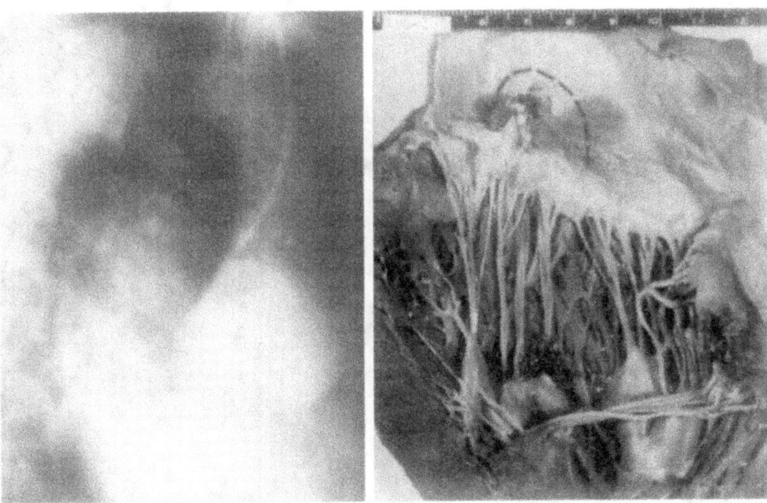

Fig. 3. Case No. 6. Aortogram *(left)* and opened mitral valve *(right)* in a 31-year-old man (A56-132) who had alpha streptococcus endocarditis 2 years before death. The aortic root is dilated. A large calcified mass (enclosed by *dashed line*) arises from the posterior mitral leaflet and several chordae from the anterior leaflet were ruptured. The chordae were greatly elongated. The calcified mass appears to represent a healed vegetation.

necropsy patients with the Marfan syndrome,[1-91] the mean age at death was 23 years and ranged from stillbirth to 65 years (Table II).

A variety of cardiovascular lesions has been observed in the great arteries and hearts of patients with the Marfan syndrome. Our 18 necropsy patients with this syndrome readily separated into three distinct groups on the basis of their cardiovascular lesions. Group I included 13 patients with *fusiform aneurysms of the ascending aorta.* All 13 patients had AR and six of them also had associated MR. In each the aneurysm involved the sinus and the proximal tubular portions of ascending aorta. Two also had fusiform aneurysms in the descending thoracic aorta. Histologic study of the wall of the ascending aorta disclosed the typical lesion of this syndrome, i.e., massive loss of elastic fibers and increased amounts of mucoid material in the media (Fig. 14). Group II included three patients with *dissection of the entire aorta.* Before dissection, the aorta in each was of normal size and histologically the wall of aorta was normal. None of these three patients had either AR or MR before the aortic dissection. Two, however, had had systemic hypertension. Group III included two patients with *isolated mitral regurgitation* with floppy mitral leaflets and markedly dilated mitral anuli. In each the aortic lumen was of normal size and its wall was normal histologically.

Previously reported patients. In contrast to the predominant occurrence of fusiform ascending aortic aneurysm in our patients (13 of 18) and the relative infrequent occurrence of aortic dissection (3 of 18), aortic dissection was the most frequent gross cardiovascular abnormality observed in the previously reported necropsy patients with the Marfan syndrome (57 [38%] of 151 patients), followed by aortic root aneurysm without dissection (53 [35%] patients), then MR without aortic root aneurysm or dissection (33 [22%] patients), and finally eight patients (5%) did not have aortic dissection or root aneurysm or MR and were placed in a miscellaneous group (Table II). Analysis of the previously reported necropsy patients disclosed that those with either fusiform ascending aortic aneurysm or aortic dissection had similar mean ages (28 and 27 years), males were slightly more frequent in both groups (3:2), and only 10% of the 110 patients were aged 15 years or under (Table II). In contrast, the 33 previously reported necropsy patients with isolated or predominant MR and the eight patients classified as miscellaneous had a much younger mean age (12 and 14 years), virtually equal numbers of males and females, and a very high percentage of patients aged 15 and younger (nearly 70%) (Table II).

AR related to aortic root aneurysm. As did all our 13 patients with fusiform ascending aortic aneurysms (or "anuloaortic ectasia"), evidence of AR was present in almost all (95%) of the previously reported necropsy patients with fusiform ascending aortic aneurysm. As an indication of the severity of the AR in the reported patients with fusiform ascending aortic aneurysm, the average indirect peak systolic systemic arterial pressure in the 29 (of

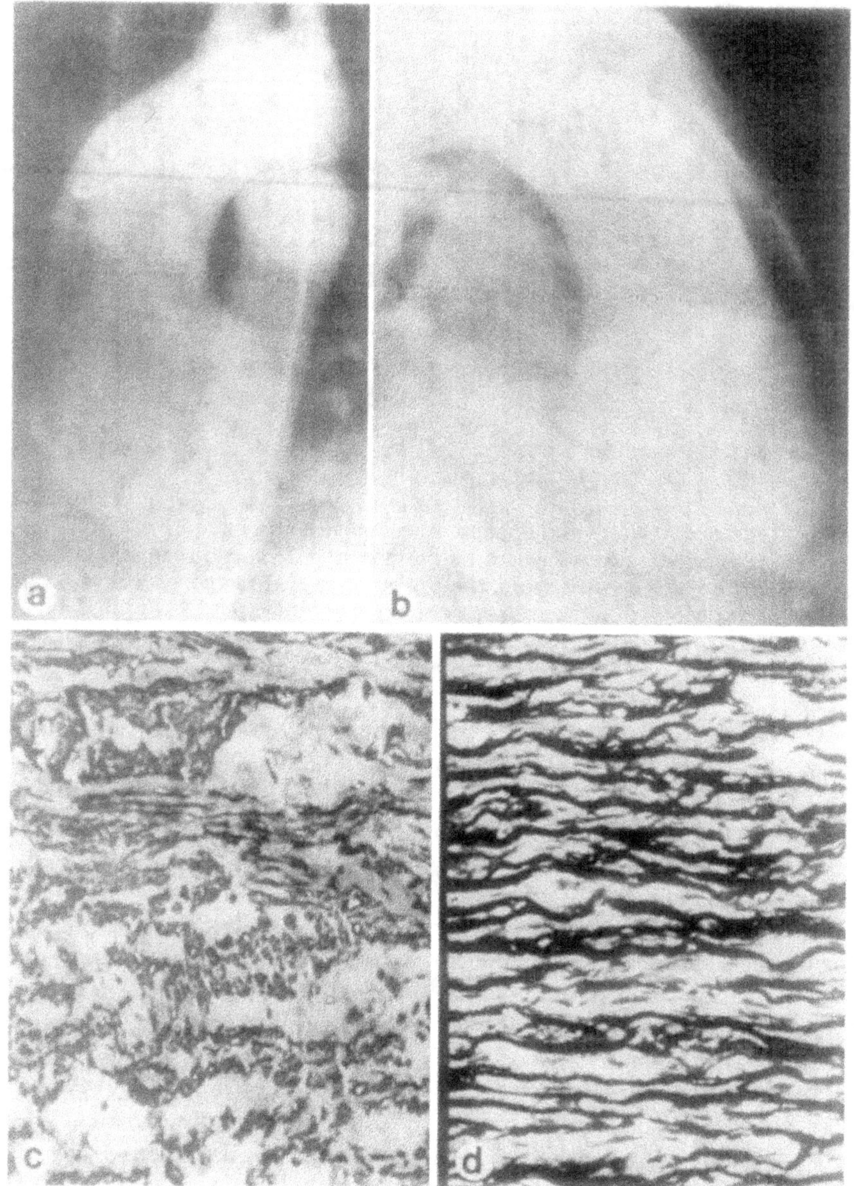

Fig. 4. Case No. 7. Aortogram (*a* and *b*) and photomicrograph of segment of dilated ascending aorta (*c*) compared to control (*d*) in a 35-year-old mentally retarded woman (MWV A77-11) whose arms and legs were disproportionally (to trunk) long (although she was short), her fingers and toes were long, multiple eye problems were present, and several siblings had typical skeletal features of the Marfan syndrome. At age 6 years, a patent ductus arteriosus was closed by suture obliteration. Substernal chest pain appeared periodically at age 26 years and the heart was enlarged at that time. During the next few years she had several episodes of rapid heart action with ventricular tachycardia documented and evidence of chronic congestive heart failure (to functional class 3/4). Shortly before replacement of the aortic valve for aortic regurgitation and of a portion of ascending aorta for the aortic root aneurysm (*a* and *b*), the aortic pressure was 120/50 mm Hg. Histologic study of the wall of the aortic aneurysm showed virtual absence of elastic fibers (compared to normal = *d*) and increased mucoid material. (Movat stains; each original magnification ×330.)

the 53) patients in whom this information was available was 146 mm Hg (range 100 to 195 mm Hg) and the average end-diastolic systemic arterial pressure was 43 mm Hg (range 0 to 90 mm Hg), yielding an average pulse pressure of just over 100 mm Hg (range 40 to 170 mm Hg). Of the 29 patients with fusiform root aneuryms and reported blood pressure measurements, 18 (62%) had systemic arterial systolic pressures greater than 140 mm Hg, 26 (90%) had systemic diastolic pressures 60 mm Hg or less,

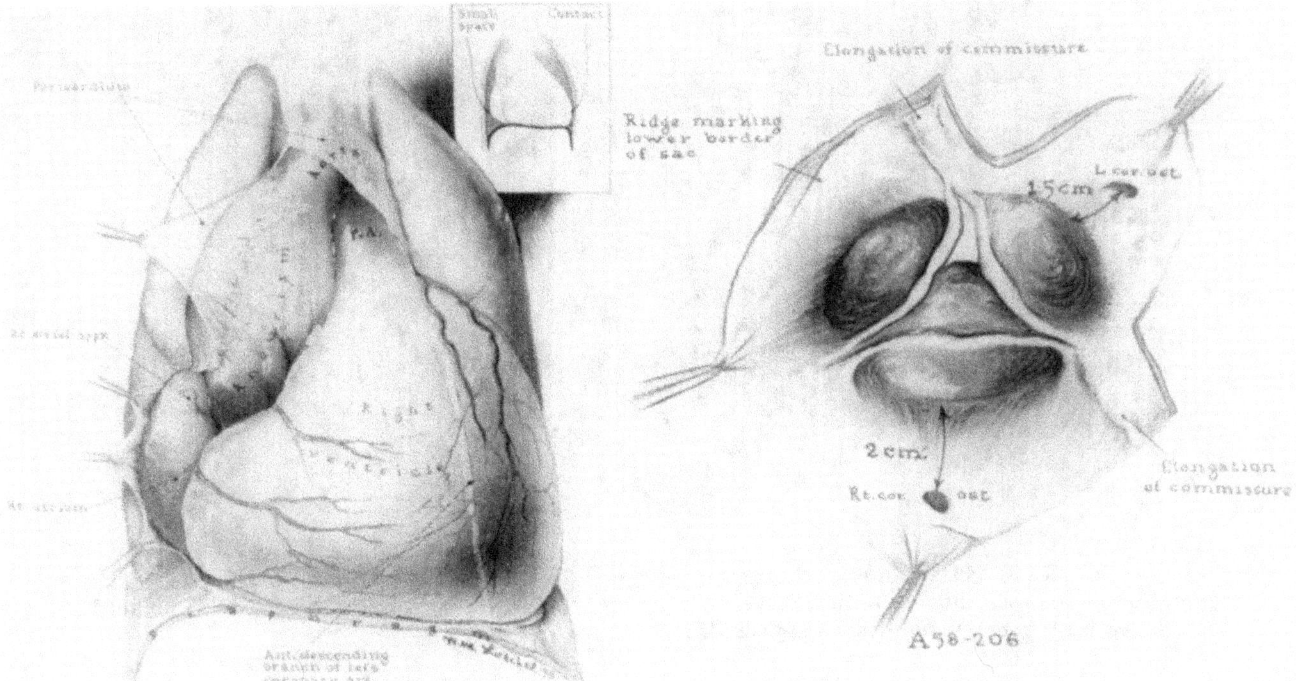

Fig. 5. Case No. 8. Drawing of heart, great arteries, and lungs *(left)* and aortic valve from above *(right)* in a 36-year-old woman (A58-206) with severe aortic regurgitation and a hugely dilated ascending aorta and heart. The aortic valve cusps protrude excessively toward the left ventricle. Chronic congestive cardiac failure began 2 years before death.

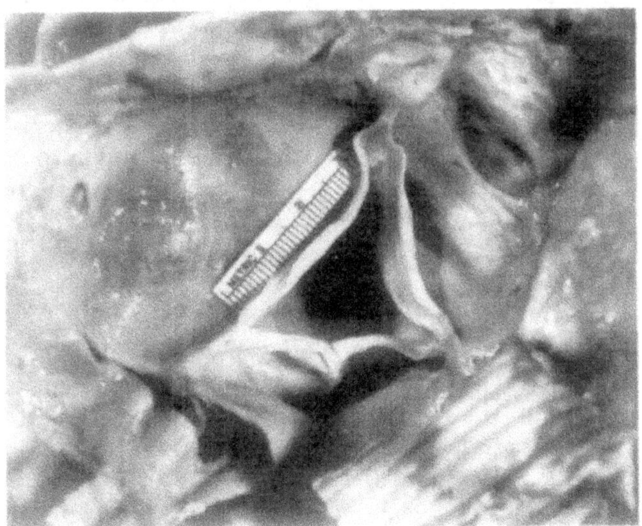

Fig. 6. Case No. 9. Aortic valve seen from above in a 38-year-old woman (A-66-76), the daughter of case No. 15. The aortic root is enormously dilated and this resulted in straightening of the cusps between the commissures, which in turn prevented coaptings of the cusps during ventricular diastole and severe aortic regurgitation. The aneurysmally dilated ascending aorta was partially resected and replaced by a graft 10 years before death. The patient died of progressive congestive heart failure from the aortic regurgitation.

and 23 (79%) had pulse pressures greater than 60 mm Hg.

Aortic dissection occurs in previously normal-sized aortas. In contrast to their frequent recording in the reported necropsy patients with fusiform ascending aortic aneurysms, blood pressure values *before the dissection occurred* were virtually unreported in the 57 previously reported necropsy patients with aortic dissection. Nevertheless, evidence of the presence of AR before the aortic dissection was rare.[17,51] The *reason that AR before dissection is rare in the* patients with aortic dissection is because dissection is infrequent in the patients with fusiform ascending aortic aneurysm, and it is the latter which primarily is responsible for the severe AR (in the absence of healed dissection). With few exceptions, aortic dissection in patients with the Marfan syndrome tends to affect the previously normal-sized aorta or the one only slightly dilated. None of our 13 patients with fusiform ascending aortic aneurysms had aortic dissection, and none of our three patients with dissection of the entire aorta had evidence of fusiform ascending aortic aneurysm or AR before the dissection. Of the reported patients with aortic dissection, those with dilated ascending aortas over

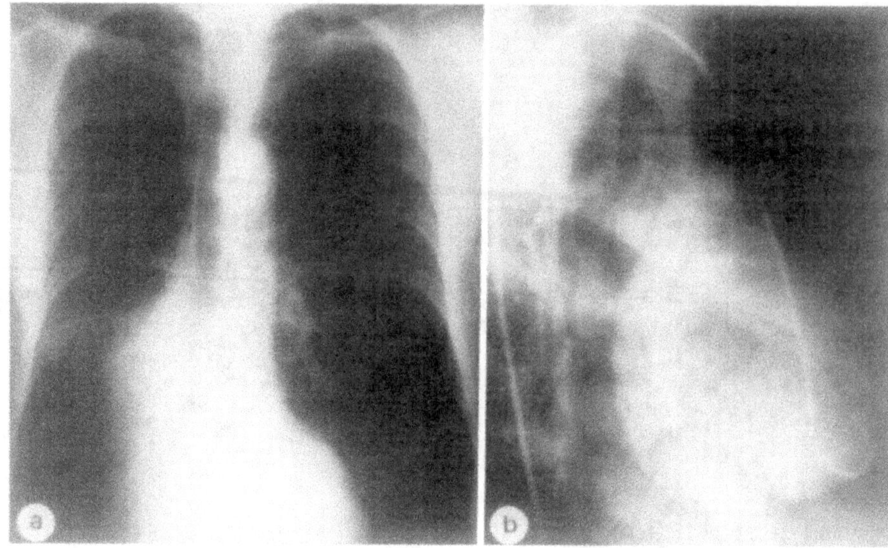

Fig. 7. Case No. 10. Posteroanterior chest roentgenogram *(a)* and lateral aortogram *(b)* showing massive dilatation of the ascending aorta in a 38-year-old man (A73-84) who was asymptomatic until 5 months before death when exertional dysnea appeared.

a long period of time usually had healed dissections and the dilatation in them appeared to be the result of aneurysm of the false channel. In at least 14[7, 19, 25, 29, 33, 40, 42, 48, 74, 76, 82] of the 57 previously reported patients with aortic dissection, the dissection had healed. In our patient No. 16 (Table I), severe AR developed during the 8 years following the dissection and the size of the aorta, of course, during that period dilated considerably (from a predissection normal size).

Severe cystic medial necrosis related to aortic aneurysm rather than to aortic dissection. The reason that fusiform ascending aortic aneurysm occurs in some patients with the Marfan syndrome and aortic dissection occurs in others appears to lie in the status of the aortic media. In each of our 13 patients with fusiform aneurysm of the ascending aorta, histologic study of the wall of the aorta disclosed severe degrees of "cystic medial necrosis." In contrast, none of our three patients with dissection involving the entire aorta had cystic medial necrosis by histologic examination. Furthermore, in 44 of the 53 previously reported necropsy patients with fusiform ascending aortic aneurysm, cystic medial necrosis was described and in the other nine patients its presence or absence was simply not mentioned. It was not mentioned as being absent in any patient, and in those in whom photomicrographs were illustrated, the degree of cystic medial necrosis was nearly always severe. Among the 57 previously reported necropsy patients with aortic dissection,

cystic medial necrosis was described as being present in 35 and as being absent in seven.[40, 42, 78] In the patients, however, in whom photomicrographs of aorta were illustrated, the degree of cystic medial necrosis was usually minimal or mild and rarely was the degree of cystic medial necrosis as severe as that observed routinely in the patients with fusiform ascending aortic aneurysm.

Thus the aortic media appears to be quite different in the patients with fusiform ascending aortic aneruysms and in those with aortic dissection, particularly when the latter involves the entire aorta. In the patients with fusiform ascending aortic aneurysm, there is usually "massive" degeneration or loss of the elastic fibers of the media and increased quantities of collagen and mucoid material. The increased quantities of collagen would appear to prevent longitudinal aortic dissection. The aortic media in the patients with aortic dissection, in contrast, tends to be normal or to show only mild degrees of cystic medial necrosis, just as in patients with aortic dissection and systemic hypertension who do not have the Marfan syndrome.[93-95] Two of our three patients with aortic dissection had evidence of diastolic systemic hypertension, whereas none of the other 16 patients had diastolic hypertension.

Aortic dissection related to systemic hypertension. In none of the previous reports describing necropsy patients with the Marfan syndrome was the degree of cystic medial necrosis graded. In 1970, however,

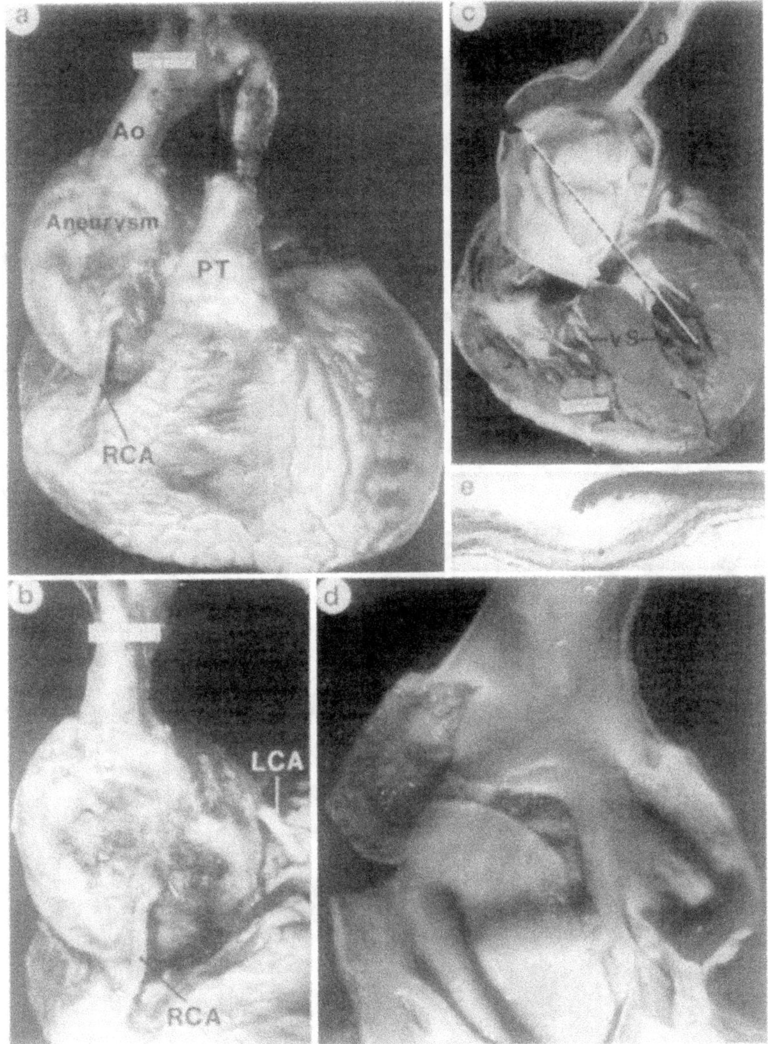

Fig. 8. Case No. 10. Heart and aorta in the patient whose radiographs are shown in Fig. 7. *a*, Exterior view. *Ao* = ascending aorta; *RCA* = right coronary artery; *PT* = pulmonary trunk. *b*, Closer view of the massive aortic aneurysm after retracting the pulmonary trunk. *LCA* = left main coronary artery. The aneurysm does not involve the distal portion of ascending aorta. *c*, View of heart and aorta after removing its anterior half. Death resulted from rupture of the right lateral wall of aorta at a point where blood ejected from left ventricle contacts the aortic wall *(arrow)*. The aneurysmal bulge is mainly to the right. *d*, Close-up view of the multiple healed tears in ascending aorta. One of the previously incomplete tears ruptured through and through. *e*, Photomicrograph of tear with portion of wall overhanging the portion of wall depleted of elastic fibers, which stain black. (Movat stain; original magnification ×7.)

Carlson et al.[93] graded the severity of cystic medial necrosis from 1 to 4 among patients with systemic hypertension and among others with normotension. They found that the frequency of cystic medial necrosis increased progressively from 10% in the first two decades of life to 60% and 64% in the seventh and eighth decades, respectively. The frequency and extent of cystic medial necrosis was higher in the hypertensive than in the normotensive patients of similar age. Schlatmann and Becker[94] confirmed the observation that certain degrees of cystic medial necrosis are observed in the normal aorta and that the degrees of cystic medial necrosis increase with age. Schlatmann and Becker[95] also compared the ascending aortic media in patients with dilated aortas to those with complete or incomplete dissection, and found only quantitative differences between the normal aging aorta and the overtly abnormal aorta. Thus these newer observations regarding the frequency, extent, and significance of cystic medial necrosis must be taken into account when evaluating its presence in the patients with the Marfan syndrome. We believe that many of the Marfan patients with aortic dissection have no

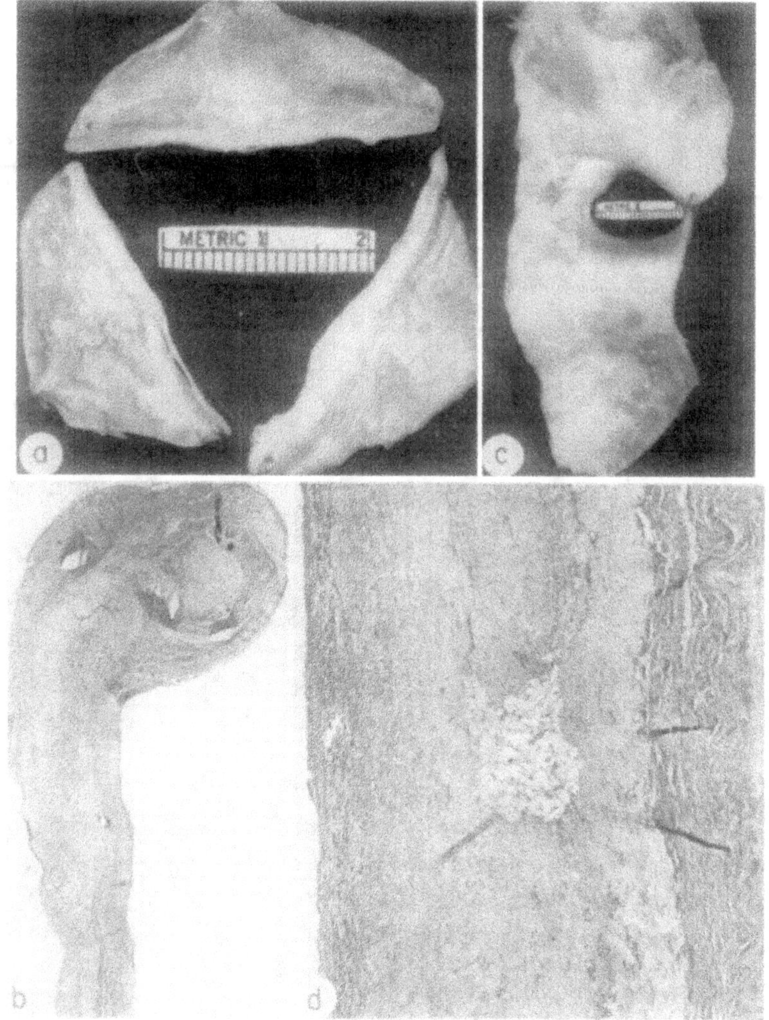

Fig. 9. Case No. 11 Operatively excised aortic valve (*a* and *b*) and ascending aorta (*c* and *d*) in a 41-year-old man (A65-64) who was asymptomatic until 7 months before death when he had the sudden onset of dyspnea which rapidly progressed to overt congestive heart failure. Examination disclosed *evidence of severe aortic regurgitation and aortic valve replacement with partial resection of the ascending aorta was carried out. a,* The aortic valve cusps were thickened on their margins. *b,* Photomicrograph of one cusp. The margin is thickened. (Hematoxylin-eosin stain; original magnification ×24.) *c,* Portion of ascending aorta excised. No tears are present. *d,* Section of ascending aorta showing striking loss of elastic fibers (stained black) and a "puddle" of acid mucopolysaccharide material. (Elastic van Gieson stain; original magnification ×58.)

more cystic medial necrosis than might be expected for the patient's age or level of systemic arterial pressure.

True nature of "cystic medial necrosis." The term "cystic medial necrosis" incidentally has certain defects because "cysts" are relatively infrequent and "necrosis" is difficult to identify. Furthermore, the striking histologic aortic lesion when full-blown is massive degeneration of elastic fibers and this feature is ignored by the term "cystic medial necrosis." When Gsell[96] first used the term "medionecrosis" in 1928 and a year later Erdheim[97,98] employed the term "cystic medial necrosis," stains for elastic

fibers were apparently infrequently employed, and we have seen that loss or degeneration of elastic fibers may be difficult to appreciate on hematoxylin-eosin stained sections.

When elastic fibers disappear from the aortic wall in this condition, the space previously occupied by them appears to be replaced by collagen fibrils and mucoid material. Although the increased acid mucopolysaccharide material has been considered an inherent defect in this condition, it is just as reasonable to believe that this material serves simply as "a filler" for the lost elastic fibers. Normally, the media of aorta in the ascending portion contains approxi-

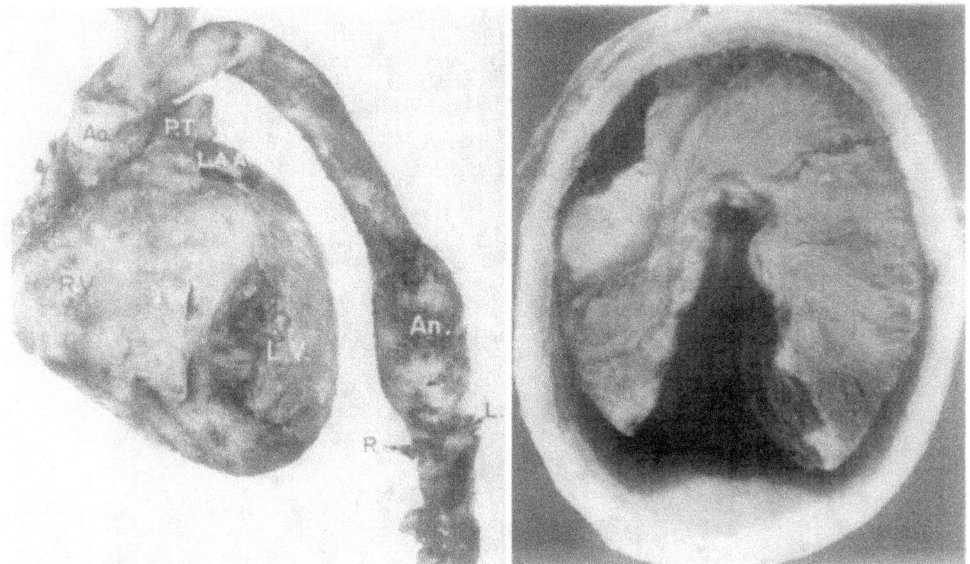

Fig. 10. Case No. 11. Heart and aorta in same patient described in Fig. 9. The ascending aorta *(Ao)* contains a graft and a fusiform aneurysm *(An)* is present in the *descending* thoracic aorta. *L.A.A.* = left atrial appendage; *R.* and *L.* = right and left renal arteries; *L.V.* = left ventricle; *P.T.* = pulmonary trunk; *R.V.* = right ventricle. *Right,* Cross-section of descending thoracic aortic aneurysm with intra-aneurysmal thrombus. This patient died 75 days after the cardiac operation with typical features of the nephrotic syndrome.

mately 58 elastic lamellae.[99] It is not clear whether or not the numbers of the elastic lamellae are normal or decreased at the time of birth in patients with the Marfan syndrome. Whether normal or decreased, however, fusiform ascending aortic aneurysm, with or without tears, has not been described in newborns with this syndrome. Thus, it appears that although the composition of the aortic media may be defective at birth, the aneurysms form later, presumably the consequence of the intra-aortic pressure's effect on an inherently weak wall. The possible consequences of the inherently or congenitally weakened aortic media are shown in Fig. 15.

Aneurysm and dissection of the descending thoracic and abdominal aorta. Although most fusiform aneurysms in the Marfan syndrome involve the ascending aorta (both sinus and tubular portions), aneurysm also may involve the descending thoracic aorta (as it did in our patients No. 4 and 11 and as reported by others[78, 82]) and the abdominal aorta, as reported by others.[13, 37, 44, 70, 82, 100-103] Because the numbers of elastic fibers in the abdominal aorta are only about one half of those present in the ascending aorta with immediate numbers in between, and because the major histologic finding in the medial portion of the aneurysmal wall is massive loss of elastic fibers, it is logical of course that the ascending aorta is the most common location of fusiform aneurysms in the Marfan syndrome. The ascending portion also moves ("stretches") the most with each heart beat ("hypermobile aorta"),[104] and this factor also may play a role in this preferential location of aneurysms in this syndrome.

Although dissection limited to the ascending aorta has been considered by some to be characteristic of the Marfan syndrome, the descending thoracic and abdominal aorta are often involved in the dissection in these patients. In each of our three patients with aortic dissection, the dissection involved the entire aorta. In the 36 (of 57) previously reported necropsy patients with aortic dissection, the location of the dissection was described: it involved the entire aorta or at least down to the abdominal aorta in 19 (53%); in five (14%)[18, 33, 47, 51, 76] it extended to the aortic isthmus; in seven (19%) it appeared to involve only the ascending portion; and in five (14%)[10, 17, 55, 68, 74] it involved only the descending thoracic aorta with or without involvement of the abdominal portion. When the dissection is limited to ascending aorta, there may be confusion with rupture of a fusiform aneurysm without actual longitudinal dissection. In at least two previously reported necropsy patients, the authors described dissection limited to the ascending aorta, but the description was far more typical of rupture of a fusiform aneurysm without dissection.[58, 69] Dissection, however, may occur in the descending thoracic and abdominal aorta without dissection in the

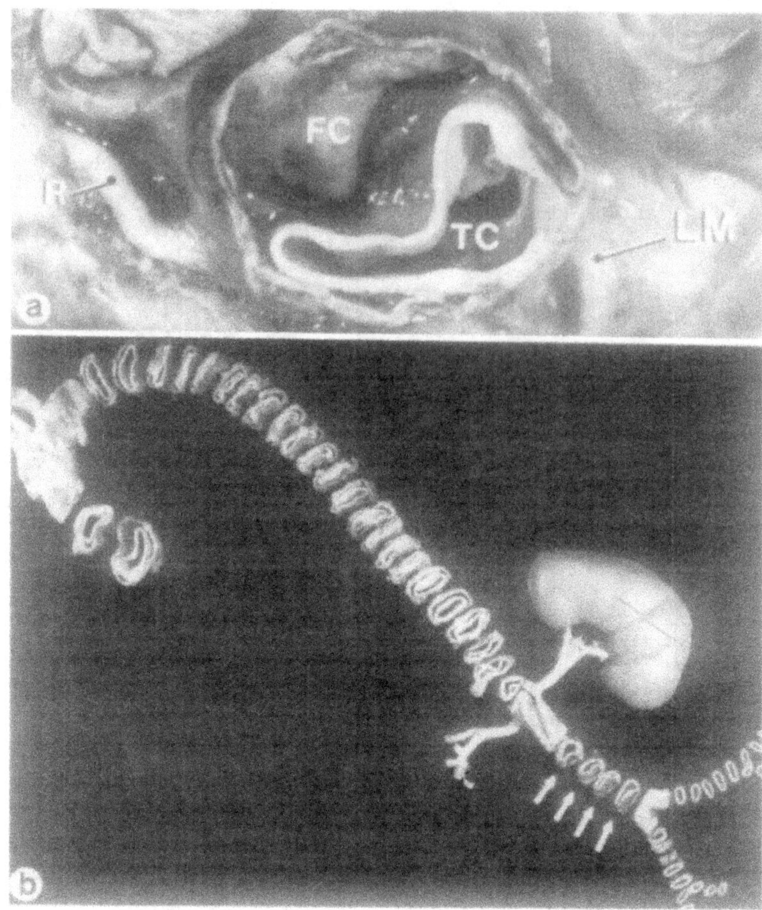

Fig. 11. Case No. 14. Dissection of the entire aorta in a 33-year-old man (76A-48) who had been asymptomatic until 15 days before death when he had the onset of severe chest pain and an aortogram showed dissection of the entire aorta. He died of rupture of the outer partition of the false channel into the pericardial sac. *a,* Aorta seen from above showing a large false channel *(FC)* and the true channel *(TC).* The ostium of the right coronary artery *(R)* has been completely separated from the true channel. *LM* = left main coronary artery. *b,* Cross-sections of the aorta. Thrombus is present in the false channel of the abdominal aorta *(arrows).* The aorta is not dilated.

ascending portion but with a fusiform aneurysm in the ascending portion.[71, 77, 84, 85]

Factors predisposing to aortic aneurysm or dissection. Certain conditions superimposed on the Marfan syndrome appear to predispose the fusiform ascending aortic aneurysm to rupture or to further dilation (thereby worsening or initiating AR) and the aorta to dissect. Of our 16 patients with aortic fusiform ascending aneurysm or dissection, one had *coarctation of the aorta* and of the 110 previously reported necropsy patients with fusiform aneurysm or dissection, 10 had aortic isthmic coarctation,[10, 15, 19, 26, 27, 34, 39, 56, 86] but in each the degree of aortic narrowing appeared to be mild. Fourteen (13%) of the 110 previously reported necropsy patients with either fusiform ascending aortic aneurysm or dissection were *pregnant* or in labor only a short period before the fatal catastrophic event

occurred,[11, 18, 39, 40, 49, 62, 64, 66, 70, 71, 76, 80, 82] and one[27] (3%) of the 33 patients with isolated MR was pregnant. Some type of *trauma* may have predisposed the aorta to rupture or to further dilation in five previously reported necropsy patients with either fusiform ascending aortic aneurysm or dissection.[27, 32, 33, 51, 54]

Rupture of aortic root aneurysm. Although the major consequence of fusiform ascending aortic aneurysm in the Marfan syndrome is aortic regurgitation (100% of our 13 patients and 95% of 42 previously reported patients where this information was recorded), rupture of the aneurysm, of course, is also a danger. This event occurred in 2 of our 13 patients and in at least 14 (25%)[7, 19, 25, 29, 33, 42, 48, 74, 76, 82] of the 57 previously reported necropsy patients with aortic dissection. Thus treatment of Marfan patients with fusiform ascending aortic aneurysms

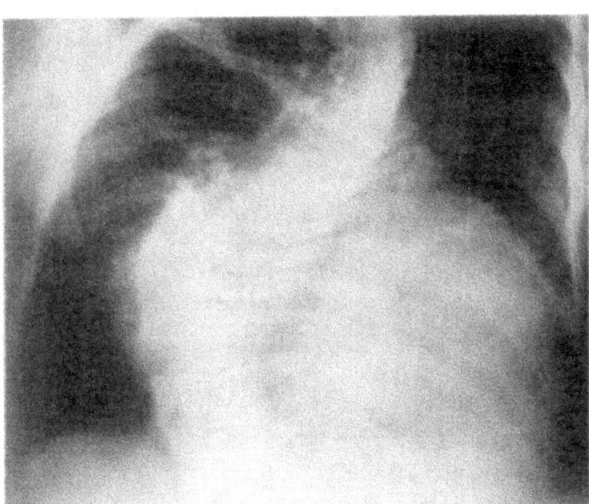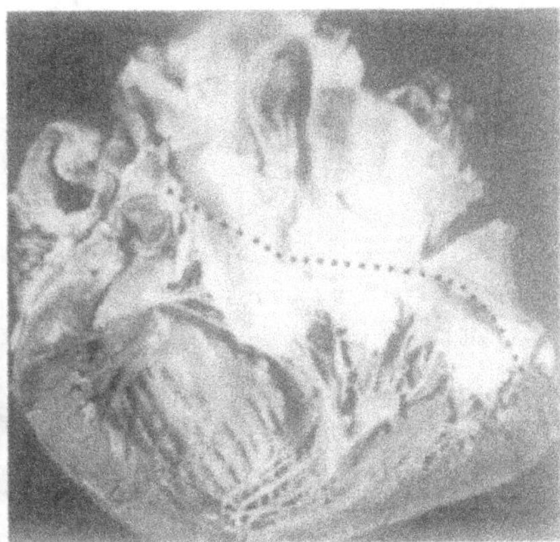

Fig. 12. Case No. 17. Posteroanterior chest roentgenogram *(left)* and opened left atrium, mitral valve, and left ventricle *(right)* in a 28-year-old man (A63-25) who had the onset of exertional dyspnea 4 years before death and evidence of overt congestive heart failure for 1 year before death. He never had a murmur of aortic regurgitation. At necropsy, the aorta was normal both grossly and histologically. The mitral valve anulus *(dotted line)* is greatly dilated (17 cm) and the length of the cusps from basal attachment to distal margin is elongated without elongation of the chordae tendineae. The vertebral column is greatly deformed *(left)*.

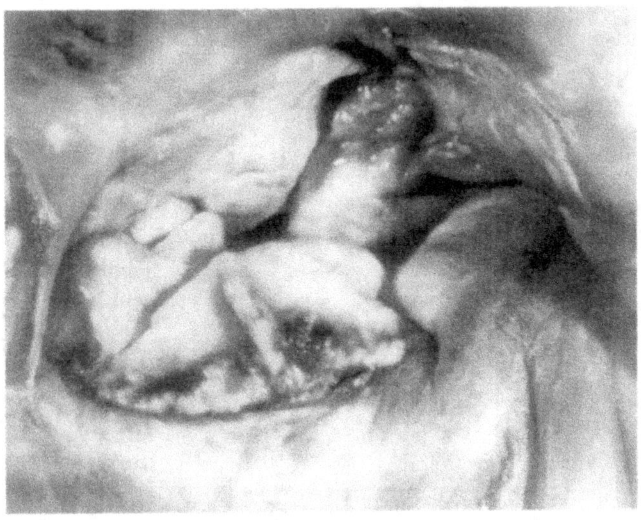

Fig. 13. Case No. 18. Mitral valve seen from above in a 35-year-old woman (A77-49) who had been asymptomatic until about age 27 when "palpitations" appeared and ECG showed sinus tachycardia and frequent ventricular extrasystoles. At age 33 years, 2 years before death, exertional dyspnea and subcutaneous edema appeared. Examination at that time disclosed a grade 4/6 murmur typical of mitral regurgitation, no precordial diastolic murmur, and the blood pressure was 120/80 mm Hg. Left ventriculogram disclosed moderate mitral regurgitation, calcium in the *mitral anulus,* and a huge left atrium. Aortic root cineangiogram disclosed a normal-sized aorta and no aortic regurgitation. She suddenly developed severe dyspnea 2 years later while eating and died, and necropsy disclosed a bolus of food in her trachea. She had been seen by her physician a day earlier and was free of evidence of congestive heart failure. At necropsy, the *mitral anulus* was huge (17 cm in circumference), the leaflets were floppy, and heavy calcific deposits were present in the anulus. A linear calcific deposit beneath one large scallop of posterior leaflet extended from the anulus toward the margin of the cusp.

must be directed at elimination or preventing AR and in preventing aneurysmal rupture, not at preventing dissection, because the latter is an infrequent complication in such patients.

Abnormalities causing MR. MR also is frequent in patients with the Marfan syndrome. At least six factors may be important in causing MR: (1) diiatation of mitral anuli, (2) floppiness or prolapse of mitral leaflets and/or elongation of chordae tendineae, (3) calcification of mitral anuli, (4) rupture of mitral chordae tendineae, (5) infective endocarditis, and (6) papillary muscle dysfunction. Of these six factors, numbers one, two, three, and five appear most important in causing severe degrees of MR. Of our 18 necropsy patients, nine had MR, isolated in two and combined with AR in seven. Of these nine patients, four had floppy mitral valves, whereas none of the nine patients without MR had floppy valves. The "floppiness" involved the posterior mitral leaflet in all four patients. The LV mural endocardium just beneath the prolapsed portion of mitral leaflet was thickened in each of the four patients. These fibrous lesions have been called "friction lesions" by Salazar and Edwards,[105] who also observed them in the hearts of patients with the Marfan syndrome. Of the nine patients with MR, the circumference of the mitral anulus ranged from 10 to 17 cm (mean = 15; normal = 9) and of the nine patients without MR, the circumference ranged from 9 to 13 cm (mean 11). Thus the mean circumference of the mitral anulus in the nine patients with MR was dilated 67% over normal (15 compared to 9) and that in the nine patients without MR, only 22% over normal (12 compared to nine). Therefore both mitral leaflet prolapse and anular dilatation play

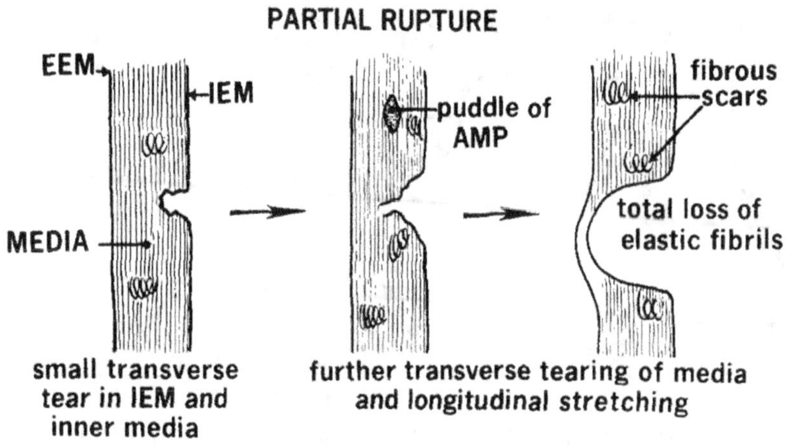

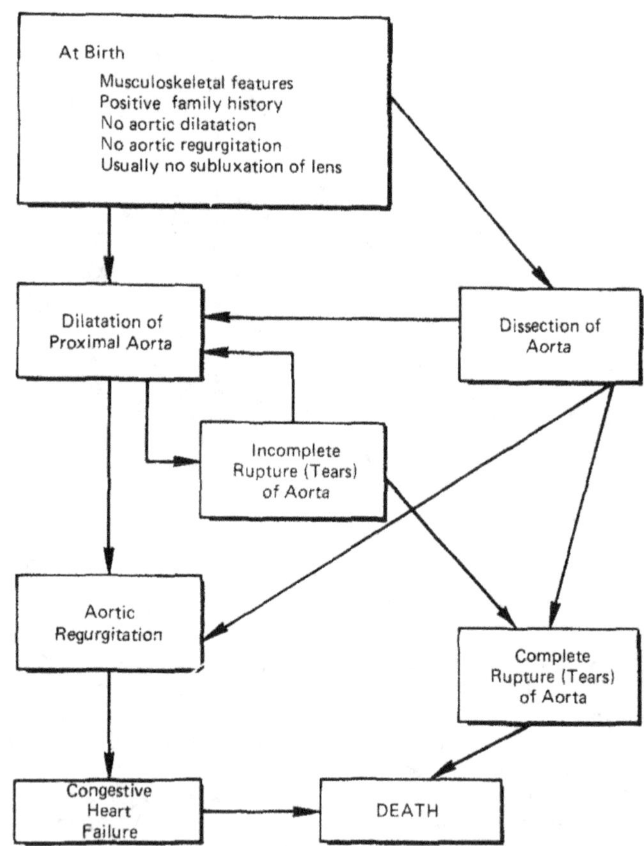

Fig. 14. Diagram showing the probable mechanism of the aortic tears. A small intimal tear begins at the internal elastic membrane *(IEM)* and inner media. The adjacent portion of aorta expands longitudinally from that point *(middle panel)* and eventually the wall of aorta thins considerably at the site of the initial tear *(right panel)*. *EEM* = external elastic membrane; *AMP* = acid mucopolysaccharide material.

significant roles in causing MR in these patients.

Calcification of the mitral anulus is known to cause or at least to be associated with MR. The degree of MR produced by this mechanism alone, however, is nearly always mild or minimal and, in addition, the mitral anuli in non-Marfan patients with mitral anular calcification is nearly always of normal or near normal circumference.[106] Of our 18 necropsy patients, five had mitral anular calcific deposits: all five had associated MR but, in addition, four had prolapsing mitral leaflets and in four the circumference of the mitral anulus was quite dilated (range 13 to 17 cm [mean = 15]). Evidence for rupture of mitral chordae tendineae was found in five of our nine patients with and in none of the nine patients without MR. Two of these five patients had histories of infective endocarditis which had healed.[107] All five patients with evidence of mitral chordal rupture had prolapsing mitral leaflets and four had dilated mitral anuli (range 15 to 17 cm [mean = 16]). The role played by "papillary muscle dysfunction" in causing MR in these patients is less clear. Among our 18 patients, the LV was dilated in each and the LV mass was increased in each. The hearts of our 18 patients ranged in weight from 375 to 850 gm (mean = 654). In 13 of the 18 patients, the mitral leaflets from their basal attachments to their distal margins were increased in length. This "stretching" probably in part was the result of the elongation (apex to base) of the LV cavities, resulting primarily from the associated AR. The resulting LV dilatation may have altered the normal angulation between the papillary muscles and mitral leaflets.[105] Whether or not MR was increased in any patient by this mechanism, however, is uncertain.

In contrast to fusiform ascending aortic aneurysm

Fig. 15. Schema of development of cardiovascular complications in the Marfan syndrome.

and dissection which generally became manifest after childhood, mitral valve abnormalities in the Marfan syndrome may be present at birth. We have studied at necropsy the heart of a 2-day-old child who at birth was found to have a loud murmur typical of MR and at necropsy, floppy mitral and tricuspid valve leaflets (Fig. 16). Although this child

Table II. Observations in 151 previously reported necropsy patients with the Marfan syndrome

C-V category	References	No. pts	Age (yr) range (mean)
1. Fusiform ascending aortic aneurysm	6,8,9,12-15,21,22,23,27(LK,WW),28,32,34,35, 37,38,41,52(No.2,No.4), 53(No.1-No.3) 55(BK,LZ), 56,58,64(No.2),67(No.12), 69,70(No.1), 71,77,78(No.2),82(MB,IMG,AD), 84,85(No. 1),86,90,91	53 (35%)	7 mo-62 (28)
2. Aortic dissection	7,9-11,17-20,24-26,27(RLL,KB),29-31,33,39, 40,42,46,47-49,50(No.3),52(No.1),54,55 (OS),61,62,66,68,74,76-78,80,82 (JR,BR,LFY),83,86(No.3),89,90	57 (38%) (healed = 14)	13-52 (27)
3. Mitral regurgitation without No. 1 or No. 2	1,2,5,16,22,27(BJP,MER),36,37,43,45,52,55 (JR,CR),59(No.1),60,63,65,72,73,75,79,81, 82(MMcG,PR,MEC,JS),83,87,88,90	33 (22%)	2 mo-6 (12)
4. Miscellaneous (not No. 1, 2, or 3)	3,4,16,37,44,55(PB),57,82	8 (5%)	stillborn-35 (14)
Totals	1-91	151 (100%)	Stillborn-65 (23)

Abbreviations: AR = aortic regurgitation; CA = coarctation of aorta; C-V = cardiovascular; F = female; M = male; mo = month; No. = number; P = pregnancy; pts = patients; T = trauma; Op = operation.

had the typical musculoskeletal features of the Marfan syndrome, the eyes were not examined and there was no family history of the Marfan syndrome in other family members and, therefore, this child was not included among our 18 necropsy patients because the definition of the syndrome was not fulfilled. Nevertheless, it is likely that the child did have the Marfan syndrome and his heart is illustrated for comparison in Fig. 16. Others[1, 22, 55, 63, 72, 81, 83] also have described abnormalities of the mitral or tricuspid valves in patients less than 1 year of age with the Marfan syndrome.

Prevalence of MR. Although most reports describing necropsy observations in patients with the Marfan syndrome have not mentioned the status of the mitral or tricuspid valves, it must be recalled that the floppy or prolapsing mitral valve was not recognized clinically until 1963[108] and at necropsy not until a year or so later. Thus, morphologic descriptions of floppy or prolapsing mitral or tricuspid valves would not be expected in the Marfan patients until about 1965, and most of the detailed reported necropsy descriptions were before that date. Nevertheless, it is now clear that prolapse of one or both mitral leaflets is common at necropsy in the Marfan syndrome and that clicks, late systolic murmurs, and echocardiographic evidence of prolapse is very common in these patients.[109, 110] Spangler et al.[109] found mitral valvular abnormalities by echocardiogram in 16 (62%) of 26 patients with the Marfan syndrome, and late or pansystolic apical murmurs and/or clicks or both in 16 (62%). Of 50 consecutive patients with the Marfan syndrome examined and reported recently by Pyeritz and McKusick,[110] 24 (48%) had midsystolic clicks with or without late systolic murmurs and 29 (58%) had echocardiographic evidence of mitral valve prolapse. Although necropsy studies demonstrate abnormalities of the aorta with or without AR to be the most frequent cardiovascular abnormality in the Marfan syndrome, recent clinical and echocardiographic studies show that mitral valve dysfunction is even more common. Even among the previously reported necropsy patients aged 15 years or younger, however, MR was the most frequent type of cardiovascular dysfunction (Table II). The MR on rare occasion may require operative treatment early in life. Pifarré et al.[111] reported severe MR requiring mitral valve replacement in a 21-month-old girl with the Marfan syndrome.

Relatively little information on the circumference of the mitral and tricuspid valve anuli has been provided in the previously reported necropsy patients with the Marfan syndrome with or without MR. Of the reported patients with MR, the mitral or tricuspid anular circumference was described as "increased" in several patients.[27, 45, 59, 73, 81] In the 21-year-old man with severe MR reported by Van Buchem,[37] the mitral anulus was reported to be 18 cm and the tricuspid 23 cm in circumference. These are the largest anular circumferences that we have encountered.

MR more related to aortic aneurysm than to aortic dissection. Marfan patients with fusiform ascending aortic aneurysms of course may also have mitral

$M:F$ (%:%)	No. age ≤ 15 years	AR	CA	P	T	C-V Op
30:23 (57:43)	8 (15%)	40/42 (95%)	5 (9%)	4 (7%)	2 (4%)	5 (9%)
35:21 (63:37).	4 (7%)	3/30 (10%)	5 (9%)	10 (18%)	3 (5%)	4 (7%)
15:16 (48:52)	24 (73%)	1 (3%)	0	1 (3%)	0	2 (6%)
3:4	4	0	0	0	0	2
83:64 (56:44)	40 (26%)	—	10 (7%)	15 (10%)	5 (3%)	13 (9%)

valvular abnormalities with or without MR. Seven of our 13 patients with fusiform ascending aortic aneurysms had MR, but none of our three patients with aortic dissection had MR. Of the 53 previously reported necropsy patients with fusiform ascending aortic root aneurysms (Table II), at least nine (17%)[6, 8, 34, 35, 41, 53, 55, 77] had anatomic mitral valve abnormalities but only one[55] definitely had evidence of MR, and that patient was only 7 months old, by far the youngest of any of the reported patients with aortic root aneurysm and the Marfan syndrome. Of the 57 reported necropsy patients with aortic dissection, nine (16%)[9, 17, 26, 39, 50[case No. 3], 68, 76, 83] had anatomic abnormalities of the mitral valve with MR in at least three.[50, 68, 83]

The Marfan syndrome may be associated with mitral anular calcification at a young age.[106, 112-115] Mitral anular calcific deposits were described in five[5, 9, 17, 30, 45] of the 151 previously reported necropsy patients with the Marfan syndrome and their ages ranged from 15 to 35 years (mean 27). Three were female and two were male. Only two of the five definitely had evidence of MR. Infective endocarditis involving the mitral valve was described in six[27, 53, 60, 73, 79, 88] and possibly seven[45] of the 151 previously reported necropsy patients with the Marfan syndrome. Five of the six definite cases were among the 33 patients in the MR group (Table II). In five patients the infection was active: the infecting bacterium was alpha streptococcus in four[27, 60, 73, 79] and *Staphylococcus aureus* in one.[88] In all seven patients the infection involved the mitral valve and in one[88]

also the aortic valve. Thus the mitral valve is the usual site of vegetations when infective endocarditis occurs in patients with the Marfan syndrome.[116] The floppy or prolapsing valve, of course, is the one most likely to be the site of infection. Because rupture of chordae tendineae is a frequent complication of infection involving the mitral valve, the degree of MR resulting from the infection can be severe.[107, 117, 118]

Of the eight previously reported necropsy patients with the Marfan syndrome classified in the miscellaneous group (Table II), three died from pulmonary infections,[3, 4, 16] two from rupture of abdominal aortic aneurysms,[37, 44] two from consequences of ventricular septal defect,[55, 57] and one was stillborn. Except for the two with ventricular septal defect, the other six appear to have had normal hearts and normal ascending aortas.

Although the above discussion concerned only patients with typical features of the Marfan syndrome, the cardiovascular features described in them also occur, of course, in patients without skeletal or ocular features of this syndrome or histories of this syndrome in other family members.[119] In addition, the characteristic histologic features in the wall of ascending aorta also have been observed in the aorta of patients with congenitally malformed aortic valves, particularly the bicuspid condition,[120] and in patients with aortic stenosis when superimposed on a congenitally malformed valve.[120, 121]

CONCLUSIONS

Among 18 necropsy patients aged 15 to 52 years (mean 34) with the Marfan syndrome, 13 had *fusiform aneurysms* of the sinus and proximal tubular portions of ascending aorta, severe AR, and severe aortic medial degeneration; three had *dissection* involving the entire aorta which was not dilated previously and the aortic media was normal histologically; and two patients had *isolated mitral regurgitation* with grossly and histologically normal aortas. Of the 13 with fusiform ascending aortic aneurysms, two ruptured spontaneously; of the remaining 11, 9 died after operations to correct the severe AR. Of the three with aortic dissection, two had systemic hypertension before the dissection. Although the only cardiovascular manifestation of the Marfan syndrome was MR in two patients, 7 of the other 16 patients also had clinical evidence of MR and 11 of the total 18 had anatomic mitral abnormalities including dilated (> 11 cm) anuli (11 patients), prolapse (seven patients), ruptured chor-

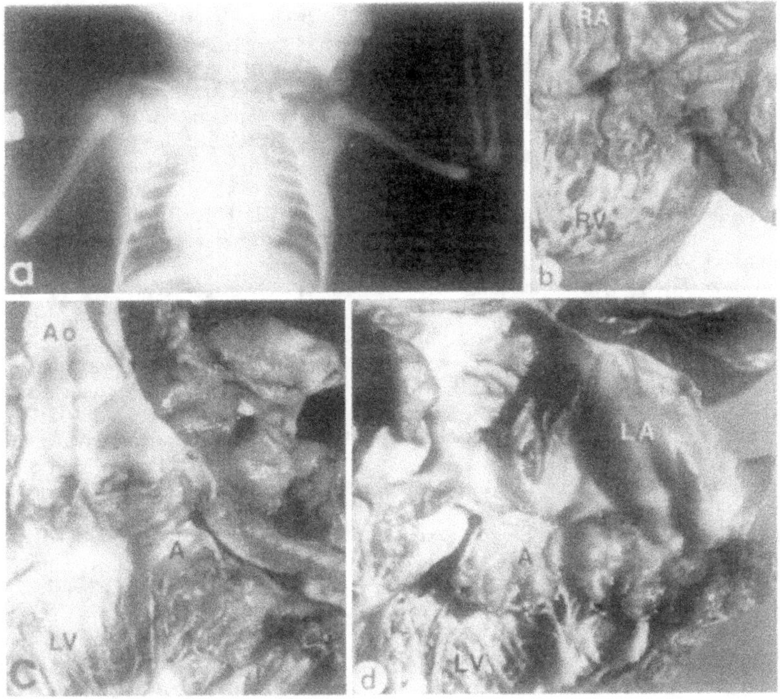

Fig. 16. Congenital floppy mitral valve and floppy tricuspid valve in a 2-day-old boy (A67-236) who had long toes and fingers, a high-arched palate, and a grade 3/6 precordial systolic murmur typical of mitral regurgitation when examined by Dr. Joseph K. Perloff. The heart was enlarged *(a)* and he died of congestive cardiac failure. At necropsy, the intima of the ascending aorta *(Ao)* was wrinkled *(c)*, suggesting that the underlying media was abnormal at this early stage. Shown here are the opened aorta, aortic valve, and left ventricle *(LV)* (A = anterior mitral leaflet). *d*, Opened left atrium *(LA)*, mitral valve, and left ventricle *(LV)*. The mitral leaflets are considerably elongated in both longitudinal and transverse dimensions. The left atrium is dilated. *b*, The tricuspid valve leaflets also are elongated in both transverse and longitudinal dimensions. *RA* = right atrium; *RV* = right ventricle.

dae tendineae (five patients), and mitral anular calcium (five patients).

Analysis of 151 previously reported necropsy patients with the Marfan syndrome disclosed that 53 (35%) had fusiform ascending aortic aneurysms, 57 (38%) had aortic dissection, 33 (22%) had isolated or predominant MR, and eight (5%) had miscellaneous conditions (mainly normal hearts and ascending aortas). The mean age at death in the patients with either fusiform ascending aortic aneurysm or dissection was similar (28 years) and the mean age of the patients with MR was much younger (12 years). Nearly three fourths of the patients with MR were aged 15 years or younger, whereas the percentage of young patients with aneurysm or dissection was much less (15% and 7%, respectively). As with our patients, the occurrence of dissection was infrequent in the previously reported patients with fusiform ascending aortic aneurysm. Dissection appeared to involve aortas which previously were of normal size or only mildly dilated, and the degree of "cystic medial necrosis" in them appeared to have been relatively mild. Thus the aneurysmally dilated ascending aorta, the most common cause of AR in these patients, is generally not a candidate for dissection but it is prone to complete rupture. And finally, mitral anular dilation with or without leaflet prolapse appears to be the major cause of MR in patients with the Marfan syndrome.

REFERENCES

1. Salle V: Ueber einen Fall von angeborener abnormen Grosse der Extremitaten mit einen an Akronemegalia erinnerden Symptomenkomplex. Jahrb Kinderheilk **75**:540, 1912.
2. Börger F: Über zwei Fälle von Arachnodaktylie. Z Kinderh **12**:161, 1915.
3. Piper RK, Irvine-Jones E: Arachnodactylia and its association with congenital heart disease. Report of a case and review of the literature. Am J Dis Child **31**:832, 1926.
4. Rambar AC, Denenholz EJ: Arachnodactyl. Report of a case with autopsy, including histologic examination. J Pediatr **15**:844, 1939.
5. Olcott CT: Arachnodactyly (Marfan's syndrome) with severe anemia. Am J Dis Child **60**:660, 1940.
6. Baer RW, Taussig HB, Oppenheimer EH: Congenital aneurysmal dilatation of the aorta associated with arachnodactyly. Bull Johns Hopkins Hosp **72**:309, 1943.
7. Etter LE, Glover LP: Arachnodactyly complicated by dislocated lens and death from rupture of dissecting aneurysm of aorta. JAMA **123**:88, 1943.

8. Stravhorn D, Wells EB: Arachnodactyly with aneurysmal dilatation of the aorta. Trans Am Clin Climatol Assoc **59**:205, 1947.

9. Tobin JR Jr, Bay EB, Humphreys EM: Marfan's syndrome in the adult. Dissecting aneurysm of the aorta associated with arachnodactyly. Arch Intern Med **80**:475, 1947.

10. Uyeyama H, Kondo B, Kamins M: Arachnodactylia and cardiovascular disease—report of an autopsied case with a summary of previously autopsied cases. Am Heart J **34**:580, 1947.

11. Lindeboom GA, Bouwer WF: Dissecting aneurysm (and renal cortical necrosis) associated with arachnodactyly (Marfan's disease). Cardiologia **15**:12, 1949.

12. Case records (Case #36351) of the Massachusetts General Hospital. N Engl J Med **243**:346, 1950.

13. Moses MF: Aortic aneurysm associated with arachnodactyly. Br Med J **2**:81, 1951.

14. Marvel RJ, Genovese PD: Cardiovascular disease in Marfan's syndrome. Am Heart J **42**:814, 1951.

15. Fischl AA, Ruthberg J: Clinical implications of Marfan's syndrome. JAMA **146**:704, 1951.

16. Tung H-L, Liebow AA: Marfan's syndrome. Observations at necropsy: With special reference to medionecrosis of the great vessels. Lab Invest **1**:382, 1952.

17. Thomas J, Brothers GB, Anderson RS, Cuff JR: Marfan's syndrome. A report of three cases with aneurysm of the aorta. Am J Med **12**:613, 1952.

18. Spenser JT: Post-mortem caeserean delivery after rupture of dissecting aortic aneurysm. Lancet **2**:565, 1952.

19. Gore I: Dissecting aneurysms of the aorta in persons under forty years of age. Arch Pathol **55**:1, 1953.

20. Goyette EM, Palmer PW: Cardiovascular lesions in arachnodactyly. Circulation **7**:373, 1953.

21. Sloper JC, Storey G: Aneurysms of the ascending aorta due to medial degeneration associated with arachnodactyly (Marfan's disease). J Clin Pathol **6**:299, 1953.

22. Traisman HS, Johnson FR: Arachnodactyly associated with aneurysm of the aorta. Am J Dis Child **87**:156, 1954.

23. Maier C, Rubli JM, Schaub F, Hedinger C: Cardiale Störungen beim Marfanschen Syndrom. Cardiologia **24**:106, 1954.

24. Faive G, Frenkiel P, Pernot C, Hueber: Le coeur des depressions sternales congénitales. Arch Mal Coeur **47**:322, 1954.

25. Pygott F: Arachnodactyly (Marfan's syndrome) with a report of two cases. Br J Radiol **28**:26, 1955.

26. Coffey JH, Barker DE, Friedlander JH: Dissecting aneurysm with Marfan's syndrome. Texas State J Med **51**:79, 1955.

27. McKusick VA: The cardiovascular aspects of Marfan's syndrome: A heritable disorder of connective tissue. Circulation **11**:321, 1955.

28. MacLeod M, Williams AW: The cardiovascular lesions in Marfan's syndrome. Arch Pathol **61**:143, 1956.

29. Hirst AE Jr, Bailey HL: Arachnodactyly with associated healed dissecting aneurysm. California Med **84**:355, 1956.

30. Neilson GH, Sullivan JJ: Dissecting aneurysm of the aorta associated with Marfan's syndrome. Med J Aust **43**:925, 1956.

31. Carpent G, Enderle J, Duret R: Syndrome de Marfan et anevrysme, dissequant de l'aorte thoracique. Acta Cardiol **11**:384, 1956.

32. Diamond EG, Larsen WE, Johnson WB, Kittle CF: Post-traumatic aortic insufficiency occurring in Marfan's syndrome, with attempted repair with a plastic valve. N Engl J Med **256**:8, 1957.

33. Case Records of the Massachusetts General Hospital. N Engl J Med **256**:30, 1957.

34. Fabre J, Veyrat R, Jeanneret O: Syndrome de Marfan avec anévrysme et coarctation de l'aorte. Schweiz Med Wochenschr **87**:49, 1957.

35. Bingle J: Marfan's syndrome. Br Med J **1**:629, 1957.

36. Austin MG, Schaefer RF: Marfan's syndrome, with unusual blood vessel manifestations. Primary medionecrosis dissection of right innominate, right carotid, and left carotid arteries. Arch Pathol **64**:205, 1957.

37. Van Buchem FSP: Cardiovascular disease in arachnodactyly. Acta Med Scand **161**:197, 1958.

38. Griffin JF, Koman GM: Severe aortic insufficiency in Marfan's syndrome. Ann Intern Med **48**:174, 1958.

39. Novell HA, Asher LA Jr, Lev M: Marfan's syndrome associated with pregnancy. Am J Obstet Gynecol **75**:802, 1958.

40. Husebye KO, Wolff HJ, Friedman LL: Aortic dissection in pregnancy: A case of Marfan's syndrome. Am Heart J **55**:662, 1958.

41. Roark JW: The Marfan syndrome. Report of one case with autopsy, special histological study, and review of the literature. Arch Intern Med **103**:123, 1959.

42. Hurley JV: Marfan's syndrome: The nature of the aortic defect. Australas Ann Med **8**:45, 1959.

43. Golden RL, Lakin H: The formes frustes in Marfan's syndrome. N Engl J Med **260**:797, 1959.

44. Harden CA: Ruptured abdominal aneurysm occurring in Marfan's syndrome. Attempted repair with the use of a Nylon prosthesis. N Engl J Med **260**:821, 1959.

45. Miller R Jr, Pearson RJ Jr: Mitral insufficiency simulating aortic stenosis: Report of an unusual manifestation of Marfan's syndrome. N Engl J Med **260**:1210, 1959.

46. Ferguson MJ, Clemente AR: Rupture and dissection of aorta in Marfan's syndrome. Am J Cardiol **4**:543, 1959.

47. Reid RTW: Marfan's syndrome complicating by dissecting aneurysm of the aorta. Med J Aust **46**:848, 1959.

48. Knight AM, Clark SW, Terry DB: Case presentation: Marfan syndrome, dissecting aneurysm, intermittent occlusion of both coronary arteries. J Med Assoc Ga **49**:222, 1960.

49. Borglin NE, Bach G: Marfan's syndrome and pregnancy. Acta Obstet Gynecol Scand **40**:271, 1961.

50. Tuna N, Thai AP: Some unusual features of the Marfan syndrome. Report of four cases. Circulation **24**:1154, 1961.

51. Atta AG, Hoch J: Marfan's syndrome and dissecting aneurysm of aorta. Arch Intern Med **108**:781, 1961.

52. Wagenvoort CA, Neufeld HN, Edwards JE: Cardiovascular system in Marfan's syndrome and in idiopathic dilatation of the ascending aorta. Am J Cardiol **9**:496, 1962.

53. Segal BL, Tabesh E, Imbriglia JE, Likoff W: The Marfan Syndrome. Necropsy findings in three patients with a review of the cardiovascular complications. Angiology **13**:444, 1962.

54. Schatz IJ, Yaworsky RG, Fine G: Myocardial infarction and unusual myocardial degeneration in the Marfan's syndrome. With dissection of the right coronary artery and aorta. Am J Cardiol **12**:553, 1963.

55. Bolande RP, Tucker AS: Pulmonary emphysema and other cardiorespiratory lesions as part of the Marfan abiotrophy. Pediatrics **33**:356, 1964.

56. Eldridge R: Coarctation in the Marfan syndrome. Arch Intern Med **113**:342, 1964.

57. Childers RW, McCrea PC: Absence of the pulmonary valve. A case occurring in the Marfan syndrome. Circulation **29**:598, 1964.

58. Wong FL, Friedman S, Yakovac W: Cardiac complications of Marfan's syndrome in a child. Report of a case with rapidly progressive course terminating with rupture of a dissecting aneurysm. Am J Dis Child **107**:404, 1964.

59. James TN, Frame B, Schatz IJ: Pathology of cardiac conduction system in Marfan's syndrome. Arch Intern Med **114**:339, 1964.

60. Wunsch CM, Steinmetz EF, Fisch C: Marfan's syndrome and subacute bacterial endocarditis. Am J Cardiol **15**:102, 1965.

61. Boijsen E, Weiland P-O: Dissecting aneurysm of the aorta in Marfan's syndrome. Acta Radiol **3**:89, 1965.

62. Moore HC: Marfan syndrome, dissecting aneurysm of the aorta, and pregnancy. J Clin Pathol **18**:277, 1965.

63. Bowden DH, Favara DE, Donahoe JL: Marfan's syndrome. Accelerated course in childhood associated with lesions of mitral valve and pulmonary artery. AM HEART J **69**:96, 1965.

64. Tricomi V: The Marfan syndrome and pregnancy. Clin Obstet Gynecol **8**:334, 1965.

65. Raghib G, Jue KL, Anderson RC, Edwards JE: Marfan's syndrome with mitral insufficiency. Am J Cardiol **16**:127, 1965.

66. Donaldson LB, de Alvarez RR: The Marfan syndrome and pregnancy. Am J Obstet Gynecol **92**:629, 1965.

67. Keech MK, Wendt VE, Read RC, Bistue AR, Bianchi FA: Family studies of the Marfan syndrome. J Chronic Dis **19**:57, 1966.

68. Kumar V, Berenson GS: The Marfan syndrome: Report of an interesting case with unusual anatomic findings. J La State Med Soc **118**:511, 1966.

69. Matsui E, Ito T: Marfan's syndrome complicated by huge hydropericardium. Jpn Heart J **8**:98, 1967.

70. Massumi RA, Lowe EW, Misanik LF, Just H, Tawakkol A: Multiple aortic aneurysms (thoracic and abdominal) in twins with Marfan's syndrome: Fatal rupture during pregnancy. J Thorac Cardiovasc Surg **53**:223, 1967.

71. Rivlin ME: Marfan's syndrome and pregnancy. J Obstet Gynecol Br Commonwealth **74**:143, 1967.

72. Shankar KR, Hultgren MK, Lauer RM, Diehl AM: Lethal tricuspid and mitral regurgitation in Marfan's syndrome. Am J Cardiol **20**:122, 1967.

73. Hiejima K, Tsuchiya S, Sakamoto Y, Shiina S: Two cases of Marfan's syndrome associated respectively with subacute bacterial endocarditis and the Wolff-Parkinson-White syndrome. Jpn Heart J **9**:208, 1968.

74. Alarcón-Segovia D, Fierro FJ, Villalobos J le J, Dies F: Bilateral renal vein thrombosis and nephrotic syndrome in a patient with the Marfan syndrome. Dis Chest **54**:73, 1968.

75. Simpson JW, Nora JJ, McNamara DG: Marfan's syndrome and mitral valve disease: Acute surgical emergencies. AM HEART J **77**:96, 1969.

76. Grondin CM, Steinberg CL, Edwards JE: Dissecting aneurysm complicating Marfan's syndrome (arachnodactyly) in a mother and son. AM HEART J **77**:301, 1969.

77. Young D: Familial dissecting aneurysm complicating Marfan's syndrome. AM HEART J **78**:577, 1969.

78. Voigt J, Hansen JPH: Spontaneous rupture of the aorta in young people. Its relation to so-called medionecrosis cystica and Marfan's syndrome. Three medicolegal cases. Acta Pathol Microbiol Scand (suppl) **212**:143, 1970.

79. Di Matteo J, Vacheron A, Sabaut D, Delvaux JC, Audoin J: Anévrysmes multiples de la valve mitrale endocardite bacterienne et syndrome de Marfan. Coeur Med Interne **10**:519, 1971.

80. Sutinen S, Piiroinen O: Marfan syndrome, pregnancy, and fatal dissection of aorta. Acta Obstet Gynecol Scand **50**:295, 1971.

81. Hohn AR, Webb HM: Cardiac studies of infant twins with Marfan's syndrome. Am J Dis Child **122**:526, 1971.

82. McKusick VA: Heritable disorders of connective tissue. 4th ed. St. Louis, 1972, The C.V. Mosby Co, p 878.

83. Phornphutkul C, Rosenthal A, Nadas AS: Cardiac manifestations of Marfan syndrome in infancy and childhood. Circulation **47**:587, 1973.

84. Takebayashi S, Kubota I, Takagi T: Ultrastructural and histochemical studies of vascular lesions in Marfan's syndrome, with report of 4 autopsy cases. Acta Pathol Jpn **23**:847, 1973.

85. Srinivasan S, Sankaran K, Chandrasekar S, Rema P, Madhavan M: Marfan's syndrome. Indian Heart J **25**:349, 1973.

86. Melsen F: Spontaneous rupture of the aorta in Marfan's syndrome. Z Rechtsmed **73**:53, 1973.

87. Glaser J, Whitman V, Liebman J: Aortic regurgitation in a young girl with severe form of Marfan syndrome (Letter to Editor). J Pediatr **83**:685, 1973.

88. Soman VR, Breton G, Hershkowitz M, Mark H: Bacterial endocarditis of mitral valve in Marfan syndrome. Br Heart J **36**:1247, 1974.

89. Leitch AG, Caves PK: A case of Marfan's syndrome with absent right coronary artery complicated by aortic dissection and right ventricular infarction. Thorax **30**:352, 1975.

90. Sayers CP, Goltz RW, Mottaz J: Pulmonary elastic tissue in generalized elastolysis (cutis laxa) with Marfan's syndrome. A light and electron microscopic study. J Invest Dermatol **65**:451, 1975.

91. Rabkin SW, Corbett BN, Benediktsson H: Marfan syndrome with coronary artery lesions in a North American Indian. Can Med Assoc J **115**:651, 1976.

92. Murdoch JL, Walker BA, Halpern BL, Kuzma JW, McKusick VA: Life expectancy and causes of death in the Marfan syndrome. N Engl J Med **286**:804, 1972.

93. Carlson RG, Lillehei CW, Edwards JE: Cystic medial necrosis of the ascending aorta in relation to age and hypertension. Am J Cardiol **25**:411, 1970.

94. Schlatmann TJM, Becker AE: Histologic changes in the normal aging aorta: Implications for dissecting aortic aneurysm. Am J Cardiol **39**:13, 1977.

95. Schlatmann TJM, Becker AE: Pathogenesis of dissecting aneurysm of aorta. Comparative histopathologic study of significance of medial changes. Am J Cardiol **39**:21, 1977.

96. Gsell O: Wandnekrosen der Aorta als selbständige Erkrankung und ihre Beziehung zur Spontanruptur. Virchows Arch Pathol Anat Physiol **270**:1, 1928.

97. Erdheim J: Medionecrosis aortae idiopathica. Virchows Arch Pathol Anat Physiol **273**:454, 1929.

98. Erdheim J: Medionecrosis aortae idiopathica cystica. Virchows Arch Pathol Anat Physiol **276**:187, 1930.

99. Wolinsky H, Glagov S: A lamellar unit of aortic medial structure and function in mammals. Circ Res **20**:99, 1967.

100. Langeron L, Giard P, Liefooghe JR, Masson C: Maladie de Marfan et anévrysme abdominal. Bull Mem Soc Med Hop Paris **70**:374, 1954.

101. Hardin CA: Successful resection of carotid and abdominal aneurysm in two related patients with Marfan's syndrome. N Engl J Med **267**:141, 1962.

102. Yu SC: Marfan's syndrome with spontaneous pneumothorax and abdominal aortic aneurysm. Int Surg **61**:30, 1976.

103. Houston HE: Abdominal aortic aneurysm in Marfan's syndrome. J Ky Med Assoc **71**:391, 1978.

104. Benchimol A, Dresser KB, Neese TC: Hypermobility of the aorta in Marfan's syndrome. Angiology **23**:103, 1972.

105. Salazar AE, Edwards JE: Friction lesions of ventricular endocardium. Relation to chordae tendineae of mitral valve. Arch Pathol **90**:364, 1970.

106. Roberts WC, Perloff JK: Mitral valvular disease. A clinicopathologic survey of the conditions causing the mitral valve to function abnormally. Ann Intern Med **77**:939, 1972.

107. Roberts WC, Buchbinder NA: Healed left-sided infective endocarditis: A clinicopathologic study of 59 patients. Am J Cardiol **40**:876, 1977.

108. Barlow JB, Pocock WA, Marchand P, Denny M: The significance of late systolic murmurs. AM HEART J **66**:443, 1963.

109. Spangler RD, Nora JJ, Lortscher RH, Wolfe RR, Okin JT: Echocardiography in Marfan's syndrome. Chest **69**:72, 1976.

110. Pyeritz RE, McKusick VA: The Marfan syndrome: Diagnosis and management. N Engl J Med **300**:772, 1979.

111. Pifarré R, Caralps JM, Sinha SN: Mitral valve replacement for regurgitation in an infant with Marfan's syndrome. J Thorac Cardiovasc Surg **67**:233, 1974.

112. Grossman M, Knott AP Jr, Jacoby WJ Jr: Calcified annulus fibrosus with mitral insufficiency in the Marfan syndrome. Arch Intern Med **121**:561, 1968.

113. Boone JA, Clowes GHA Jr: Calcified annulus fibrosus with mitral insufficiency in the Marfan syndrome: With prosthetic replacement of the mitral valve. South Med J **62**:682, 1969.

114. Goodman HB, Dorney ER: Marfan's syndrome with massive calcification of the mitral annulus at age twenty-six. Am J Cardiol **24**:426, 1969.

115. Thornsvard C, Wolcott BW, D'Ambrosio U: Mitral annulus calcification in Marfan's syndrome. Report of a case. Med Ann DC **41**:451, 1972.

116. Bowers D, Lim DW: Subacute bacterial endocarditis and Marfan's syndrome. Can Med Assoc J **86**:455, 1962.

117. Roberts WC, Braunwald E, Morrow AG: Acute severe mitral regurgitation secondary to ruptured chordae tendineae. Clinical, hemodynamic, and pathologic considerations. Circulation **33**:58, 1966.

118. Roberts WC: Characteristics and consequences of infective endocarditis (active or healed or both) learned from morphologic studies. *In* Rahimtoola SH, editor: Infective endocarditis. New York, 1978, Grune & Stratton, Inc, p 55.

119. Waller BF, Reis RL, McIntosh CL, Epstein SE, Roberts WC: Marfan cardiovascular disease without the Marfan syndrome. Fusiform ascending aortic aneurysm with aortic and mitral valve regurgitation. Chest **77**:533, 1980.

120. Edwards WD, Leaf DS, Edwards JE: Dissecting aortic aneurysm associated with congenital bicuspid aortic valve. Circulation **57**:1022, 1978.

121. Roberts WC: Aortic dissection: Anatomy, consequences, and causes. Am Heart J **101**:195, 1981.

Severe Aortic Regurgitation from Systemic Hypertension[*]

*Bruce F. Waller, M.D., F.C.C.P.; Joan C. Kishel, M.D.; and
William C. Roberts, M.D., F.C.C.P.*

Although about 10 percent of patients with systemic hypertension have a basal diastolic blowing murmur indicating aortic regurgitation (AR) (Fig 1),[1-7] the degree of aortic regurgitation is usually minimal or mild. The occurrence of severe aortic regurgitation from systemic hypertension unassociated with aortic dissection is rare,[8] but herein we describe such a patient who had aortic regurgitation severe enough to require aortic valve replacement.

Case Report

A 64-year-old woman, who died on August 3, 1981, had systemic arterial hypertension noted for the first time at age 36 years (1953). At age 40, she began antihypertensive treatment (reserpine). At age 50 (1967), a grade 2/6 diastolic blowing murmur of aortic regurgitation was noted

*From the Pathology Branch, National Heart, Lung and Blood Institute, National Institutes of Health, Bethesda.
Reprint requests: Dr. Roberts, Bldg 10A, Rm 3E30, NHLBI, National Institutes of Health, Bethesda 20205

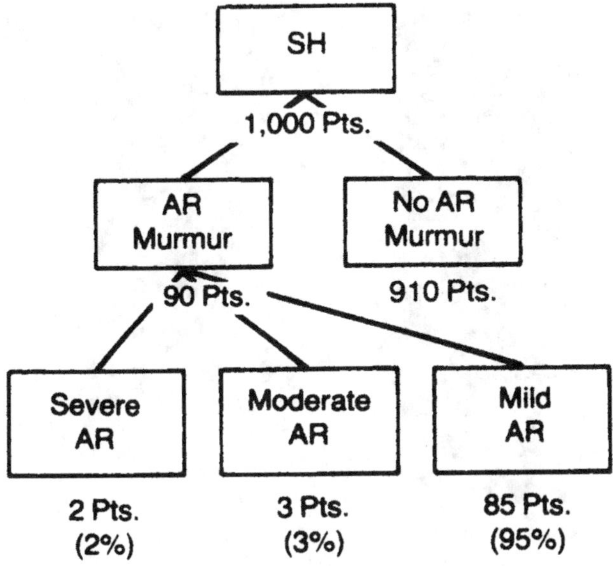

FIGURE 1. Frequency and severity of aortic regurgitation (AR) in patients (pts) with systemic hypertension (SH) based on previously reported data.[1-7]

and the blood pressure was 240/120 mm Hg (Fig 2). During the next seven years, the blood pressure remained elevated despite administration of diuretics, reserpine and alpha-methyldopa. At age 55 years (1973), angina pectoris appeared and thereafter it progressed. On examination at age 56, the intensity of the aortic regurgitation murmur was grade 3/6. The ECG (Fig 3) showed sinus bradycardia and left ventricular hypertrophy, and the chest radiograph (Fig 4), an enlarged cardiac silhouette. On M-mode echocardiogram (Fig 5), the left ventricular free wall and ventricular septum were of similar thickness and the ascending aorta was dilated. The results of the cardiac catheterization are summarized in Table 1. She underwent aortic valve replacement with a tilting-disc prosthesis and had two aortocoronary bypass conduits placed to the left anterior descending coronary system. The aortic valve was three-cuspid; each cusp was freely mobile, but mildly thickened by fibrous tissue without calcific deposits, and no commissure was fused.

The blood pressure in the first six weeks postoperation was reduced compared to the preoperation and late postoperation values (Fig 2). Later she was treated with beta-blocking and vasodilating agents. A murmur of aortic regurgitation was absent postoperatively. At age 62 (1980), angina pectoris and exertional dyspnea reappeared. The blood pressure was 210/100 mm Hg. She took warfarin only intermittently, and in July, 1981 she developed acute pulmonary edema without audible prosthetic aortic valve sounds, and died several days later.

At necropsy, the heart weighed 530 g. The orifice of the aortic-valve prosthesis was severely narrowed by thrombus which made the occluder immobile. A healed transmural left ventricular infarct was present (Fig 6) and the left main, left anterior descending, and right coronary arteries were each narrowed >75 percent in cross-sectional area by atherosclerotic plaques.

Comments

The patient described above had systemic hypertension and aortic regurgitation severe enough to warrant aortic-valve replacement without clinical or morphologic explanation for the aortic regurgitation other than systemic hypertension. Recently, we reported four other patients, all men aged 43-59 years (mean 50), with severe systemic hypertension, chronic congestive heart failure, and aortic

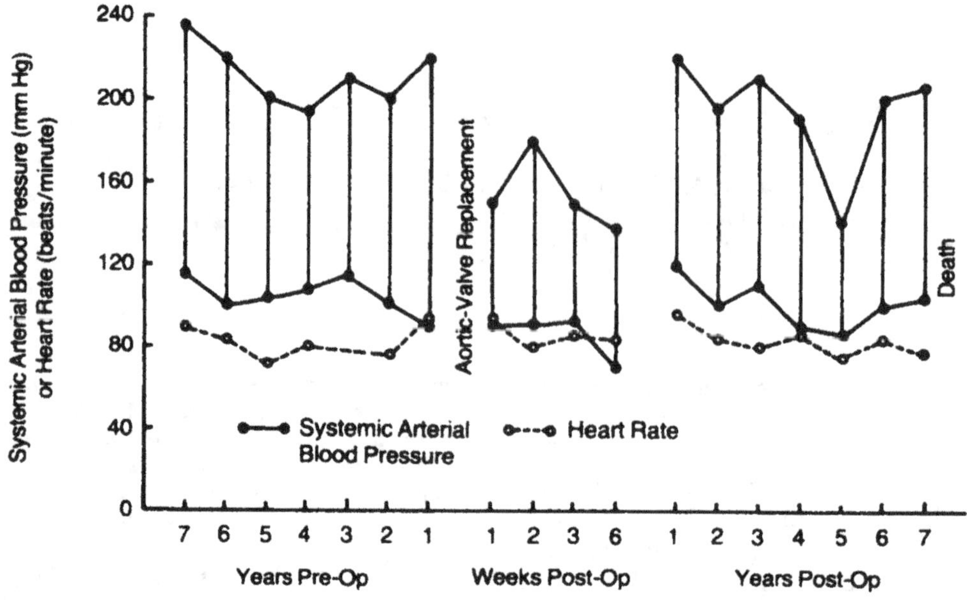

FIGURE 2. Systolic and diastolic systemic arterial pressures before and after aortic-valve replacement.

regurgitation severe enough to warrant aortic-valve replacement.[8] The hypertension had been present from 1-30 years (mean 13). In each of the four previous patients and in the present patient, the aortic valve was three-cuspid; each cusp was free of calcific deposits and freely mobile.

Until these five patients were encountered, we had not observed severe aortic regurgitation from systemic hypertension alone and are unaware of any reports describing aortic valve replacement for aortic regurgitation in such patients. At least 79 patients with systemic hypertension and aortic regurgitation (by auscultation), however, were reported between 1940 and 1971, but none had aortic valve replacement.[1-7] Of the 79 patients, the aortic regurgitation was severe in 17 (22 percent) and mild or moderate in 62 (78 percent). Each of the 17 patients with severe aortic regurgitation had fatal congestive heart failure, but another definite, probable or possible cause of the failure other than aortic regurgitation appears to have been present in six. Of the remaining 11 patients, necropsy information was available in seven. The aortic valve and ascending aorta were reported to be normal in all seven. The aortic valve "ring" was dilated in only one (7-12 cm [mean 9]), the left ventricle was dilated in only three patients, but the heart weight

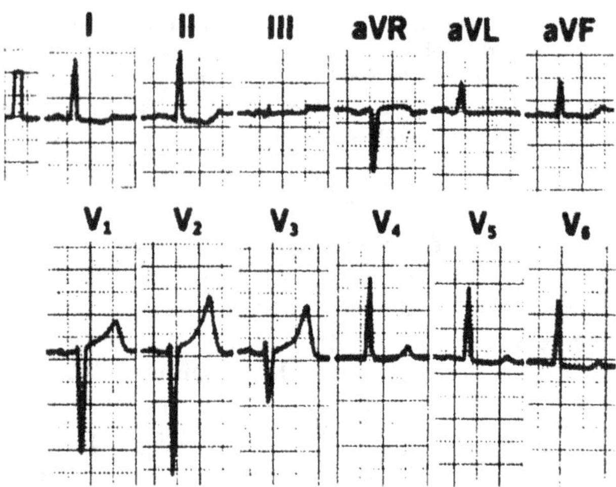

FIGURE 3. Electrocardiogram in patient at age 56 years (eight years before death) showing left ventricular hypertrophy and nonspecific ST segment and T wave changes. The total QRS amplitude is 195 mm.

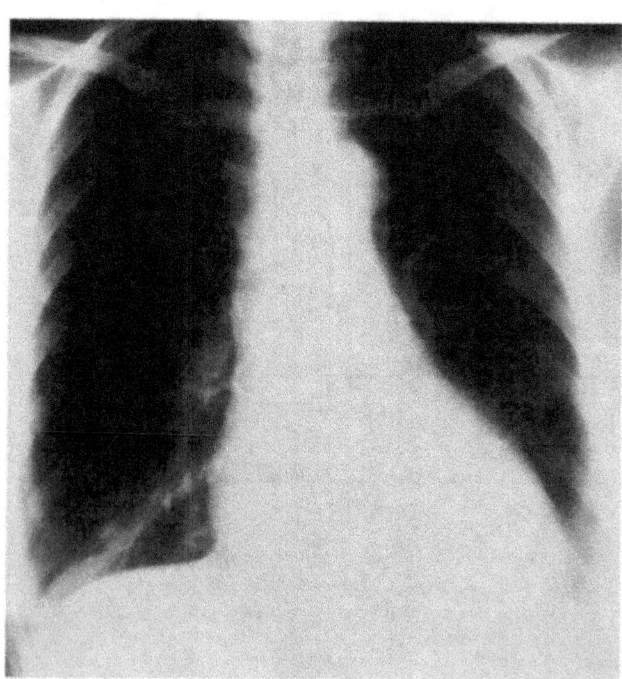

FIGURE 4. Posteroanterior chest roentgenogram obtained before aortic valve replacement eight years before death showing an enlarged cardiac silhouette.

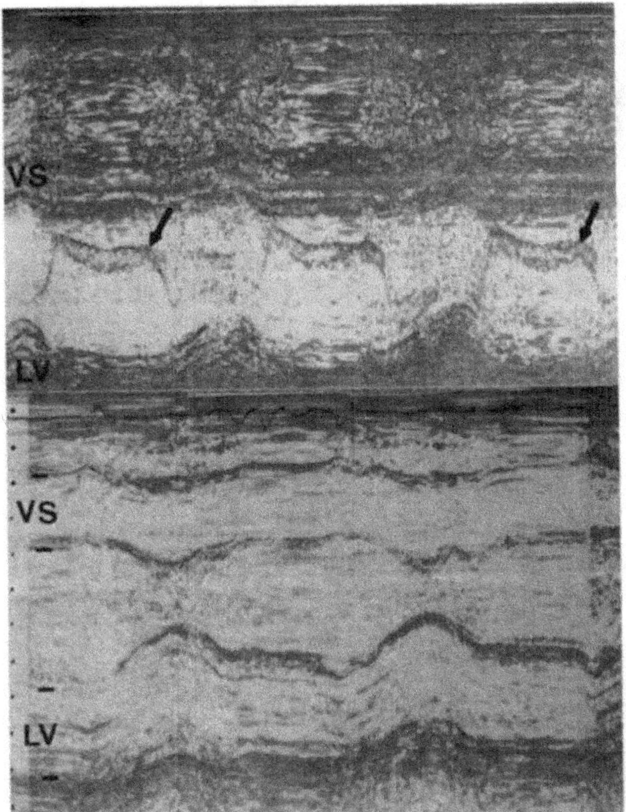

FIGURE 5. M-mode echocardiograms recorded just before aortic valve replacement. The anterior mitral valve leaflet flutters *(arrow)*, *(upper)*. The ventricular septum (VS) and left ventricular free wall (LV) are of similar thickness *(lower)*.

was increased in all seven (460-700 g [mean 565 g]).

Certain factors increase the possibility of develop-

Table 1—*Hemodynamic Data (Pressures in mm Hg)*	
Left ventricle (LV) (s/d)	160/11
Femoral artery (FA) (s/d)	160/60
Pulmonary arterial wedge (mean)	7
Right ventricle (s/d)	20/5
Right atrium (mean)	3
Cardiac index (L/min/M²)	1.6
AR by aortogram (1+-4+)	3+
Coronary arterial narrowing (% diameter reduction)	
Left main	70
Left anterior descending	50
Left circumflex	50
Right	0

s/d = peak systole/end diastole

ing aortic regurgitation in patients with systemic hypertension.[1-7] 1) *Magnitude of systemic arterial pressure.* The higher the pressure, the greater the chance of aortic regurgitation. 2) *Age of patient.* Of patients with similar levels of systemic arterial pressure, *older patients* have a higher frequency of aortic regurgitation than do younger patients. 3) *Duration of systemic hypertension.* Of patients of similar age and similar pressure, those with systemic hypertension of longer duration have a higher frequency of aortic regurgitation than do those of shorter duration. The mechanism by which severe aortic regurgitation develops in some patients with systemic hypertension is unclear.

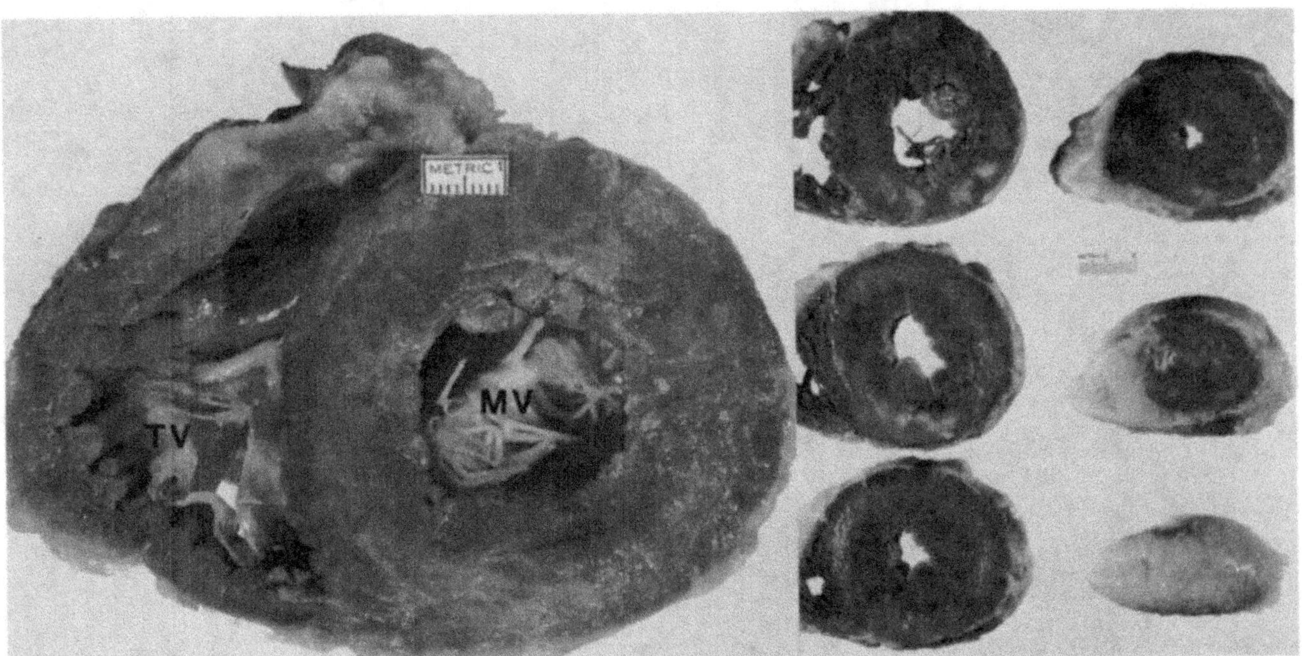

FIGURE 6. *Left:* Basal portion of the cardiac ventricles. MV=mitral valve leaflets and TV=tricuspid valve leaflets. *Right:* Transverse sections of both cardiac ventricles from base-to-apex showing nondilated cavities, thickened ventricular walls and a healed myocardial infarct.

REFERENCES

1 Barlow J, Kincaid-Smith P. The auscultatory findings in hypertension. Br Heart J 1960; 22:505-14

2 Garvin CF. Functional aortic insufficiency. Am J Med 1940; 13:1799-04

3 Gouley BA, Sickel EM. Aortic regurgitation caused by dilatation of the aortic orifice and associated with a characteristic valvular lesion. Am Heart J 1943; 26:24-38

4 Hammon L. Diagnostic implications of aortic insufficiency. Cincinnati J Med 1944: 25:95-125

5 Fenichel NM. Arteriosclerotic aortic insufficiency. Am Heart J 1950; 40:117-24

6 Puchner TC, Huston JH, Hellmuth GA. Aortic valve insufficiency in arterial hypertension. Am J Cardiol 1960; 5:758-60

7 Matalon R, Moussalli ARJ, Nidus BD, Katz LA, Eisinger RP. Functional aortic insufficiency—a feature of renal failure. N Engl J Med 1971; 285:1522-23

8 Waller BF, Zoltick JM, Rosen JH, Katz NM, Gomes MN, Fletcher RD, et al. Severe aortic regurgitation from systemic hypertension without aortic dissection requiring aortic valve replacement. Analysis of 4 patients. Am J Cardiol 1982; 49:473-77

Severe Aortic Regurgitation Secondary to Systemic Hypertension (Without Aortic Dissection)

BRUCE F. WALLER, MD, WILLIAM C. ROBERTS, MD

*C*linical and morphologic observations are described in five patients who had severe aortic regurgitation (AR) from severe systemic hypertension unassociated with aortic dissection; each patient underwent aortic valve replacement. Although it is well recognized that minimal or mild AR occurs in patients with systemic hypertension, severe AR in such patients is rare, and aortic valve replacement in such cases has not been reported in other centers. Why such severe AR developed in our five patients, however, was not determined. Although a rare cause, systemic hypertension must nevertheless be added to the list of causes of severe pure AR.

INTRODUCTION

It is well recognized that a small (about 10%[1]) percentage of patients with systemic hypertension have a basal diastolic blowing murmur indicative of aortic regurgitation (AR), which is usually of minimal or mild degree (Figure 1). The development of severe AR purely on the basis of elevated intra-aortic pressure in the absence of aortic dissection is extremely rare; and to our knowledge, aortic valve replacement for pure AR secondary to systemic hypertension unassociated with dissection has only recently been reported.[2,3] This paper summarizes available information on cases of severe AR secondary to systemic hypertension.

PATIENTS STUDIED

Pertinent clinical and morphologic observations in five patients are summarized in Figures 2 through 12 and Tables I through IV. Each had systemic hypertension treated with combinations of antihypertensive drugs including afterload-reducing agents. Patient #2 had the shortest duration of clinically recognized systemic hypertension (one year) and patient #5 the longest (30 years). Systemic hypertension was present clinically from six months to 24 years before a murmur of aortic regurgitation was recognized. The highest indirect, systemic and systolic brachial arterial pressures in the five patients ranged from 195 to 270 mm Hg (average 235) and the lowest from 140 to 195 mm Hg (average 165). The highest indirect, systemic and diastolic brachial arterial pressures in the five patients ranged from 85 to 150 mm Hg (average 117) and the lowest from 35 to 85 mm Hg (average 64). Preoperative and postoperative systemic arterial pressures in the five patients are summarized in Figures 2 through 6. The cause of the systemic hypertension in patients #1 and #5 was renal disease—bilateral polycystic disease (each kidney weighed 400 g) in patient #1 and probably congenital hypoplasia (each kidney weighed 70 g) in patient #5; the cause was considered essential or idiopathic in patients #2, #3, and #4.

All five patients had precordial diastolic blowing murmurs typical of AR. By aortic root angiography, the degree of AR was either 3+ or 4+ on a 1+ to 4+ scale (Table II, Figures 7 and 8). Hemodynamic data in the five patients are summarized in Table II. The left ventricular end-diastolic pressure was above normal in only patient #5. None of the five patients had clinical or anatomic evidence of mitral valve dysfunction.

From the Pathology Branch, National Heart, Lung and Blood Institute, National Institutes of Health, Bethesda.

Address for reprints: Bruce F. Waller, MD, and William C. Roberts, MD, Pathology Branch, National Heart, Lung and Blood Institute, NIH, Bethesda, MD 20205.

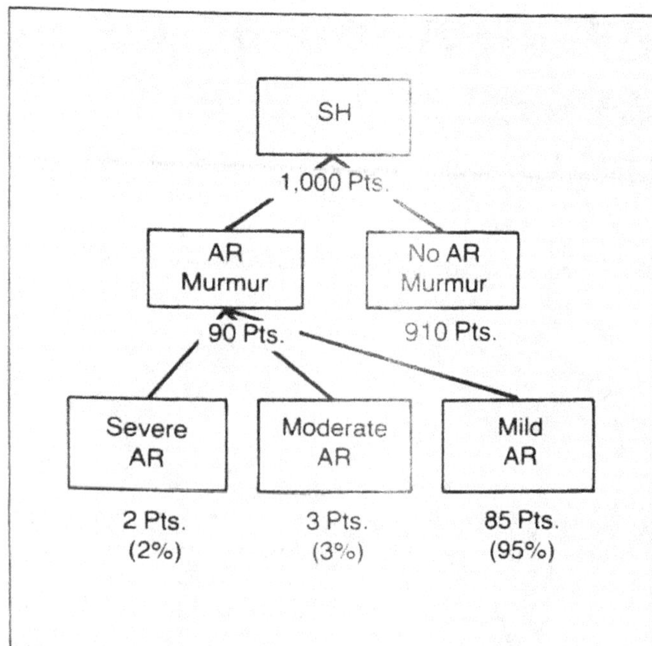

Figure 1. Frequency and severity of aortic regurgitation (AR) in patients (pts.) with systemic hypertension (SH) based on previously reported data.[1,4–9]

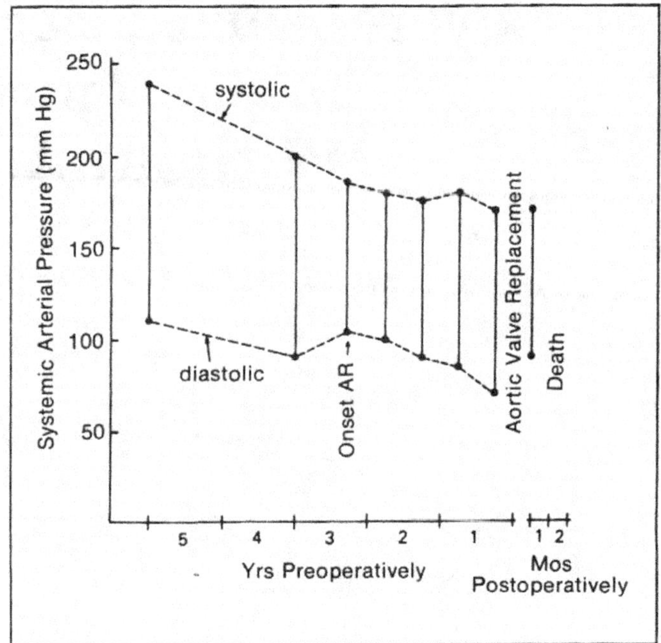

Figure 2. Patient #1. Indirect systolic and diastolic systemic arterial pressures before and shortly after aortic valve replacement.

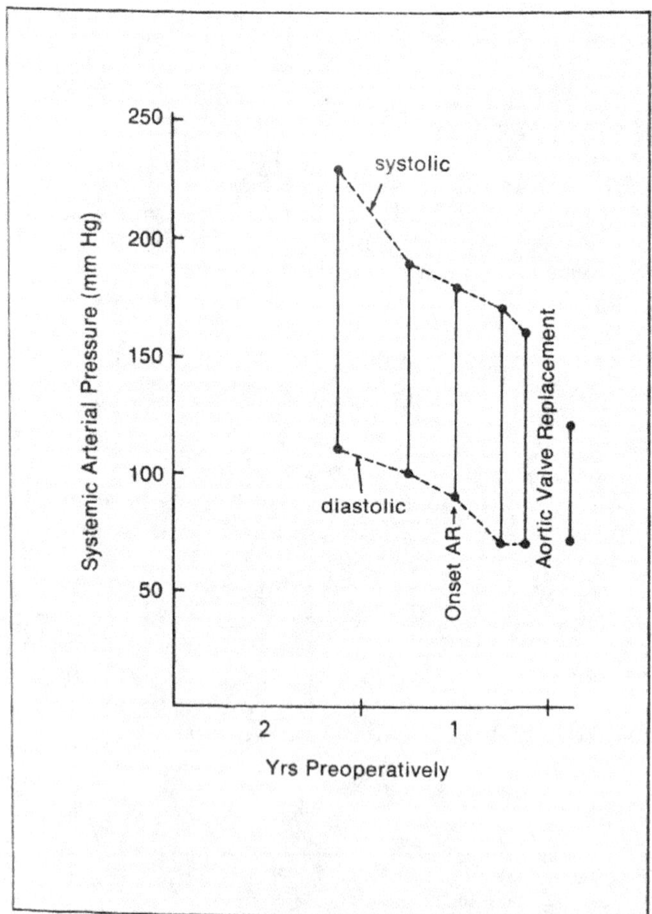

Figure 3. Patient #2. Indirect systolic and diastolic systemic arterial pressures before and shortly after aortic valve replacement.

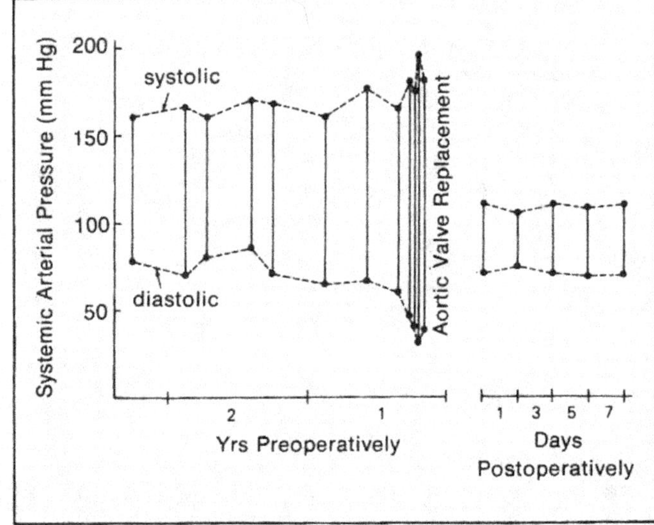

Figure 4. Patient #3. Indirect systolic and diastolic systemic arterial pressures before and shortly after aortic valve replacement.

Four patients had evidence of chronic congestive heart failure: in three for six months or less and in one for 24 months. Preoperatively, all five were considered to be in functional class (New York Heart Association) III or IV. The congestive heart failure progressed rapidly in patients #1, #2, and #5 and more slowly in patient #3. Patients #3, #4, and #5 had at least one episode of acute pulmonary edema. One patient (#4) had chest pain (typical angina pectoris).

TABLE I

**CLINICAL OBSERVATIONS IN 5 PATIENTS UNDERGOING AORTIC VALVE REPLACEMENT (AVR) FOR
PURE AR SECONDARY TO SYSTEMIC HYPERTENSION (SH) AND MORPHOLOGIC OBSERVATIONS
IN THREE NONSURVIVORS**

Observation	#1 (43 M)	#2 (48 M)	#3 (55 M)	#4 (56 F)	#5 (59 M)
Before Valve Replacement					
Duration (yrs) of SH	12	1	7	17	30
Duration (mos) of AR	24	6	36	72	10
Duration (mos) of CHF	6	2	24	0	4
Grade (1–6) murmur of AR	3	3	4†	3	4
Indirect systemic pressure	170–240 (193)	160–230 (188)	160–195 (182)	195–238 (220)	140–270 (176)
(s/d) (mm Hg) before AVR	70–120 (110)	70–110 (116)	35–85 (66)	85–118 (100)	60–150 (105)
Serum creatinine (mg/dl)	2.4‡	1.1	1.2	0.9	1.8
Blood-urea nitrogen (mg/dl)	28	17	23	22	38
Indirect systemic pressure	170/90	120/70	110/55	150/100	—
(s/d) (mm Hg) 1 mo after AVR					
Length of survival (mo) after AVR	1.5	12	11	84	0
Necropsy					
Heart weight (g)	595	—	—	530	810
Circumference of aortic sinotubular junction (cm)	11	—	—	8	11
LV wall fibrosis or necrosis	0	—§	—§	+	0
One or more major coronary arteries narrowed >75% in cross-sectional area	0	0	+**	+††	0

* By age (yrs) at AVR and sex.
† Diastolic thrill along left sternal border.
‡ Mean of three values.
§ By angiography, no left ventricular (LV) segmental wall-motion abnormalities were present.
** Right coronary artery was severely narrowed and an aortocoronary arterial bypass conduit was inserted.
†† Left main, left anterior descending, left circumflex, and right coronary arteries were severely narrowed, and two aortocoronary bypass
conduits were placed into the left anterior descending system.
CHF = congestive heart failure; s/d = systolic/diastolic (mm Hg).

TABLE II

**HEMODYNAMIC DATA IMMEDIATELY PREOPERATIVELY IN 5 PATIENTS UNDERGOING AORTIC VALVE
REPLACEMENT FOR PURE AR SECONDARY TO SYSTEMIC HYPERTENSION**

Measurement	#1 (43 M)	#2 (48 M)	#3 (55 M)	#4 (56 F)	#5 (59 M)
Right ventricle (s/d)	24/3	50/8	20/3	20/5	42/6
Pulmonary artery (PA) (s/d) (mean)	24/12 (16)	50/18 (38)	20/8 (12)	20/8 (12)	42/22 (29)
PA wedge (A:V:mean)	–:–:8	18:20:20	4:6:5	11:10:7	29:27:22
Left ventricle (s/d)	150/8	160/12	184/12	160/11	170/22
Aorta (s/d) (mean)	150/65 (110)	160/75 (—)	184/45 (118)	160/60 (105)	170/70 (115)
Amount AR (1+–4+) by angiography	3+	4+	4+	3+	4+
Cardiac index (L/min/m²)	4.4	2.1	3.2	1.6	2.8

* By age (yrs) at AVR and sex.
s/d = systolic/diastolic (mm Hg).

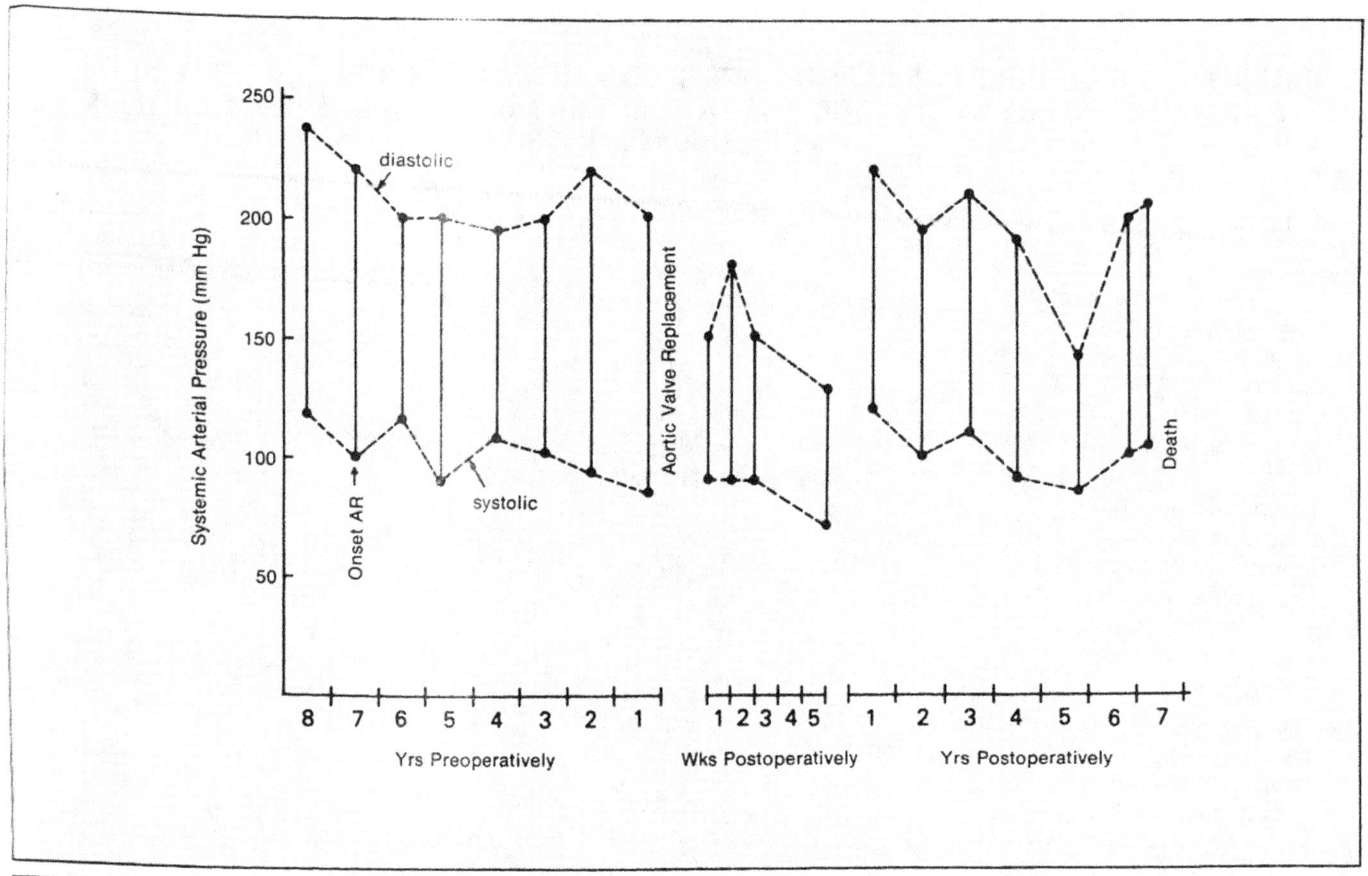

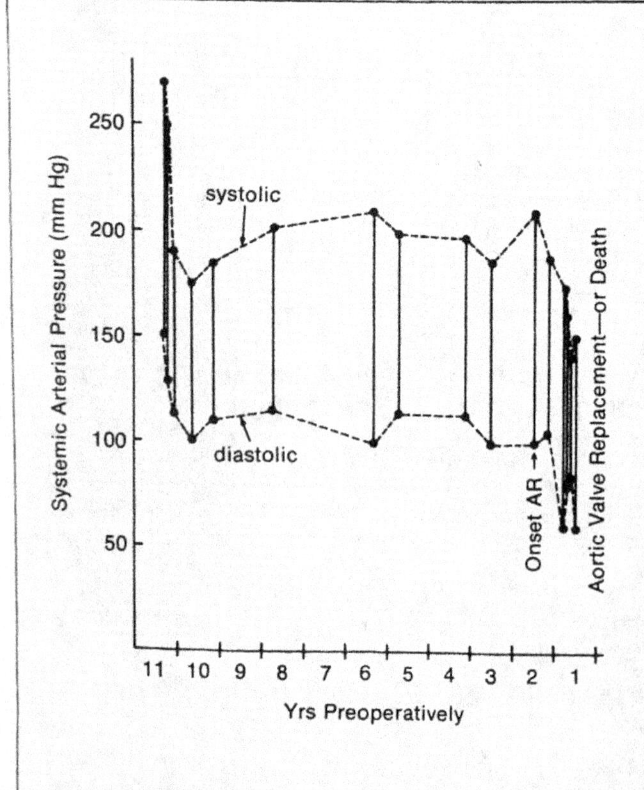

Figure 5. Patient #4. Indirect systolic and diastolic systemic arterial pressures years before and after aortic valve replacement.

Figure 6. Patient #5. Indirect systolic and diastolic systemic arterial pressures before aortic valve replacement.

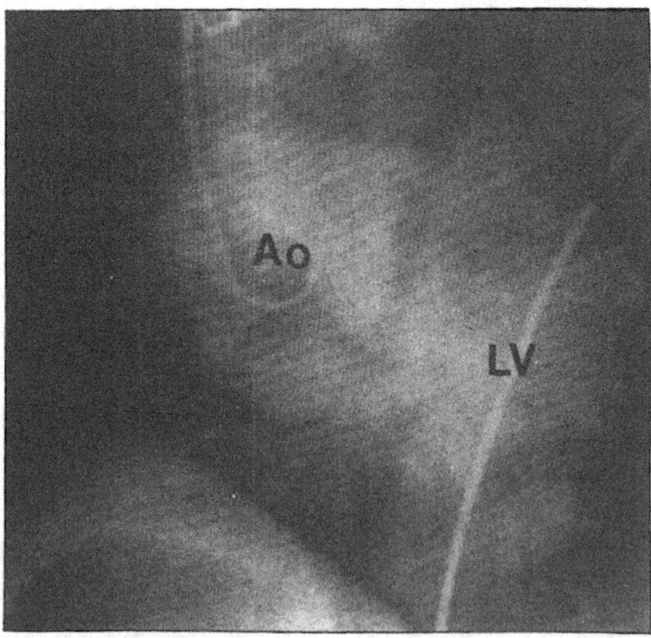

Figure 7. Patient #2. Frame of aortic "root" angiogram showing a dilated ascending aorta (Ao) and severe aortic regurgitation into the left ventricle (LV).

TABLE III
CERTAIN ELECTROCARDIOGRAPHIC FINDINGS PREOPERATIVELY IN 5 PATIENTS UNDERGOING AORTIC VALVE REPLACEMENT FOR PURE AR SECONDARY TO SYSTEMIC HYPERTENSION

Finding	Patients*				
	#1 (43 M)	#2 (48 M)	#3 (55 M)	#4 (56 F)	#5 (59 M)
Sinus rhythm (beats/min)	100	94	63	55	83
PR interval (sec)	0.18	0.14	0.16	0.18	0.18
QRS duration (sec)	0.12	0.08	0.08	0.08	0.08
QRS axis (degrees)	−45	+20	+20	+30	−20
Left atrial abnormality	0	+	+	±	±
Left ventricular hypertrophy	±	+	+	+	+
Strain pattern	+	+	+	±	+
Complete left bundle branch block	+	0	0	0	0

* By age (yrs) at AVR and sex.

TABLE IV
M-MODE ECHOCARDIOGRAPHIC MEASUREMENTS PREOPERATIVELY IN 5 PATIENTS UNDERGOING AORTIC VALVE REPLACEMENT FOR PURE AR SECONDARY TO SYSTEMIC HYPERTENSION

Measurement (mm)	Normal Subjects (av)	Patients*				
		#1 (43 M)	#2 (48 M)	#3 (55 M)	#4 (56 F)	#5 (59 M)
Ventricular septum						
End systole	—	30	24	20	24	25
End diastole	6−11 (9)	22	18	16	22	14
LV free wall						
End systole	—	26	22	21	27	24
End diastole	6−11 (9)	14	16	15	24	12
LV cavity						
End systole	—	60	59	46	22	38
End diastole	37−56 (47)	80	75	71	36	67
Left atrial cavity						
End systole	—	38	37	40	44	40
End diastole	19−40 (29)	35	34	32	40	35
Aorta						
End systole	—	47	48	46	44	49
End diastole	20−37 (27)	41	42	41	38	40

* By age (yrs) at AVR and sex.
LV = left ventricular.

Electrocardiographic and echocardiographic findings are summarized in Tables III and IV. The ascending aorta was dilated (Figures 7, 8, 10) by both echocardiography and angiography.

At operation, the aortic valve was tricuspid in all five cases. Each cusp was delicate, freely mobile, and free of calcific deposits; none of the three commissures was fused (Figure 11). The wall of the ascending aorta in all five patients was normal, and necropsy studies in patients #1, #4, and #5 also disclosed the wall to be normal, both grossly and histologically. In the three autopsied subjects (#1, #4, and #5) (Figure 12), the left ventricular walls were free of foci of fibrosis and necrosis in two (#1 and #5) but had a transmural scar in one patient (#4). Patient #1 died of aortic dissection 45 days after operation. The cause of the dissection was never established, but it involved the entire aorta

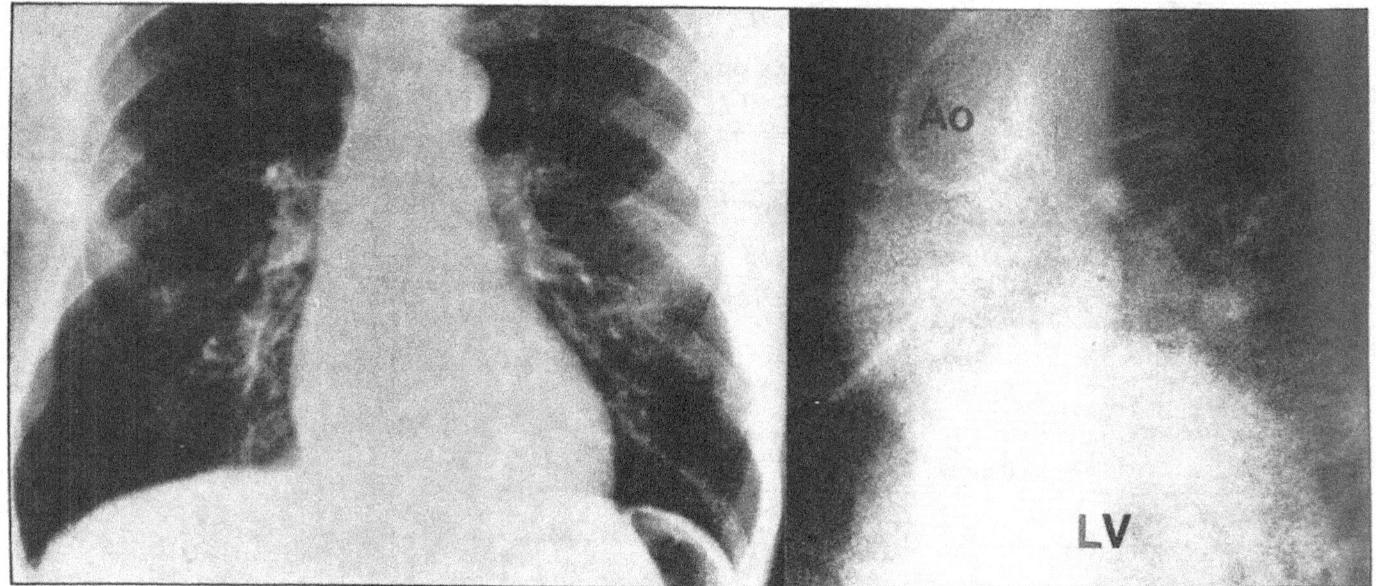

Figure 8. Patient #5. *Left:* Posteroanterior chest radiograph, which is normal. *Right:* Frame from aortic "root" (Ao) angiogram showing severe aortic regurgitation into the left ventricle (LV).

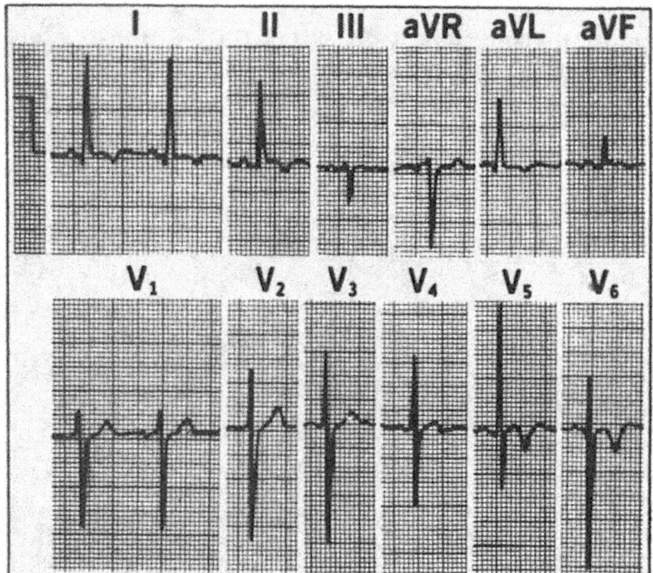

Figure 9. Patient #4. Electrocardiogram showing left ventricular hypertrophy with strain pattern.

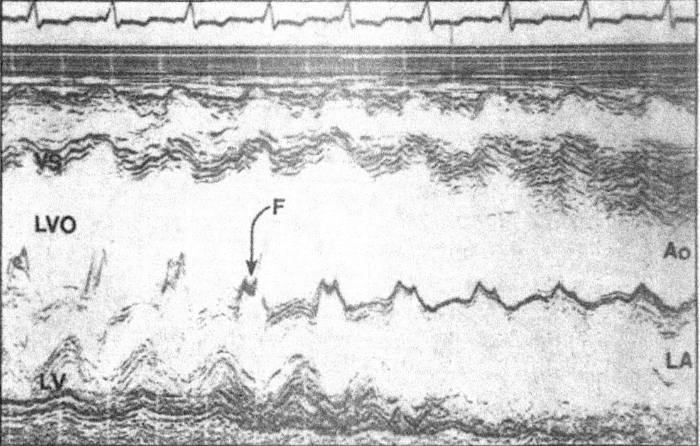

Figure 10. Patient #5. M-mode echocardiogram showing a sweep from left ventricular outflow (LVO) to aorta (Ao). The left ventricular cavity is dilated, and the mitral valve is fluttering (F). LA = left atrium; VS = ventricular septum.

from ascending portion to beyond the abdominal aortic bifurcation. Other than the dissection, which was acute, the wall of the aorta in patient #1 was normal. Patient #4 died from thrombus obstructing the tilting-disc prosthesis eight years after operation, and patient #5 died of excessive bleeding 36 hours after operation.

The major epicardial coronary arteries in patients #1, #2, and #5 examined preoperatively by selective angiography were free of significant narrowings. The right coronary artery in patient #3 and the left main, left anterior descending, left circumflex, and right coronary arteries in patient #4 were narrowed >75% in diameter. Aortocoronary

bypass conduits were inserted at the time of aortic valve replacement in both patients. In addition, necropsy disclosed severe narrowing of the major epicardial coronary arteries.

COMMENTS

Each of the five patients described had severe AR and severe systemic hypertension; four had chronic congestive heart failure. None had an explanation for the AR other than systemic hypertension, and the cause of chronic congestive heart failure appears to have been the severe AR. All five underwent aortic valve replacement: one died of exces-

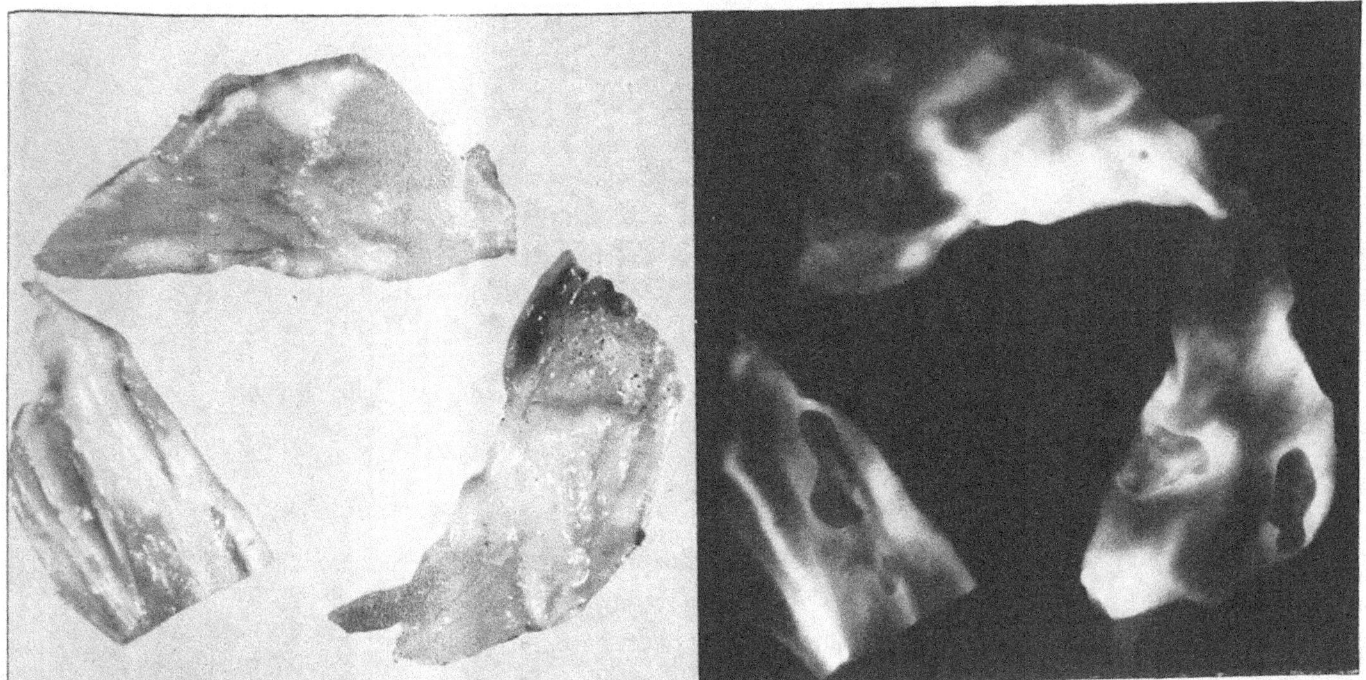

Figure 11. Patient #3. *Left:* Normal operatively excised aortic valve. *Right:* radiograph.

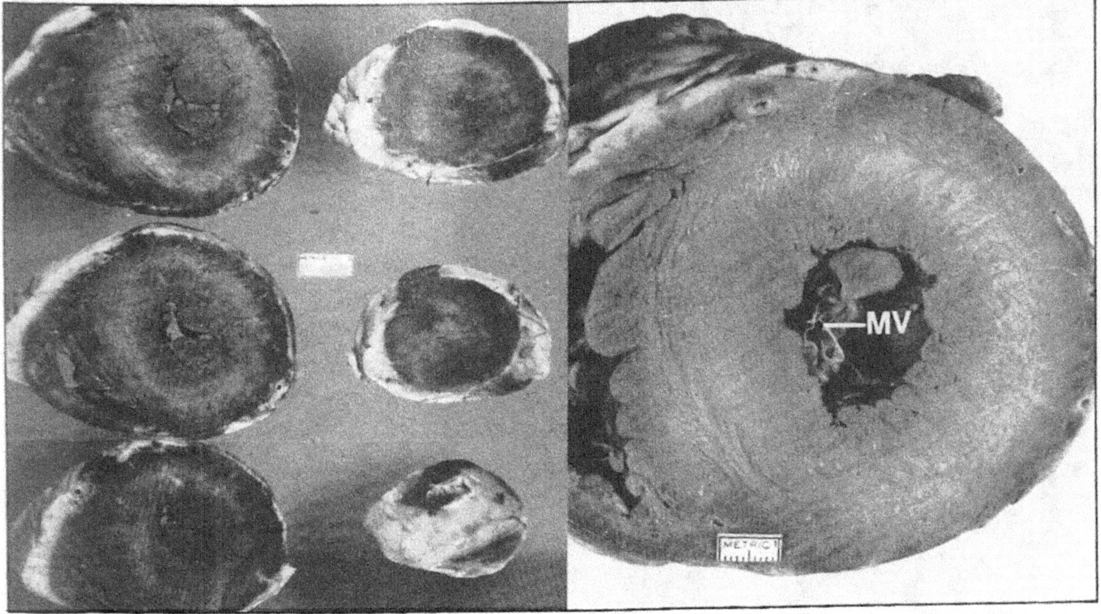

Figure 12. Patient #5. *Left:* Transverse sections of both cardiac ventricles from base to apex showing nondilated cavities and thickened ventricular walls. *Right:* Close-up of left ventricular basal portion showing a part of the mitral valve (MV).

sive bleeding soon after surgery; one of an aortic dissection 45 days postoperatively; and one from a thrombosed tilting-disc prosthesis eight years postoperatively. In the remaining two, evidence of congestive failure disappeared in the early postoperative period. The systemic arterial pressures remained elevated for about a month postoperatively in two of the three survivors. Until these five patients were encountered (they were all seen within an 18-month period), we had not observed a patient with severe AR stemming from systemic hypertension alone, and we are not aware of any report describing aortic valve replacement in such patients.

The frequency with which severe AR develops in patients with systemic hypertension is unclear. In Table V, we tabulated previous reports describing precordial murmurs consistent with AR in the presence of systemic hypertension. Of the 79 patients analyzed from these seven studies,[1,4-9] 17 patients (all from three studies reported in 1940, 1943, and 1950[4,5,7]) appear to have had severe AR. All 17

TABLE V

SUMMARY OF PREVIOUSLY REPORTED PATIENTS WITH SYSTEMIC HYPERTENSION AND PURE AR

Author (yr)	Garvin (1940)	Gouley (1943)	Hamman (1944)	Fenichel (1950)	Puchner (1960)	Barlow (1960)	Matalon (1971)	Total
No. of patients	9	8	1	16	27	9	9	79
Ages (yrs)	38–78 (59)	45–72(–)	54	59–75 (67)	— (54)	—	23–71 (–)	23–78 (59)
Men to women ratio	5:4	8:0	0:1	10:6	—	—	8:1	31:12
Systemic arterial pressure (s/d) (mm Hg) [range (av)]	$\frac{160-250\ (194)}{50-160\ (103)}$	$\frac{150-190\ (-)}{35-100}$	$\frac{220}{120}$	$\frac{150-240\ (203)}{60-120\ (107)}$	$\frac{180-260\ (216)}{110-160\ (131)}$	$\frac{>180(-)}{-}$	—	$\frac{150-260\ (204)}{35-160\ (114)}$
Pulse pressure (mm Hg) [range (av)]	60–120 (80)	85–128 (105)		60–170 (115)	40–130 (85)	—	—	40–130 (96)
No. of patients with severe AR	7	8	0	2	0	0	0	17
No. of patients with chronic congestive heart failure	9	8	0	8	0	0	9	34*
No. of deaths	9	8	1	4	0	3	4	29*
No. of autopsies confirming anatomically normal ascending aorta and aortic valve	9	8	1	0	0	3	4	25
Heart weight (g) [range (mean)]	450–700 (550)	400–700 (590)†		—	—	—	— (418)	400–700 (570)
Circumference of aortic "ring" (cm) [range (mean)]	7–10 (8.3)	8–12 (–)‡	9	—	—	↑	↑§	7–12 (8.3)

* Includes all 17 patients with severe aortic regurgitation.
† 4 patients.
‡ 6 patients.
§ 1 patient.

TABLE VI

CLINICAL AND AUTOPSY FINDINGS IN 7 PREVIOUSLY REPORTED PATIENTS WITH SEVERE AR AND CHRONIC AND EVENTUALLY FATAL CHF PRODUCED BY SEVERE SYSTEMIC HYPERTENSION

Author (yr)	Age (yrs)	Sex	Duration (mos) CHF	Indirect SAP (mm Hg) (s/d)	PP (mm Hg)	HW (g)	Normal AA and AV at Autopsy	C of Ao "Ring" (cm)	Dilated LV Cavity
Garvin	53	F	13	180/60	120	575	+	9	+
(1940)	41	F	12	220/100	122	525	+	7	—
	58	M	6	160/100	100	460	+	8	—
	78	M	8	190/70	120	625	+	9	+
	68	F	18	210/100	110	510	+	10	—
Gouley	70	M	"mos"	160/45	115	560	+	8	+
(1943)	66	M	10	225/80	145	700	+	12	0

AA = ascending aorta; Ao = aorta; AV = aortic valve; C = circumference; HW = heart weight; LV = left ventricular; PP = pulse pressure; s/d = systolic/diastolic; SAP = systemic arterial pressure; CHF = congestive heart failure. + = positive or present; 0 = negative or absent; — = no information available.

had evidence of congestive heart failure and all died. Of this subgroup, however, another definite, probable, or possible cause of the congestive heart failure other than AR appears to have been present in six patients. Of the remaining 11, information on necropsy was provided in seven cases (Table VI). Thus, these seven would appear to be similar to our four cases, although of course none of the seven had undergone aortic valve replacement or had received antihypertensive medications.

The mechanism by which severe AR develops in a few patients with systemic hypertension is unclear. The aorta was dilated in all five of our patients and in six of the seven autopsied subjects (Table VI). We presume that because dilatation of the aortic root causes stretching of the aortic valve cusps they fail to coapt during ventricular diastole resulting in a central leak, which is the cause of the AR. However, the aorta appears to dilate to a similar degree in many other patients without development of AR.

Although severe AR appears to be rare in patients with systemic hypertension, minimal and mild degrees of AR are common in hypertensive patients. Of 100 patients with systemic arterial systolic pressures >180 mm Hg reported by Barlow and Kincaid-Smith,[1] diastolic blowing murmurs consistent with AR were found in nine. Their report and those of others[4-9] have pointed out that among hypertensive persons, the higher the systemic arterial pressure, the greater the chance that AR will develop. Among patients with similar levels of systemic arterial pressure, *older patients* have a higher frequency of AR than do younger patients. Furthermore, of those of similar age and pressure, those with systemic hypertension of *longer duration* have a higher frequency of AR than do those of shorter duration. Of the few patients with severe AR from systemic hypertension, the systemic arterial diastolic pressure usually is >60 mm Hg; nevertheless, the pulse pressure is >100 mm Hg.

REFERENCES

1. Barlow J, Kincaid-Smith P: The auscultatory findings in hypertension. *Br Heart J* 1960; 22:505.

2. Waller BF, Zoltick JM, Rosen JH, et al: Severe aortic regurgitation from systemic hypertension (without aortic dissection) requiring aortic valve replacement: Analysis of 4 patients. *Am J Cardiol* 1982; 49:473.

3. Waller BF, Kishel JC, Roberts WC: Severe aortic regurgitation from systemic hypertension. *Chest* (in press).

4. Garvin CF: Functional aortic insufficiency. *Am J Med* 1940; 13:1799.

5. Gouley BA, Sickel EM: Aortic regurgitation caused by dilatation of the aortic orifice and associated with a characteristic valvular lesion. *Am Heart J* 1943; 26:24.

6. Hamman L: Diagnostic implications of aortic insufficiency. *Cincinnati J Med* 1944; 25:95.

7. Fenichel NM: Arteriosclerotic aortic insufficiency. *Am Heart J* 1950; 40:117.

8. Puchner TC, Huston JH, Hellmuth GA: Aortic valve insufficiency in arterial hypertension. *Am J Cardiol* 1960; 5:758.

9. Matalon R, Moussalli ARJ, Nidus BD, et al: Functional aortic insufficiency a feature of renal failure. *N Engl J Med* 1971; 285:1522.

Amounts of Coronary Arterial Narrowing by Atherosclerotic Plaques in Clinically Isolated, Chronic, Pure Aortic Regurgitation: Analysis of 37 Necropsy Patients Older than 30 Years

PAUL J. DAY,* BRUCE M. McMANUS, MD, PhD, and WILLIAM C. ROBERTS, MD

The degree of cross-sectional area (XSA) narrowing by atherosclerotic plaque in each of the 4 major epicardial coronary arteries (right, left main, left anterior descending and left circumflex) was determined at necropsy in 37 patients (30 men and 7 women) aged 34 to 77 years (mean 54) with severe, isolated, chronic, pure aortic regurgitation (AR). In 7 patients (19%), ≥ 1 major coronary artery was narrowed 76 to 100% in XSA at some point. Of the 148 major coronary arteries examined in the 37 patients, 12 arteries (8%) were narrowed at some point 76 to 100% in XSA. Each of the 148 major coronary arteries were divided into 5-mm-long segments (average 53 per patient) and a histologic section from each segment was examined. Of the 1,977 segments, 1,087 were narrowed 0 to 25%, 669 (34%) 26 to 50%, 170 (9%) 51 to 75%, 48 (2%) 76 to 95% and 3 (0.001%) 96 to 100%. The average amount of XSA narrowing by atherosclerotic plaque per segment was about 28%. Of the 37 patients, 9 had had angina pectoris, 2 of whom had significant (>75% XSA reduction) coronary narrowing; 2 other patients had had acute myocardial infarction clinically, 1 of whom had significant coronary narrowing at necropsy. Thus, in general, the amount of coronary narrowing in our 37 adults with severe, pure, isolated, chronic AR was relatively mild. (Am J Cardiol 1984;53:173–177)

In recent years a number of articles have focused on the frequency and extent of coronary arterial narrowing and of angina pectoris in patients with aortic valve stenosis. Surprisingly, relatively little angiographic and no necropsy information about the frequency of and extent of coronary narrowing has been reported in patients with pure aortic regurgitation (AR). In this report we describe the amounts of narrowing by atherosclerotic plaques observed at necropsy in the 4 major epicardial coronary arteries in 37 patients >30 years with clinically isolated, pure, severe AR.

Patients

Certain clinical and morphologic findings in the 37 patients are summarized in Table I. For inclusion in this study the patients had to fulfill the following criteria: (1) age >30 years

From the Pathology Branch, National Heart, Lung, and Blood Institute, National Institutes of Health, Bethesda, Maryland. Manuscript received and accepted September 30, 1983.

* Student, Saint Mary's College, Saint Mary's City, Maryland 20686.

Address for reprints: William C. Roberts MD, Building 10A, Room 3E-30, National Institutes of Health, Bethesda, Maryland 20205.

at death; (2) presence of AR by auscultation with the intensity of the basal diastolic blowing murmur grade ≥ 2 on a scale of 6; (3) absence of aortic valve stenosis as determined by left-sided cardiac catheterization (20 patients) and by morphologic examination of the aortic valve (at necropsy or the operatively excised valve) (all 37 patients); (4) absence of significant mitral valve dysfunction during life and presence of an anatomically normal mitral valve at necropsy; (5) presence of cardiomegaly at necropsy (heart weight >400 g); (6) absence of active infective endocarditis; (7) if aortic valve replacement had been performed (17 patients), the patient died within 60 days of the procedure; and (8) availability of the 4 major epicardial coronary arteries so that they could be examined in their entirety as discussed herein.

In the files of the Pathology Branch, National Heart, Lung, and Blood Institute, National Institutes of Health, 143 necropsy patients >20 years have been coded as having pure AR. Most of these cases were eliminated from the present study because of the presence of active infective endocarditis, the presence of only mild degrees of AR, age 30 years and younger or the unavailability of the heart specimen with intact epicardial coronary arteries.

In each of the 37 patients included in this study, the clinical records were examined, the heart was reexamined, and the 4 major (right, left main, left anterior descending and left cir-

TABLE I Clinical and Cardiac Morphologic Observations in the 37 Necropsy Patients with Severe Chronic Aortic Regurgitation

Pt	Cause of AR	Age (yr) & Sex	AP	Clinical AMI	Pressure (mm Hg) LV	Pressure (mm Hg) SA*	AR by Cine (1+ = 4+)	AVR[†]	HW (g)	LV F	No. of 4 Major CAs >75%	No. of 5-mm Segs	No. of 5-mm Segs Narrowed 0–25%	26–50%	51–75%	76–95%	96–100%	Score[‡] Total	Mean
1	Syphilis	37M	+	0	152/50	152/55	4+	0	600	0	0	52	20	23	9	0	0	93	1.8
2	Syphilis	44M	0	0	160/5	160.85	3+	0	850	+	0	47	23	19	5	0	0	76	1.6
3	Syphilis	53M	+	0	150/20	150/40	4+	+	575	0	0	54	22	32	0	0	0	86	1.6
4	Syphilis	55M	0	0	138/37	160/51	4+	+	940	0	3	61	0	18	31	11	0	176	2.9
5	Syphilis	64M	0	0	⋯	145/55	⋯	0	540	0	0	55	22	32	1	0	0	89	1.6
6	Syphilis	64M	0	0	⋯	150/60	⋯	0	600	+	0	56	28	28	0	0	0	84	1.5
7	Syphilis	65F	0	0	170/8	184/50	4+	+	710	0	1	48	6	30	11	1	0	103	2.1
8	Syphilis	69M	+	0	⋯	170/50	⋯	0	640	0	0	61	51	10	0	0	0	71	1.2
9	Syphilis	69F	0	0	⋯	200/90	⋯	0	650	0	0	46	38	8	0	0	0	54	1.2
10	Syphilis	72F	0	0	⋯	155/95	⋯	0	500	0	0	70	41	27	2	0	0	101	1.4
11	Syphilis	75M	0	0	⋯	150/80	⋯	0	630	0	0	45	33	11	1	0	0	58	1.3
12	Syphilis	77M	0	0	⋯	200/100	⋯	0	620	0	1	64	25	26	11	2	0	118	1.8
13	IE	39M	0	0	140/20	140/38	4+	0	1010	0	0	72	45	16	11	0	0	110	1.5
14	IE	40M	0	0	⋯	120/40	⋯	0	600	0	0	54	54	0	0	0	0	54	1.0
15	IE	44M	0	0	⋯	130/40	⋯	0	610	0	0	54	50	4	0	0	0	58	1.1
16	IE	45M	0	0	120/50	120/50	⋯	+	610	0	0	36	20	16	0	0	0	52	1.4
17	IE	47M	0	0	⋯	135/45	⋯	0	590	0	0	69	44	25	0	0	0	94	1.4
18	IE	50M	0	+[§]	⋯	170/60	⋯	+	980	+[§]	0	54	54	0	0	0	0	54	1.0
19	IE	52F	0	0	130/44	150/40	4+	+	500	0	0	54	54	0	0	0	0	54	1.0
20	IE	53M	0	0	⋯	145/45	⋯	+	690	0	0	54	13	41	0	0	0	95	1.8
21	IE	55F	0	0	⋯	150/40	⋯	0	520	0	0	60	34	21	5	0	0	91	1.5
22	Anky S	34M	0	0	100/22	120/25	4+	+	700	0	0	54	50	4	0	0	0	58	1.1
23	Anky S	37M	+	0	⋯	230/125[‖]	⋯	0	765	+	2	34	1	5	15	11	2	108	3.2
24	Anky S	38M	0	0	170/16	175/50	4+	+	1100	0	0	60	53	7	0	0	0	67	1.1
25	Anky S	52M	+	0	160/18	168/30	4+	+	850	0	0	44	24	19	1	0	0	65	1.5
26	Anky S	55M	0	0	114/40	124/38	4+	0	680	0	0	54	7	31	16	0	0	117	2.2
27	Anky S	57M	+	0	⋯	170/60	⋯	0	500	0	0	52	43	8	1	0	0	62	1.2
28	Marfan	41M	0	0	100/30	100/40	3+	+	750	0	0	58	36	20	2	0	0	82	1.4
29	Marfan	48F	0	0	150/12	150/40	3+	+	520	0	0	32	16	16	0	0	0	48	1.5
30	Marfan	62M	0	0	105/32	105/50	4+	+	856	0	0	53	29	24	0	0	0	77	1.5
31	Marfan	69M	0	+	110/40	110/60	3+	+	650	+	2	43	12	16	9	6	0	95	2.2
32	Uncertain	34M	0	0	105/–	122/–	4+	+	460	0	1	56	4	18	20	14	0	156	2.8
33	Uncertain	41M	+	0	88/19	96/20	4+	+	920	0	0	54	41	12	1	0	0	68	1.3
34	Uncertain	58M	0	0	⋯	155.45	⋯	0	640	0	0	59	11	46	2	0	0	109	1.8
35	Trauma	71M	+	0	130/30	130/60	4+	0	470	+	2	50	0	31	15	3	1	123	2.5
36	SH	71M	0	0	160/30	160/80	3+	0	845	0	0	54	38	16	0	0	0	70	1.3
37	Congenital	51F	+	0	⋯	210/80	⋯	+	550	0	0	54	45	9	0	0	0	63	1.2

* When a left ventricular pressure is recorded, the SA pressure is direct; when not, it is indirect.
[†] Performed within 60 days of death.
[‡] The score is derived by assigning a number to each 5-mm segment according to its degree of luminal narrowing by atherosclerotic plaque: 1 = 0–25% cross- sectional area narrowing; 2 = 26–50%; 3 = 51–75%; and 4 = 76–100%. The *total score* was obtained for each patient by adding up the numbers for all 5-mm segments. The *mean score* was calculated by dividing the total score per patient by the number of 5-mm segments examined from that patient.
[§] Probably embolic in origin (during active infective endocarditis).
[‖] Recorded 5 years before death.
AMI = acute myocardial infarction; Anky S = ankylosing spondylitis; AP = angina pectoris; AR = aortic regurgitation; AVR = aortic valve replacement; CAs = coronary arteries; F = transmural fibrosis; HW = heart weight; IE = healed infective endocarditis; LV = left ventricle; SA = systemic artery; Segs = segments; SH = systemic hypertension.

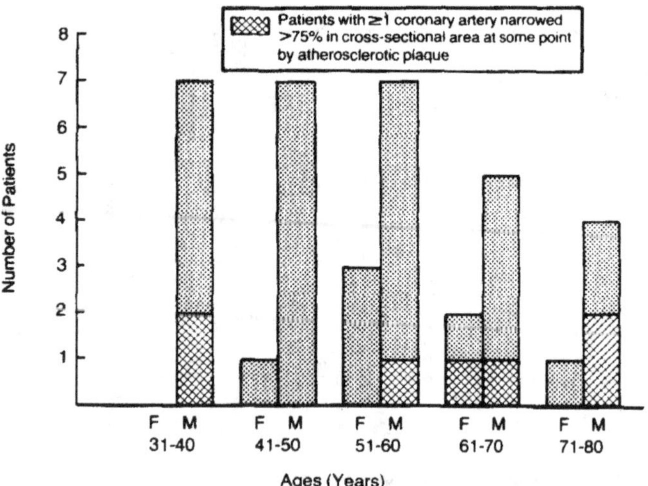

FIGURE 1. Number of necropsy patients by age decade and sex with severe pure aortic regurgitation in whom ≥ 1 major epicardial coronary artery (right, left main, left anterior descending and left circumflex) was narrowed 76 to 100% in cross-sectional area at some point by atherosclerotic plaques.

cumflex) epicardial coronary arteries were excised intact from the heart, decalcified if necessary, divided into 5-mm-long segments, cut transversely to the long axis of the artery, labeled sequentially from the origin of the artery from either the aorta or left main coronary artery, processed in alcohols and xylene, embedded in paraffin, cut 6 μ thick, and at least 1 histologic section from each 5-mm segment was stained by the Movat method[1] and examined. The degree of cross-sectional area (XSA) narrowing by atherosclerotic plaques was determined by examining the Movat-stained sections, which clearly delineate the internal elastic membrane. The amount of XSA luminal narrowing was determined by magnifying each cross section of coronary artery approximately 40 times via microscopy and estimating the degrees of luminal obliteration by dividing visually the XSA of the coronary artery into 4 quadrants, each comprising 25% of the total XSA luminal area. The degrees of XSA narrowing were categorized initially into 4 groups: 0 to 25, 26 to 50, 51 to 75 and 76 to 100%. Any section narrowed >75% was further classified into a group with narrowing 76 to 95% or into a group with narrowing 96 to 100%. Both the inter- and intraobserver error by this technique are <5%.[2]

Of the 37 patients, the cause of the AR was cardiovascular syphilis[3] in 12, infective endocarditis that healed[4] in 9, ankylosing spondylitis[5] in 6, the Marfan syndrome[6] (2 patients) or the Marfan cardiovascular disease without the skeletal features[7] (2 patients) in 4, undetermined in 3, and trauma,[3] systemic hypertension[8,9] and congenital (quadricuspid aortic valve) in 1 each, respectively. The 37 patients ranged in age from 34 to 77 years (mean 54) (Fig. 1); 30 (81%) were men and 7 (19%) were women. Ischemic-type chest pain occurred in 11 patients (30%): angina pectoris in 9 (24%) and clinical features diagnostic of acute myocardial infarction in 2 (5%). Of the 37 patients, 20 (54%) had left-sided cardiac catheterization, including aortic "root" angiography in 19 and selective coronary angiography in 5. The left ventricular (LV) peak systolic pressures ranged from 88 to 170 mm Hg (average 135) and the direct systemic arterial pressures from 96 to 184 mm Hg (average 140); the LV end-diastolic pressures ranged from 5 to 50 mm Hg (average 26) and the direct systemic arterial end-

diastolic pressures from 20 to 85 mm Hg (average 48). The degree of AR by cineangiography was graded 3+ or 4+ on a scale of 1 to 4+ in all 19 patients.

The cause of death in the 37 patients was variable: 17 (46%) died of complications of aortic valve replacement performed within 60 days of death; 13 (35%) died from chronic congestive heart failure secondary to the severe AR; 3 (8%) (Patients 11, 12 and 27) from cancer; 1 (3%) (Patient 9) from stroke; 1 (3%) (Patient 23) from associated severe coronary atherosclerosis; 1 (3%) (Patient 5) from chronic renal disease requiring chronic dialysis; and 1 (2%) (Patient 17) from an accident (kicked in the head by a horse). Thus, although all 37 patients had clinical evidence of severe AR, 30 (81%) died directly from consequences of the severe AR.

At necropsy, the hearts in the 30 men weighed 460 to 1100 g (mean 727) (normal ≤400 g); only 5 men (17%) had hearts that weighed <600 g. The hearts in the 7 women weighed 500 to 750 g (mean 564; normal weight ≤350 g); 5 of the 7 had hearts that weighed <600 g.

A grossly visible transmural LV scar (healed myocardial infarction) was found in 6 patients (16%), and none had scars limited to the LV subendocardium (inner half of the myocardial wall). Of the 6 patients, only 2 had a clinical event compatible with acute myocardial infarction, and in 1 of them (Patient 18) (Table I) the infarct occurred during active infective endocarditis and was most likely embolic in origin[10]; 2 others with LV scars had angina pectoris. Of the 6 patients with LV scars, 3 had significant and 3 had insignificant coronary narrowing at necropsy.

Results

Of the 37 patients, 7 (19%) had ≥1 of their 4 major epicardial coronary arteries narrowed >75% in XSA by atherosclerotic plaques (Fig. 1): in 3 patients, 1 of the 4 arteries was so narrowed; in 3 patients, 2 such arteries, and in 1 patient, 3 such arteries. In all 37 patients, the left main coronary artery was narrowed ≤50% in XSA. Of the 148 major epicardial coronary arteries examined in the 37 patients, 12 (8%) were narrowed at some point >75% in XSA by atherosclerotic plaque.

A total of 1,977 of the 5-mm segments of the 148 major coronary arteries were examined in the 37 patients. Of these, 1,087 segments (55%) were narrowed 0 to 25% in XSA by atherosclerotic plaque, 669 (34%) were narrowed 26 to 50%, 170 (9%) 51 to 75%; 48 (2%) 76 to 95%, and 3 (0.001%) 96 to 100%. The amount of narrowing by the patients' sex and age decade is summarized in Figure 2. Of the 7 patients in whom ≥1 major coronary artery was narrowed at some point >75% in XSA, 356 of the 5-mm segments of coronary artery were examined. Of these, 48 (13%) segments were narrowed 0 to 25%, 144 (41%) 26 to 50%, 113 (32%) 51 to 75%; 48 (13%) 76 to 95%, and 3 (1%) 96 to 100%. Of the 30 patients in whom none of the 4 major coronary arteries was narrowed >75%, 1,621 of the 5-mm segments were examined: 1,039 (64%) were narrowed 0 to 25%, 525 segments (32%) 26 to 50% and 57 (4%) 51 to 75%.

A scoring system was used to indicate the severity and extent of coronary arterial narrowing. Every 5-mm segment of coronary artery from each patient was assigned a score of 1 to 4, based on the amount of XSA narrowing by atherosclerotic plaque: 1 = 0 to 25% narrowing; 2 = 26 to 50%; 3 = 51 to 75%, and 4 = 76 to 100%. A total score was determined for each patient and the

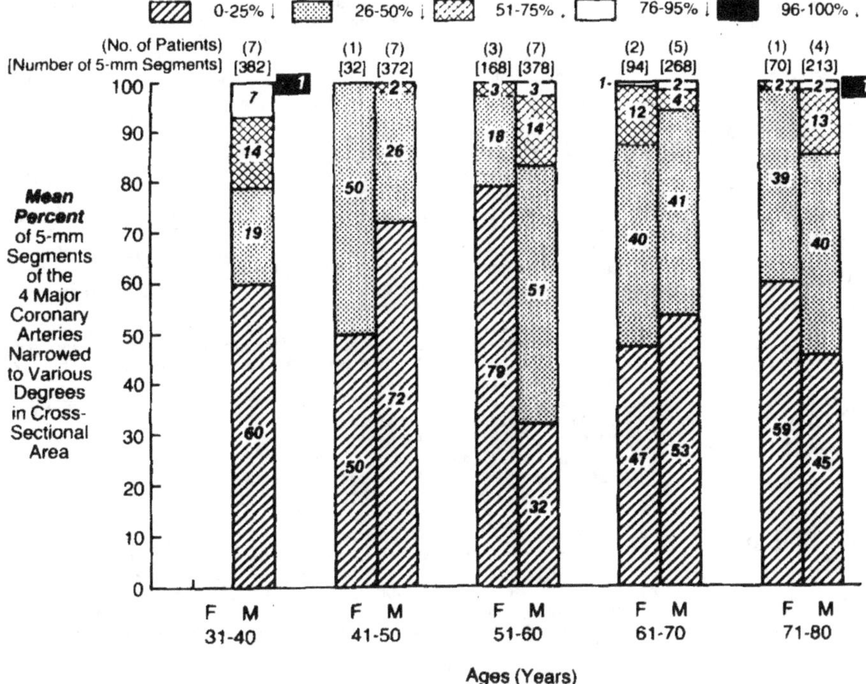

FIGURE 2. Number and percent of 1,977 five-millimeter segments of the 4 major epicardial coronary arteries narrowed to various degrees by atherosclerotic plaques in 37 patients (30 men, 7 women) aged 34 to 77 years with severe pure aortic regurgitation.

score per segment was then calculated by dividing the total score per patient by the number of segments examined from that patient. Of the 2,139 segments examined from the 37 patients, the total score was 3,352 and the mean score 1.6, indicating that the amount of XSA narrowing for each of the 2,139 segments was approximately 28%.

Of the 7 patients in whom ≥1 major coronary artery was narrowed 76 to 100% in XSA by atherosclerotic plaque, 2 had had angina pectoris, 1 had had a clinical event characteristic of acute myocardial infarction, and 3 had grossly visible LV scars, transmural in each; the mean score for the group of 7 patients was 2.1, indicating that each 5-mm segment from these patients was narrowed approximately 42%. In contrast, of the 30 patients with insignificant (≤75% reduction in XSA) coronary narrowing, 7 (23%) had had angina pectoris, 1 (3%) had had a clinical event diagnosed as acute myocardial infarction (probably embolic in origin), and 3 (10%) had grossly visible LV scars. The mean score for the 30 patients was 104, indicating that each 5-mm coronary segment in these patients was narrowed approximately 23%, or just over half that of the other group.

Thus, of the 9 patients considered to have angina pectoris, 2 had significant and 7 had insignificant coronary narrowing. Of the 2 patients with acute myocardial infarction clinically, 1 had significant coronary narrowing at necropsy and the other patient did not. The latter patient (Patient 18) had an acute myocardial infarction during active infective endocarditis, and therefore, the cause of the infarct likely was an embolus that subsequently lysed or organized, and at necropsy the narrowing was insignificant.[11]

Coronary angiography had been performed during life in 5 patients, 3 (Patients 7, 31 and 35) of whom had significant (>50% diameter reduction) and 2 (Patients 2 and 36) of whom had insignificant coronary narrowing.

Discussion

This study demonstrates that 7 (19%) of our 37 patients >30 years old with severe, chronic, pure isolated AR had narrowing >75% in XSA of ≥1 of the 4 major epicardial coronary arteries by atherosclerotic plaque. The extent of the severe (>75% XSA) coronary narrowing in these 7 patients, however, was relatively mild compared with the extent of severe narrowing observed in necropsy patients with fatal coronary heart disease unassociated with aortic valve dysfunction.[12–25] Of the 7 patients with AR and significant coronary narrowing, 14% of the 5-mm-long segments of the 4 major coronary arteries (average of 53 segments per patient) were narrowed >75%, whereas in patients with fatal symptomatic coronary heart disease unassociated with AR or aortic valve stenosis, an average of 33% of the coronary segments are narrowed >75%.[12–25]

The frequency of angina pectoris did not appear to be different in the 7 patients with compared to the 30 patients without significant coronary narrowing; angina was present in 2 of the 7 with and in 7 of the 30 without significant narrowing. Furthermore, the frequency of clinical acute myocardial infarction and LV scars was similar in the 7 patients with and in the 30 patients without significant coronary narrowing.

No previous study has examined the status of the epicardial coronary arteries in necropsy patients with pure AR, and indeed coronary angiographic data focusing exclusively on patients with pure AR is virtually nonexistent. Several reports,[26–33] however, have described coronary angiographic features of patients with aortic valve disease, and a number of them included findings in patients with severe AR. Of 20 patients (mean age 40 years, 10 with angina) with severe AR and peak gradients <30 mm Hg described by Basta et al,[26] 3 (10%) had significant (>50% diameter reduction) coronary narrowing (1 vessel in each) by angiography. Of 30 patients with "predominant" AR studied by Lacy et al,[27] 9 (30%) had significant coronary narrowing (1 vessel in 5) by angiography. Of 29 patients (mean age 49 years, 18 with angina) with severe AR (3+ or 4+/4+ AR by aortic angiography and <10 mm Hg peak pressure gradient) studied by Grayboys and Cohn,[28] 5 (17%) had significant coronary narrowing. Of 17 patients (mean age 42 years) with severe AR (peak pressure gradients <20 mm Hg) reported by Clark et al,[30] 3 (18%) had significant coronary narrowing (1 vessel in 1). Of 31 patients (mean age 55 years) with severe AR (pressure gradients <10 mm Hg) reported by Hakki et al,[31] 11 (35%) had significant coronary narrowing (1 vessel in 4). Of 17 patients with severe AR (pressure gradients <30 mm Hg) reported by Saltups,[32] 5 (29%) had significant coronary narrowing (1 vessel in 1). Of the 11 patients (mean age 48 years) with pure AR reported by Pichard and associates,[33] none had significant coronary narrowing by angiography.

References

1. **Movat HZ.** Demonstration of all connective tissue elements in a single section: pentachrome stains. Arch Pathol 1955;60:289–295.
2. **Isner JM, Wu M, Virmani R, Jones AA, Roberts WC.** Comparison of degrees of luminal narrowing determined by visual inspection of histologic sections under magnification among three independent observers and comparison to that obtained by video planimetry. An analysis of 559 five-millimeter segments of 61 coronary arteries from eleven patients. Lab Invest 1980; 42:566–570.
3. **Roberts WC, Dangel JC, Bulkley BH.** Non-rheumatic valvular cardiac disease: a clinicopathologic survey of 27 different conditions causing valvular dysfunction. Cardiovasc Clinics 1973;5:333–446.
4. **Roberts WC, Buchbinder NA.** Healed left-sided infective endocarditis: a clinicopathologic study of 59 patients. Am J Cardiol 1977;40:876–888.
5. **Bulkley BH, Roberts WC.** Ankylosing spondylitis and aortic regurgitation. Description of the characteristic cardiovascular lesion from study of eight necropsy patients. Circulation 1973;48:1014–1027.
6. **Roberts WC, Honig HS.** The spectrum of cardiovascular disease in the Marfan syndrome: a clinico-morphologic study of 18 necropsy patients and comparison to 151 previously reported necropsy patients. Am Heart J 1982;104:115–135.
7. **Waller BF, Reis RL, McIntosh CL, Epstein SE, Roberts WC.** The Marfan cardiovascular disease without the Marfan syndrome. Chest 1980;77: 533–540.
8. **Waller BF, Zoltick, JM, Rosen JH, Katz NM, Gomes MN, Fletcher RD, Wallace RB, Roberts WC.** Severe aortic regurgitation from systemic hypertension (without aortic dissection) requiring aortic valve replacement. Analysis of four patients. Am J Cardiol 1982;49:473–477.
9. **Waller BF, Roberts WC.** Severe aortic regurgitation secondary to systemic hypertension (without aortic dissection). Cardiovasc Rev Rep 1982;3: 1504–1518.
10. **Roberts WC.** Coronary embolism: a review of causes, consequences, and diagnostic considerations. Cardiovasc Med 1978;3:699–710.
11. **Arnett EN, Roberts WC.** Acute myocardial infarction and angiographically normal coronary arteries. An unproven combination. Circulation 1976; 53:395–400.
12. **Roberts WC, Jones AA.** Quantitation of coronary arterial narrowing at necropsy in sudden coronary death. Analysis of 31 patients and comparison with 25 control subjects. Am J Cardiol 1979;44:39–45.
13. **Roberts WC, Virmani R.** Quantification of coronary arterial narrowing in clinically-isolated unstable angina pectoris. An analysis of 22 necropsy patients. Am J Med 1979;67:792–799.
14. **Roberts WC, Jones AA.** Quantification of coronary arterial narrowing at necropsy in acute transmural myocardial infarction: analysis and comparison of findings in 27 patients and 22 controls. Circulation 1980;61:786–790.
15. **Virmani R, Roberts WC.** Quantification of coronary arterial narrowing and of left ventricular myocardial scarring in healed myocardial infarction with chronic eventually fatal, congestive cardiac failure. Am J Med 1980;68: 831–838.
16. **Cabin HS, Roberts WC.** True left ventricular aneurysm and healed myocardial infarction. Clinical and necropsy observations including quantification of degrees of coronary arterial narrowing. Am J Cardiol 1980;46:754–763.
17. **Waller BF, Roberts WC.** Amount of narrowing by atherosclerotic plaque in 44 nonbypassed and 52 bypassed major epicardial coronary arteries in 32 necropsy patients who died within 1 month of aortocoronary bypass grafting. Am J Cardiol 1980;46:956–962.
18. **Virmani R, Roberts WC.** Non-fatal healed transmural myocardial infarction and fatal non-cardiac disease. Qualification and quantification of coronary arterial narrowing and of left ventricular scarring in 18 necropsy patients. Br Heart J 1981;45:434–441.
19. **Cabin HS, Roberts WC.** Fatal cardiac arrest during cardiac catheterization for angina pectoris: analysis of 10 necropsy patients. Am J Cardiol 1981; 48:1–8.
20. **Brosius FC III, Roberts WC.** Comparison of degree and extent of coronary narrowing by atherosclerotic plaque in anterior and posterior transmural acute myocardial infarction. Circulation 1981;64:715–722.
21. **Cabin HS, Roberts WC.** Comparison of amount and extent of coronary narrowing by atherosclerotic plaque and of myocardial scarring at necropsy in anterior and posterior healed transmural myocardial infarction. Circulation 1982;66:93–99.
22. **Cabin HC, Roberts WC.** Relations of healed transmural myocardial infarct size to length of survival after acute myocardial infarction, age at death, and amount and extent of coronary arterial narrowing by atherosclerotic plaques: analysis of 70 necropsy patients. Am Heart J 1982;104:216–220.
23. **Cabin HS, Roberts WC.** Relation of serum cholesterol and triglyceride levels to the amount and extent of coronary arterial narrowing by atherosclerotic plaque in coronary heart disease. Quantification analysis of 2,037 five mm segments of 160 major epicardial coronary arteries in 40 necropsy patients. Am J Med 1982;73:227–234.
24. **Cabin HS, Roberts WC.** Quantitative comparison of extent of coronary narrowing and size of healed myocardial infarct in 33 necropsy patients with clinically recognized and in 28 with clinically unrecognized ("silent") previous acute myocardial infarction. Am J Cardiol 1982;50:677–681.
25. **Virmani R, Roberts WC.** Extravasated erythrocytes, iron, and fibrin in atherosclerotic plaques of coronary arteries in fatal coronary heart disease and their relation to luminal thrombus: frequency and significance in 57 necropsy patients and in 2958 five mm segments of 224 major epicardial coronary arteries. Am Heart J 1983;105:788–797.
26. **Basta LL, Raines D, Najjar S, Kioschos JM.** Clinical, haemodynamic, and coronary angiographic correlates of angina pectoris in patients with severe aortic valve disease. Br Heart J 1975;37:150–157.
27. **Lacy J, Goodin R, McMartin D, Masden R, Flowers N.** Coronary atherosclerosis in valvular heart disease. Annals Thorac Surg 1977;23:429–435.
28. **Graboys TB, Cohn PF.** The prevalence of angina pectoris and abnormal coronary arteriograms in severe aortic valvular disease. Am Heart J 1977;93:683–686.
29. **Storstein O, Enge I.** Angina pectoris in aortic valvular disease and its relation to coronary pathology. Acta Med Scand 1979;205:275–278.
30. **Clark DG, McAnulty JH, Rahimtoola SH.** Valve replacement in aortic insufficiency with left ventricular dysfunction. Circulation 1980;61:411–421.
31. **Hakki A-H, Kimbiris D, Iskandrian AS, Segal BL, Mintz GS, Bemis CE.** Angina pectoris and coronary artery disease in patients with severe aortic valvular disease. Am Heart J 1980;100:441–448.
32. **Saltups A.** Coronary arteriography in isolated aortic and mitral valve disease. Aust NZ J Med 1982;12:494–497.
33. **Pichard AD, Smith H, Holt J, Meller J, Gorlin R.** Coronary vascular reserve in left ventricular hypertrophy secondary to chronic aortic regurgitation. Am J Cardiol 1983;51:315–320.

Electrocardiographic Observations in Clinically Isolated, Pure, Chronic, Severe Aortic Regurgitation: Analysis of 30 Necropsy Patients Aged 19 to 65 Years

WILLIAM C. ROBERTS, MD, and PAUL J. DAY*

Certain electrocardiographic findings are described in 30 necropsy patients with clinically isolated pure, chronic, severe aortic regurgitation. They were 19 to 65 years old (mean 45). The hearts of the 22 men ranged in weight from 430 to 1,110 g (mean 717) and of the 8 women, from 375 to 950 g (mean 638). Four had grossly visible left ventricular (LV) scars. All but 1 patient was in sinus rhythm. The PR interval was >0.20 second in 8 patients (28%) and the QRS duration was ≥0.12 second in 6 patients (20%). Only 5 patients (17%) had 1 or more ventricular premature complexes recorded on the resting electrocardiogram analyzed. The mean QRS amplitude for each of the 12 leads averaged 23 mm. The highest mean QRS voltage occurred in leads V_2 and V_3 (each 38 mm), and the lowest in lead aVR (11 mm). The mean QRS voltage in V_5 was higher than in V_6 (33 vs 28 mm) and in 22 patients (73%) the QRS voltage in V_5 was higher than in V_6. The sum of the S wave in V_1 plus the larger of the R wave in V_5 or V_6 (Sokolow-Lyon index) averaged 51 mm and in only 22 patients (73%) was it >35 mm. The Romhilt-Estes voltage criteria for LV hypertrophy was fulfilled even less frequently, despite the severe degrees of LV hypertrophy in the patients studied. The total 12-lead QRS amplitude in the 30 patients ranged from 109 to 428 mm (mean 272) (10 mm = 1 mV) and in 27 patients (90%) it was >175 mm. The ratio of total 12-lead QRS voltage to heart weight in the 30 patients with aortic regurgitation was 0.42, only slightly higher than that in previously studied adults with severe aortic stenosis (0.39), an observation indicating that cavity dilatation does not magnify the QRS voltage generated by a given mass of myocardium.

(Am J Cardiol 1985;55:431–438)

Although many studies are available on electrocardiographic findings in patients with aortic valve stenosis, few studies have described electrocardiographic findings in patients with chronic aortic regurgitation (AR). Electrocardiographic QRS voltage observations[1-7] in patients with chronic AR usually have been limited to analysis of the presence of left ventricular (LV) hypertrophy as determined by criteria proposed by Sokolow and Lyon[8] or Romhilt and Estes.[9] No studies of patients with fatal, pure, isolated AR have compared electrocardiographic findings during life to necropsy cardiac findings. Such a correlation is the purpose of this report. The amplitude of the QRS complexes in all 12 leads, in addition to that of certain R and S waves, was measured in all patients.

Definitions

The terms describing AR in the patients were defined as follows: *Clinically isolated*—valvular dysfunction limited to the aortic valve. Function of the mitral, tricuspid and pulmonic valves was normal. *Pure*—no peak systolic pressure gradient present between left ventricle and systemic artery. *Chronic*—evidence of severe AR for more than 6 months.

Severe—AR graded 3+ or 4+/4+ by aortic root angiogram or symptoms of cardiac functional class III or IV (New York Heart Association criteria) and the symptoms attributable only to AR.

Patients

Inclusion criteria for this study were (1) presence of chronic, isolated, pure, severe AR; (2) age at death older than 15 years; (3) interval between aortic valve replacement and death within 2 months; (4) availability of 12-lead electrocardiogram (ECG) recorded either preoperatively or within 1 month of death; and (5) heart weight >350 g in women and >400 g in men. The ECG analyzed was always that obtained just before aortic valve replacement (19 patients) or in the patients who did not undergo aortic valve operation,[10] the one recorded in the last month of life. The amplitude of the QRS complexes was measured from the peak of the R wave to the maximal dip of the S or Q wave, whichever was greater (Fig. 1). The cardiac catheterization data were obtained just before aortic valve replacement (16 patients) or within 6 months of death in the patients who did not undergo aortic valve operation (6 patients).

Thirty patients fulfilled the inclusion criteria. Certain clinical and morphologic findings for these patients are summarized in Table I. In all 30 patients the clinical records were examined, the heart in each was examined initially and the hearts in 25 patients were reexamined. The amounts of coronary arterial narrowing present was determined by examination of 5-mm transverse sections of the 4 major coronary arteries by a method delineated elsewhere.[11] Of the 30 patients, the cause of the AR was infective endocarditis that had healed in 8,[10] cardiovascular syphilis in 6,[12] ankylosing spondylitis in 5,[13] Marfan's syndrome in 5,[14] uncertain cause

From the Pathology Branch, National Heart, Lung, and Blood Institute, National Institutes of Health, Bethesda, Maryland. Manuscript received September 12, 1984, accepted October 2, 1984.

* Student, Saint Mary's College, Saint Mary's City, Maryland 20686.

Address for reprints: William C. Roberts, MD, Building 10A, Room 3E-30, National Institutes of Health, Bethesda, Maryland 20205.

in 4, trauma in 1[15] and systemic hypertension in 1.[16] The patients were 19 to 65 years old (mean 45); 22 (73%) were men and 8 (27%) were women. Of the 30 patients, 29 had evidence of congestive heart failure (New York Heart Association functional class III or IV); patient 2 (Table I) was asymptomatic but had aortic valve replacement because of a LV end-systolic dimension >55 mm by echocardiogram. Of the 30 patients, 22 had left-sided cardiac catheterization and aortic root angiograms. LV peak systolic pressures ranged from 88 to 190 mm Hg (mean 133), LV end-diastolic pressures from 8 to 80 mm Hg (mean 32) and systemic arterial end-diastolic pressures from 20 to 65 mm Hg (mean 42). Nineteen patients died of complications of aortic valve replacement; the other 11 died from chronic congestive heart failure secondary to the AR.

At necropsy, the hearts in the 22 men weighed 430 to 1,100 g (mean 717) (normal ≤400 g) and the hearts in the 8 women weighed 375 to 950 g (mean 638) (normal ≤350 g). These weights were total heart weights, not just LV weights. A grossly visible, transmural (involving all the inner half and a portion or all of the outer half of the wall) LV scar (healed myocardial infarct) was present in 4 patients, but none during life had a clinical event diagnosed as, or compatible with, acute myocardial infarction.

The comparison of means was done using an unpaired Student t test, the comparison of ratios was done using a chi-square test, and the correlation coefficients were calculated using a Pearson's product moment test. Significance was judged if the test yielded a p valve <0.05.

Results

General electrocardiographic observations: Electrocardiographic findings are summarized in Tables I and II. The total 12-lead QRS amplitude in the 30 patients ranged from 109 to 428 mm (mean 272) (10 mm = 1 mV), and in 27 patients (90%) it was >175 mm (Table II). The relation of the total 12-lead QRS voltage to heart weight in the 30 patients is illustrated in Figure 2. The method of measuring various QRS complexes for this measurement is illustrated in Figure 1. The mean QRS voltage for each of the 12 leads in each patient was 23 mm. The individual and mean QRS amplitudes in each of the 12 leads is displayed in Table II. The highest mean QRS voltage occurred in leads V_2 and V_3 (each 38 mm), and the lowest mean voltage in lead aVR, 11 mm. The QRS mean voltage in V_5 was higher than that in V_6 (33 mm vs 28 mm); in 22 patients (73%), the QRS voltage in V_5 was higher than that in V_6.

Various previously recommended electrocardiographic QRS voltage criteria (summarized by Murphy et al[17]) for LV hypertrophy and the frequency of their occurrence in our 30 patients with chronic AR are summarized in Table III. A few criteria have been slightly modified to allow the number designating the upper limit of normal to end in a 0 or a 5, and to allow the elevated value to always be greater than a certain number rather than equal to or greater than a certain number. Of the 18 criteria analyzed, only 1 upper-limit number was evaluated in 3, two values were analyzed in 14, and 4 values in 1. Thus, a total of 35 values were analyzed for the 18 criteria: 34 were measurements in millimeters of QRS voltage and 1 was a ratio. The 2 criteria that had the highest positive frequency were the sum of the tallest limb-lead R wave plus the deepest limb-lead S wave >15 mm (90%, 27 of 30 patients) and the sum of the voltage of the QRS complex in all 12

leads, >175 mm (90%). The sum of the S wave in lead V_1 plus the larger of the R wave in V_5 or V_6 was >35 mm in 22 patients (73%). The sum of the larger S wave of leads V_1 or V_2 plus the larger of the R wave of V_5 or V_6 was >35 mm in 26 patients (87%) and >40 mm in 22 patients (73%). The sum of the deepest S wave in leads V_1, V_2 and V_3 plus the tallest R waves in leads V_4, V_5 and V_6 was >35 mm in 26 patients (87%), >40 mm in 25 patients (83%), >45 mm in 22 patients (73%) and >50 mm in 21 patients (70%). The tallest R wave plus the deepest S wave in any single V lead was >35 mm in 19 patients (63%).

The S-wave amplitude in lead V_1 ranged from 9 to 60 mm (mean 23); the R-wave amplitude in lead V_5 ranged from 9 to 64 mm (mean 25) and in V_6, from 11 to 47 mm (mean 25). The sum of the S wave in V_1 and the larger of the R waves in either V_5 or V_6 (Sokolow-Lyon index) ranged from 22 to 110 mm (mean 51). The deepest S wave in leads V_1, V_2 and V_3 ranged from 12 to 70 mm (mean 38) and in 23 patients (77%) it was >25 mm. The largest precordial S wave was in lead V_1 in 3 patients (10%), in lead V_2 in 12 patients (40%), in lead V_3 in 13 patients (43%) and in V_4 in 2 patients (7%). The average S-wave amplitude was higher in lead V_2 than V_1 (40 vs 24 mm).

The largest R wave in leads V_4, V_5 and V_6 ranged from 12 to 64 mm (mean 30) and in 19 patients (63%) it was >25 mm; the largest precordial R wave was in lead V_4 in 2 patients (7%), in V_5 in 19 (63%) and in V_6 in 9 (30%). The mean height of the R wave in both leads V_5 and V_6 averaged 25 mm. The R wave in V_6 was larger than the R wave in V_5 in 9 patients (30%).

Of the 30 patients, 29 (97%) were in sinus rhythm. The PR interval in them ranged from 0.16 to 0.36 second (mean 0.21) and it was >0.20 second in 8 (28%) patients. The width of the QRS complex ranged from 0.06 to 0.14 second (mean 0.10); in 6 (20%) patients it was ≥0.12 second. The QRS axes are listed in Table II. Of the 30

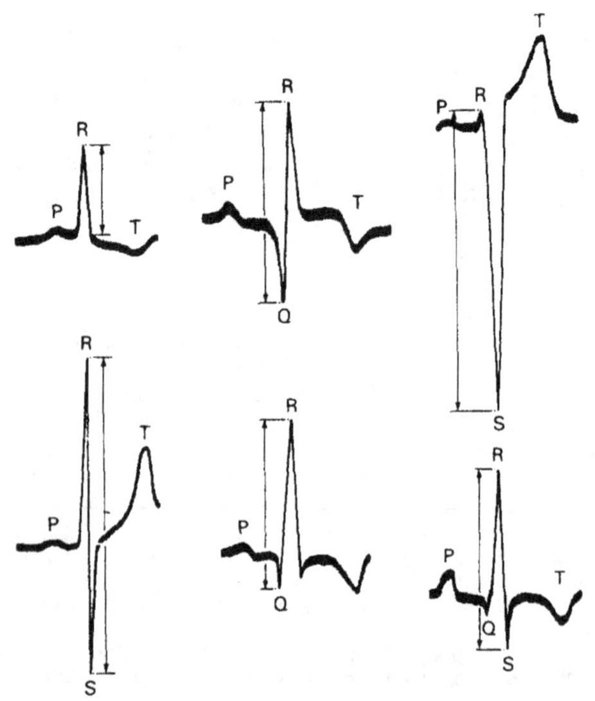

FIGURE 1. Method of measurement for various QRS complexes.

TABLE I Certain Clinical Morphologic and Electrocardiographic Features in 30 Necropsy Patients with Chronic, Severe, Pure Aortic Regurgitation

| | | | | | Pressures (mm Hg) | | | | | | | | | Electrocardiogram | | | | |
| | | | | | LV | | SA | | AR | | | | No. of | | | | Intervals (sec) | | |
Pt	Autopsy No.	Age (yr) & Sex	Cause of AR	AP	S	D	S	D	by Cine (1+–4+)	AVR	HW (g)	LV F	4 Major CA >75%	VR (bpm)	QRS axis (Degrees)	PR	QRS	VPC
1	A57-251	33M	IE	0	...	...	130	70	...	0	430	0	0	84	−40	0.27	0.14	0
2	A80-139	37M	IE	0	115	23	120	60	4+	+	610	0	0	90	−20	0.16	0.10	0
3	A69-254	39M	IE	0	140	20	140	38	4+	0	1010	0	0	68	0	0.20	0.12	0
4	71A-21	40M	IE	0	190	31	190	60	4+	+	575	+	0	72	+30	0.18	0.09	0
5	A70-117	45M	IE	0	120	50	120	50	4+	+	610	0	0	72	−15	0.20	0.11	0
6	71A-407	49M	IE	0	...	...	160	40	...	+	640	0	0	100	+30	0.18	0.11	+
7	A71-149	52F	IE	0	130	44	150	40	4+	+	500	0	0	75	0	0.15	0.10	0
8	A72-42	59M	IE	0	118	38	123	52	3+	+	840	0	0	70	+60	0.24	0.12	0
9	A58-280	19M	Syphilis	0	148	33	148	33	4+	0	750	0	0	100	+45	0.16	0.10	0
10	A61-192	37M	Syphilis	+	152	20	152	55	4+	0	600	0	0	66	+30	0.20	0.07	+
11	70A369	50M	Syphilis	+	...	...	160	60	...	0	720	+	2	90	−50	0.17	0.10	0
12	A65-106	55M	Syphilis	0	138	37	160	51	4+	+	940	0	3	75	−20	0.20	0.10	0
13	A64-223	56F	Syphilis	0	106	25	108	27	4+	+	800	+	3	72	+60	0.20	0.11	0
14	A77-241	65F	Syphilis	0	170	8	184	50	4+	+	710	0	1	81	+50	0.16	0.08	0
15	A61-274	34M	Anky Sp	0	100	22	120	25	4+	+	700	0	0	64	−30	0.26	0.10	0
16	A68-142	38M	Anky Sp	0	180	16	180	50	4+	+	1100	0	0	75	0	0.28	0.11	0
17	A61-99	52M	Anky Sp	0	160	18	168	30	4+	+	850	0	0	60	−15	0.36	0.14	0
18	A61-262	55M	Anky Sp	0	114	40	120	38	4+	0	680	0	0	82	−30	0.22	0.06	0
19	A66-127	57M	Anky Sp	0	...	...	200	80	...	0	500	0	0	110	0	0.17	0.09	0
20	A77-11	35F	Marfan	+	120	24	120	50	4+	+	375	0	0	66	−30	0.17	0.12	0
21	A58-206	36F	Marfan	0	...	...	130	40	...	0	700	0	0	95	−45	0.19	0.10	0
22	A65-64	41M	Marfan	0	100	30	100	40	3+	+	750	0	0	72	−10	0.20	0.10	+
23	A69-278	48F	Marfan	+	150	12	150	40	3+	+	520	0	0	72	+110	0.16	0.11	0
24	A59-169	59M	Marfan	0	190	25	200	80	3+	0	865	0	0	100	+20	...	0.08	+
25	71A27	34M	Uncertain	0	105	36	122	65	3+	+	460	0	0	84	−10	0.20	0.08	0
26	70A309	40F	Uncertain	0	...	...	180	60	...	0	950	0	0	70	+60	0.20	0.10	0
27	A64-102	41M	Uncertain	0	88	19	96	20	4+	+	920	0	0	75	+50	0.28	0.13	+
28	69A-135	59M	Uncertain	0	...	...	140	60	...	+	630	0	2	70	−20	0.167	0.08	0
29	A60-261	35M	Trauma	0	100	50	110	50	4+	0	550	+	0	85	+50	0.31	0.10	0
30	A68-325	51F	SH	+	...	...	210	80	...	+	600	0	0	76	−30	0.20	0.10	0
Mean or total		45 22M		5	132	28	139*	50*	22	19	696	4	5	79	+9	0.21	0.10	5

* Includes only the 23 patients in whom the systemic arterial pressure was measured directly at catheterization.

Anky Sp = ankylosing spondylitis; AP = angina pectrois; AR = aortic regurgitation; AVR = aortic valve replacement; CA = coronary artery; Cine-cineangiogram; D = end-diastole; F = grossly visible fibrosis; HW = heart weight; LV = left ventricle or left ventricular; S = peak systole; SA = systemic artery; SH = systemic hypertension; VPC = ventricular premature complex; VR = ventricular rate.

 Electrocardiographic QRS Amplitudes (in mm [10 mm = 1 mV]) in 30 Necropsy Patients with Chronic, Pure, Isolated Aortic Regurgitation

Pt	I	II	III	aVR	aVL	aVF	V_1	V_2	V_3	V_4	V_5	V_6	Total 12 Lead	S V_1	S V_2	R V_5	R V_6
1	7	7	12	5	9	9	11	33	42	42	29	34	240	10	33	22	32
2	13	20	23	14	19	19	11	14	11	12	15	11	182	10	12	12	11
3	12	8	15	9	12	10	30	56	52	37	24	50	315	27	54	23	47
4	15	15	12	15	11	10	31	33	20	48	35	28	273	29	28	35	28
5	8	30	28	18	15	26	32	72	44	58	50	29	410	25	62	48	28
6	9	12	8	7	9	7	33	37	40	41	32	28	263	27	32	31	28
7	7	8	7	7	7	7	26	48	47	28	30	20	242	24	48	27	20
8	8	9	5	7	6	7	24	25	12	17	17	16	153	23	24	16	14
9	5	18	17	11	6	17	25	53	49	55	36	19	311	17	36	21	17
10	9	7	4	8	5	4	18	29	35	14	31	29	193	20	31	32	30
11	16	5	14	8	16	11	16	31	38	34	30	15	234	16	30	23	15
12	20	7	24	10	21	15	27	58	46	17	23	31	299	28	49	29	31
13	13	18	21	10	15	19	21	28	32	29	39	36	281	20	24	27	34
14	11	14	9	11	8	9	10	12	15	20	30	20	169	9	16	18	17
15	19	17	28	13	23	19	31	64	74	24	68	48	428	30	59	64	44
16	29	13	21	22	27	9	50	58	72	42	21	50	414	50	59	9	42
17	21	11	12	14	17	4	21	18	16	8	27	27	196	15	15	26	24
18	9	4	11	6	10	8	14	18	31	31	27	24	193	13	16	15	21
19	19	21	8	21	11	12	50	54	37	70	45	26	374	39	38	37	25
20	11	8	6	8	8	5	14	34	46	40	42	24	246	7	13	15	12
21	21	18	35	12	28	26	39	44	37	39	45	37	381	31	39	37	30
22	21	14	19	18	16	10	64	74	62	20	46	27	391	60	72	50	27
23	9	32	42	13	30	37	8	23	28	38	62	62	384	9	21	12	16
24	9	9	13	5	12	12	15	29	34	16	26	22	202	17	35	16	14
25	5	5	6	5	5	4	9	22	18	6	15	9	109	8	18	14	8
26	12	9	10	9	12	5	32	39	40	27	20	35	250	29	37	10	31
27	8	11	6	8	8	9	31	52	76	52	25	29	367	22	52	11	27
28	11	15	8	11	6	11	14	19	26	33	29	19	202	13	19	20	15
29	10	8	11	6	10	9	22	22	30	24	30	25	207	21	21	29	24
30	18	20	15	18	13	17	35	25	16	15	29	28	249	33	22	28	26
Mean	13	14	15	11	13	13	25	38	38	32	33	28	272	23	34	25	25

Pt	Largest S V_1-V_3 (mm)	(Lead)	Largest R V_4-V_6 (mm)	(Lead)	Largest R 6 Limb Leads (mm)	(Lead)	Largest S 6 Limb Leads (mm)	(Lead)	R	S
1	33	V_3	32	V_6	8	aVL	11	III	5	11
2	12	V_2	12	V_5	16	aVL	17	III	12	17
3	54	V_2	47	V_6	12	I	10	III	12	10
4	29	V_1	35	V_5	15	I	15	aVR	15	7
5	62	V_2	48	V_5	18	II	17	III	9	17
6	39	V_4	31	V_5	12	II	3	aVL	7	0
7	48	V_2	27	V_5	8	I	8	aVR	8	5
8	24	V_2	16	V_5	9	I	9	aVR	9	2
9	40	V_4	21	V_5	11	II	7	AVF	3	6
10	35	V_3	32	V_5	10	I	8	AVR	10	4
11	35	V_3	23	V_5	15	I	13	III	15	13
12	49	V_2	31	V_6	23	aVL	22	III	18	22
13	29	V_3	34	V_6	19	aVF	11	aVR	11	0
14	16	V_2	18	V_5	14	II	12	aVR	10	0
15	68	V_3	64	V_5	20	aVL	22	III	18	22
16	68	V_3	42	V_6	30	I	23	aVR	30	20
17	15	V_1	26	V_5	19	I	16	aVR	19	12
18	27	V_3	21	V_6	9	I	11	III	9	11
19	38	V_2	46	V_4	20	I	19	aVR	20	7
20	16	V_3	15	V_5	11	I	8	aVR	11	5
21	39	V_2	37	V_5	29	aVL	32	III	19	32
22	72	V_2	50	V_5	23	I	18	aVR	23	15
23	27	V_3	16	V_6	37	aVF	29	aVL	2	41
24	40	V_3	16	V_5	11	aVL	11	III	10	11
25	18	V_2	14	V_5	3	I	3	aVR	3	3
26	39	V_3	31	V_6	9	I	10	aVR	9	4
27	72	V_3	27	V_6	7	I	7	aVR	7	2
28	19	V_2	25	V_4	11	I	9	aVR	11	8
29	32	V_3	29	V_5	10	I	10	III	10	10
30	34	V_1	28	V_5	20	II	17	aVR	17	0
Mean	38		30		15		14		12	10

single rest ECGs analyzed, 1 or more premature ventricular complexes were present in 5 patients (17%) (nos. 6, 10, 22, 24 and 27, Table I and II) and 1 or more premature atrial complexes in 1 patient (no. 2).

Comparison of men to women: No significant (p >0.05) differences were observed between the 22 men and 8 women in mean age; percent with significant coronary arterial narrowing, LV scarring, angina pectoris or widened ($\geq$0.12 second) QRS complexes; mean heart weight (717 vs 638 g); average total 12-lead QRS voltage (269 vs 275 mm); average Sokolow-Lyon index (52 vs 46 mm), or mean LV peak systolic pressure (134 vs 130 mm Hg).

TABLE III Recommended or Modified Electrocardiographic Criteria for Determining Left Ventricular Hypertrophy as Applied to 30 Necropsy Patients with Severe Cardiomegaly from Chronic, Pure, Severe Aortic Regurgitation

No.	QRS Complex Measured	Value Considered Upper Limit of Normal (mm)	No. (%) of 30 Patients Above Normal Limit
1a	$SV_1 + RV_5$ or V_6 (larger)	35	22 (73)
b	$SV_1 + RV_5$ or V_6 (larger)	40	18 (60)
2a	SV_1 or V_2 (larger) + RV_5 or V_6 (larger)	35	26 (87)
b	SV_1 or V_2 (larger) + RV_5 or V_6 (larger)	40	22 (73)
3a	SV_1 or V_2 (larger) + RV_6	35	25 (83)
b	SV_1 or V_2 (larger) + RV_6	40	21 (70)
4a	$SV_2 + RV_5$	35	24 (80)
b	$SV_2 + RV_5$	40	22 (73)
5a	Deepest $SV_1 - V_3$ + tallest $RV_4 - V_6$	35	26 (87)
b	Deepest $SV_1 - V_3$ + tallest $RV_4 - V_6$	40	25 (83)
c	Deepest $SV_1 - V_3$ + tallest $rV_4 - V_6$	45	22 (73)
d	Deepest $SV_1 - V_3$ + tallest $V_4 - V_6$	50	21 (70)
6a	Tallest R + deepest S in any V lead	35	19 (63)
b	Tallest R + deepest S in any V lead	40	16 (53)
7a	Deepest $SV_1 - V_3$	25	23 (77)
b	Deepest $SV_1 - V_3$	30	19 (63)
8a	Tallest $RV_4 - V_6$	25	19 (63)
b	Tallest $RV_4 - V_6$	30	14 (47)
9a	Deeper SV_1 or V_2	25	19 (63)
b	Deeper SV_1 or V_2	30	17 (57)
10a	Tallest RV_5 or V_6	25	26 (87)
b	Tallest RV_5 or V_6	30	14 (47)
11	$RV_6 > RV_5$	<1	9 (30)
12a	Tallest limb-lead R + deepest limb-lead S	15	27 (90)
b	Tallest limb-lead R + deepest limb-lead S	20	17 (57)
13a	$R_1 + S_3$	15	20 (67)
b	$R_1 + S_3$	20	14 (47)
14a	Tallest limb-lead R	10	21 (70)
b	Tallest limb-lead R	15	13 (43)
15a	Deepest limb-lead S	10	18 (60)
b	Deepest limb-lead S	15	11 (37)
16	R_1	10	15 (50)
17	S_3	10	13 (43)
18a	Total 12-lead QRS voltage	175	27 (90)
b	Total 12-lead QRS voltage	200	23 (77)

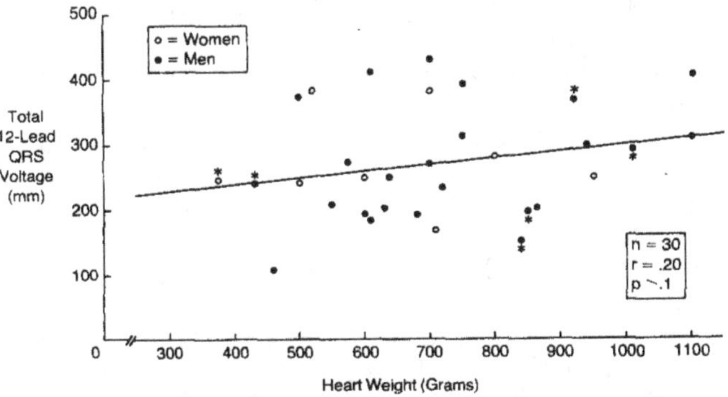

FIGURE 2. Relation of the total 12-lead QRS voltage (mm) to heart weight (grams) in the 30 patients with severe, pure aortic regurgitation. **Asterisks** designate the patients in whom the widths of the QRS complexes were at least 0.12 second.

Comparison of patients younger than 40 years and older than 40 years: No significant differences were observed between the 13 younger and the 17 older (older than 40 years) patients in sex ratio; percent with angina pectoris, widened QRS complexes or LV scarring; mean heart weight (677 vs 710 g); average Sokolow-Lyon index (50 vs 50 mm), or mean LV peak-systolic pressure (137 vs 129 mm Hg). The percent with significant (>75% cross-sectional area) coronary arterial narrowing was different (0 of 13 vs 5 of 17) (p <0.05).

Comparison of patients with and without angina pectoris: No significant differences were observed between the 6 patients with and the 24 patients without angina in mean age; sex ratio; frequency of coronary arterial narrowing or LV scarring; average total 12-lead QRS voltage (287 vs 267 mm); mean Sokolow-Lyon index (55 vs 49 mm); or LV peak systolic pressure (117 vs 138 mm Hg). The frequency of widened QRS complexes was different (3 of 6 vs 3 of 24) (p <0.05).

Comparison of patients with total 12-lead QRS voltage 250 mm or less to those with total voltage more than 250 mm: No significant differences were observed between the 17 patients with total 12-lead QRS voltage ≤250 mm and the 13 patients with larger total voltage in mean age, sex ratio, percent with significant coronary arterial narrowing, LV scarring, angina pectoris or widened QRS complexes; mean LV peak systolic pressure (135 vs 133 mm Hg), or mean heart weight (648 vs 760 g). The average Sokolow-Lyon index was different (39 vs 65 mm) (p <0.001).

Comparison of patients with normal and abnormal Sokolow-Lyon indexes: No significant differences were observed between the 8 patients with normal and the 22 patients with abnormal (>35 mm) indexes in mean age; sex ratio; percent with narrowed coronary arteries, LV scar, angina pectoris or widened QRS complexes, or mean LV peak systolic pressure (131 vs 136 mm Hg). The average total 12-lead QRS voltage was different (210 vs 296 mm) (p <0.05). The Sokolow-Lyon index in the 22 patients in whom this index was >35 mm ranged from 38 to 110 mm (mean 61) and their hearts weighed 430 to 1,100 g (mean 729); in the 8 patients in whom the Sokolow-Lyon index was <35 mm, the index ranged from 22 to 34 mm (mean 27) and their hearts weighed 375 to 865 g (mean 606).

Comparison of patients with normal and widened (more than 0.12 second) QRS complexes: No significant differences were observed between the 24 patients with QRS widths <0.12 second compared to the 6 with longer widths in mean age; sex ratio; percent with narrowed coronary arteries, LV scar or angina pectoris; mean heart weight (686 vs 738 g); average total 12-lead QRS voltage (276 vs 249 mm); mean Sokolow-Lyon index (51 vs 44 mm), or mean LV peak systolic pressure (138 vs 117 mm Hg). The frequency of angina pectoris was different (p <0.05): angina was present in 3 of 24 patients with normal-width QRS complexes and in 3 of 6 patients with widened complexes (p <0.05).

Comparison of patients with left ventricular peak systolic pressure less than 140 mm Hg to those with pressures greater than 140 mm Hg: No significant differences were observed between the 14 patients with the lower compared to the 8 patients with the higher (>140 mm) pressures in age; sex ratio; percent with angina, coronary arterial narrowing, LV scar, or widened QRS complexes; mean heart weight (696 vs 746 g), average total 12-lead QRS voltage (271 vs 267 mm), or mean Sokolow-Lyon index (52 vs 44 mm).

Comparison of patients with hearts weighing 600 g or less to those with hearts weighing more than 600 g: No significant differences were observed between the 10 patients with hearts ≤600 g compared to the 20 patients with larger hearts in mean age; sex ratio; percent with angina pectoris, coronary arterial narrowing, LV scar or widened QRS complexes; average total 12-lead QRS voltage (252 vs 280 mm); mean Sokolow-Lyon index (45 vs 53 mm), or mean LV peak-systolic pressure (130 vs 135 mm Hg).

Comparison of patients with and without coronary arterial narrowing: The mean age was older among the 5 patients with narrowing >75% in cross-sectional area of 1 or more major coronary arteries compared to that among the 25 patients without (57 vs 42 years), and the percent with LV scarring was higher (2 of 5 vs 2 of 25) (p <0.05). No significant differences were observed between the 2 groups in sex ratio; percent with angina or widened QRS complexes; mean heart weights (729 vs 688 g); average total 12-lead QRS voltage (243 vs 277 mm); mean Sokolow-Lyon index (47 vs 51 mm), or mean LV peak-systolic pressure (138 vs 140 mm Hg).

Comparison of patients with and without left ventricular scarring: Except for a higher frequency of coronary arterial narrowing in the patients with LV scars (2 of 4 vs 2 of 26) (p <0.05), no significant differences between these groups occurred in age; sex ratio; percent with angina or widened QRS complexes; mean heart weight (661 vs 701 g); average total 12-lead QRS voltage (249 vs 274 mm); mean Sokolow-Lyon index (50 vs 50 mm) or mean LV peak-systolic pressure (132 vs 135 mm Hg).

Discussion

Patients with chronic severe AR generally have hearts of greater weight than that observed in other conditions.[18] Thus, these patients should have larger QRS voltages than observed in other conditions. In addition to measuring R and S waves in 1 or more leads for LV hypertrophy as suggested by many investigators and summarized by Murphy et al[17] and in Table III, we measured the total QRS voltage in all 12 leads in each patient and compared its usefulness to that of other voltage criteria for LV hypertrophy.

Because patients with chronic, severe AR generally have the largest human hearts, these persons would appear to be the ideal group to examine the usefulness of the various QRS voltage criteria for LV hypertrophy. Many studies, of course, have compared LV mass determined at necropsy[9,19] or by angiography[20] or echocardiography[21–23] to QRS voltage, but few of the previous studies have included patients with chronic, severe, pure AR. All previous studies have demonstrated that all QRS voltage criteria for LV hypertrophy are unreliable. The present study demonstrates the same finding, but in a group of patients with larger hearts than those studied previously. Our patients as a group had hearts that weighed roughly 2 times normal.

The Sokolow-Lyon index[8] (sum of the S wave in V_1 plus the larger of the R wave in either V_5 or V_6), the most widely used QRS voltage criterion for LV hypertrophy, was >35 mm, i.e., abnormal, in only 22 of our 30 patients (73%) whose mean heart weight was 696 g. The QRS voltage for LV hypertrophy advocated by Romhilt and Estes[9] fared even worse, although these 2 investigators also incorporated non-QRS-voltage criteria for LV hypertrophy. Only 8 of our 30 patients (27%) had an R wave in the 6 limb leads ≥20 mm and only 5 (17%) had an S wave in these leads ≥20 mm (In our Table III, we use the criteria >20 mm rather than ≥20 mm to aid in comparisons to other criteria.); 23 patients (77%) had an S wave in leads V_1, V_2 and V_3 ≥25 mm and 20 (67%) had an R wave in leads V_4, V_5 and V_6 ≥25 mm. (Again, in the table we modified these voltage criteria to >25 mm rather than ≥25 mm.) A total of 25 patients (83%), however, satisfied the Romhilt-Estes QRS voltage criteria in 1 or more of the 4 lead sites (R in limb leads ≥20; S in limb leads ≥20; S in V_1, V_2 and V_3 ≥25 and R in V_4, V_5 and V_6 ≥25 mm).

A better criterion of LV hypertrophy was the sum of the tallest R wave and deepest S wave in the 6 limb leads. This sum was >15 mm in 27 (90%) of 30 patients.

In contrast to the disappointing frequency of fulfillment of the Sokolow-Lyon, Romhilt-Estes and most other criteria (Table III) for LV hypertrophy in our 30 patients with chronic, severe AR, measurement of the sum of the height and depth of the QRS complexes in all 12 leads did appear useful. Although the upper limit of normal QRS voltage in each of the 12 electrocardiographic leads in adults without evidence of cardiac disease has been well established,[17,24–27] the upper limit of total 12-lead QRS voltage has not been established in human adults whose LV mass has been determined by necropsy or by an angiographic or echocardiographic means. It is likely, however, that the total 12-lead QRS voltage in adults over 30 or so years of age with normal sized hearts is <175 mm. Indeed, Richard B. Devereux (AJC Editorial Board Member), in his review of the present manuscript, stated that 12-lead QRS voltage was <175 mm in 87 of 92 clinically normal patients (95%) studied by him, P.N. Casale and P. Kligfield (unpublished observations), indicating that this criterion has good specificity (100 times number of normal subjects with negative test divided by total number of normal subjects tested). Using 175 mm as the upper limit of normal, 27 of our 30 patients (90%) had LV hypertrophy by this criterion.

In the present study we also examined 10 other variables, further analyzing each to compare patients with to those without 1 or more variables or to compare patients with greater than to those with less than a certain figure. A total of 90 comparisons were examined among the 10 variables. Of the 90, only 8 (9%) showed a significant (p <0.05) difference in the variable analyzed. The 4 patients with transmural LV scars had a higher frequency of coronary narrowing (2 of 4 patients) than the 26 patients without LV scars (2 of 26 patients) (p <0.05) and vice versa. Patients older than 40 years had a significantly higher frequency of coronary narrowing than did the younger patients (p <0.05) and vice versa. Angina was significantly more frequent in pa-

TABLE IV Comparison of Total 12-Lead QRS Amplitude in Necropsy Patients with Chronic Aortic Regurgitation to Necropsy Patients with Aortic Valve Stenosis and Cardiac Amyloidosis

	Aortic Stenosis	p Value	Aortic Regurgitation	p Value	Cardiac Amyloidosis
No. of patients	50		30		30
Age (yr), range (mean)	16–65 (48)	NS	19–65 (45)	<0.001	21–93 (58)
Men (n)	36 (72%)	NS	22 (73%)	NS	15 (50%)
Women (n)	14 (28%)	NS	8 (27%)	NS	15 (50%)
Substernal pain (n)	34 (68%)	<0.01	11 (37%)	<0.05	4 (13%)
SA peak systole (mm Hg), range (average)	63–180 (112)	<0.001	96–200 (139)	<0.001	90–110 (104)
SA end-diastole (mm Hg), range (average)	34–88 (62)	<0.001	20–65 (42)	<0.001	60–80 (67)
Heart weight (g), range (mean)	380–880 (606)	<0.05	375–1110 (696)	<0.001	370–900 (532)
Narrowed coronary artery (n)	16 (32%)	NS	5 (17%)	NS	5 (17%)
Left ventricular scar (n)	7 (14%)	NS	4 (13%)	NS	4 (13%)
Total 12-lead QRS voltage (mm), range (average)	144–417 (257)	NS	109–428 (270)	<0.0001	58–199 (104)
Total 12-lead QRS voltage >175 mm, (n)	47 (94%)	NS	27 (90%)	<0.0001	2 (7%)

tients with QRS widths ≥0.12 second than in those with shorter QRS widths (3 of 6 vs 3 of 24) (p <0.05) and, conversely, the patients with the normal Sokolow-Lyon indices had significantly lower average total 12-lead QRS voltage than did the 21 patients with an abnormal (>35 mm) Sokolow-Lyon index (210 vs 296 mm); conversely, the 17 patients with total 12-lead QRS voltages ≤250 mm had lower mean Sokolow-Lyon indexes than did the 13 patients with total 12-lead QRS voltages >250 mm (39 vs 65 mm) (p <0.001).

Two other studies from this laboratory have used total 12-lead QRS voltage. One examined electrocardiograms in 50 necropsy patients with severe (LV systemic arterial peak systolic pressure gradients >50 mm Hg) aortic valve stenosis[28] and the other examined electrocardiograms in 30 necropsy patients with cardiac amyloidosis[29] (Table IV). Findings in these 2 groups of patients are summarized in Table IV and the findings are compared with those in the 30 patients with pure, chronic AR. The mean total QRS voltage was highest among patients with AR and lowest for those with amyloid. The percent of patients with AR or aortic stenosis having total 12-lead QRS voltage >175 mm was similar (90% and 94%), and 13 times higher than that in the amyloid group. The ratio of 12-lead QRS voltage to heart weight was slightly lower in the patients with aortic stenosis compared to those with pure AR (0.39 vs 0.42), indicating that cavity dilatation does not magnify the QRS voltage generated by a given mass of myocardium.

References

1. Spagnuolo M, Kloth H, Taranta A, Doyle E, Pasternack B. Natural history of rheumatic aortic regurgitation: criteria predictive of death, congestive heart failure, and angina in young patients. Circulation 1971;44:368–380.
2. Angioff E. Aortic incompetence: clinical haemodynamic and angiographic evaluation. IV. Physical signs and electrocardiographic findings. Acta Med Scand 1972;193:suppl 538:35–39.
3. Goldschlager N, Pfeifer J, Cohn K, Popper R, Selzer A. The natural history of aortic regurgitation: a clinical and hemodynamic study. Am J Med 1973;54:577–588.
4. Hirshfeld JW, Jr, Epstein SE, Roberts AJ, Glancy DL, Morrow AG. Indices predicting long-term survival after valve replacement in patients with aortic regurgitation and patients with aortic stenosis. Circulation 1974;50:1190–1199.
5. Henry WL, Bonow RO, Borer JS, Ware JH, Kent KM, Redwood DR, McIntosh CL, Morrow AG, Epstein SE. Observations on the optimum time for operative intervention for aortic regurgitation. I. Evaluation of the results of aortic valve replacement in symptomatic patients. Circulation 1980;61:471–483.
6. Henry WL, Bonow RO, Rosing DR, Epstein SE. Observations on the optimum time for operative intervention for aortic regurgitation. II. Serial echocardiographic evaluation of asymptomatic patients. Circulation 1980;61:484–492.
7. Carroll JD, Gaasch WH, Naimi S, Levine HJ. Regression of myocardial hypertrophy: electrocardiographic-echocardiographic correlations after aortic valve replacement in patients with chronic aortic regurgitation. Circulation 1982;65:980–987.
8. Sokolow M, Lyon TP. The ventricular complex in left ventricular hypertrophy as obtained by unipolar precordial and limb leads. Am Heart J 1949;37:161–186.
9. Romhill DW, Estes EH. A point-score system for the ECG diagnosis of left ventricular hypertrophy. Am Heart J 1968;75:752–758.
10. Roberts WC, Buchbinder NA. Healed left-sided infective endocarditis: clinicopathologic study of 59 patients. Am J Cardiol 1977;40:876–888.
11. Day PJ, McManus BM, Roberts WC. Amounts of coronary arterial narrowing by atherosclerotic plaques in clinically isolated, chronic, pure aortic regurgitation: analysis of 37 necropsy patients older than 30 years. Am J Cardiol 1984;53:173–177.
12. Roberts WC, Dangel JC, Bulkley BH. Non-rheumatic valvular cardiac disease: a clinicopathologic survey of 27 different conditions causing valvular dysfunction. Cardiovasc Clin 1973;5:333–446.
13. Bulkley BH, Roberts WC. Ankylosing spondylitis and aortic regurgitation: description of the characteristic cardiovascular lesion from study of eight necropsy patients. Circulation 1973;48:1014–1027.
14. Roberts WC, Honig HS. The spectrum of cardiovascular disease in the Marfan syndrome: a clinico-morphologic study of 18 necropsy patients and comparison to 151 previously reported necropsy patients. Am Heart J 1982;104:115–135.
15. Levine RJ, Roberts WC, Morrow AG. Traumatic aortic regurgitation. Am J Cardiol 1962;10:752–763.
16. Waller BF, Zoltick JM, Rosen JH, Katz NM, Gomes MN, Fletcher RD, Wallace RB, Roberts WC. Severe aortic regurgitation from systemic hypertension (without aortic dissection) requiring aortic valve replacement. Analysis of four patients. Am J Cardiol 1982;49:473–477.
17. Murphy ML, Thenabadu PN, Blue LR, Meade J, de Soyza N, Doherty JE, Baker BJ. Descriptive characteristics of the electrocardiogram from autopsied men free of cardiopulmonary disease—a basis for evaluating criteria for ventricular hypertrophy. Am J Cardiol 1983;52:1275–1280.
18. Roberts WC, Podolak MJ. The king of hearts: analysis of 23 patients with hearts weighing 1000 grams or more. Am J Cardiol 1985; 55:485–494.
19. Scott RC. The correlation between the electrocardiographic patterns of ventricular hypertrophy and the anatomic findings. Circulation 1960;21:256–291.
20. Baxley WA, Dodge HT, Sandler H. A quantitative angiocardiographic study of left ventricular hypertrophy and the electrocardiogram. Circulation 1968;37:509–517.
21. Bennett DH, Evans DW. Correlation of left ventricular mass determined by echocardiography with vectorcardiographic and electrocardiographic voltage measurements. Br Heart J 1974;36:981–987.
22. Reichek N, Devereux RB. Left ventricular hypertrophy: relationship of anatomic, echocardiographic and electrocardiographic findings. Circulation 1981;63:1391–1398.
23. Devereux RB, Phillips MC, Casale PN, Eisenberg RR, Kligfield P. Geometric determinants of electrocardiographic left ventricular hypertrophy. Circulation 1983;67:907–911.
24. Winsor T, ed. Electrocardiographic Textbook. Vol. 1. New York: American Heart Association, 1956: appendix pages 144–160.
25. Simonson E. Differentiation Between Normal and Abnormal in Electrocardiography. St. Louis: CV Mosby, 1961;51,132.
26. Criteria Committee of the New York Heart Association. Diseases of the Heart and Blood Vessels. Nomenclature and Criteria for Diagnosis. 6th ed. Boston: Little, Brown, 1964;437.
27. Cooksey JD, Dunn M, Massie E. Clinical Vectocardiography and Electrocardiography. 2nd ed. Chicago: Year Book Medical, 1977;81.
28. Siegel RJ, Roberts WC. Electrocardiographic observations in severe aortic valve stenosis: correlative necropsy study to clinical, hemodynamic, and ECG variables demonstrating relation of 12-lead QRS amplitude to peak systolic transaortic pressure gradient. Am Heart J 1982;103:210–221.
29. Roberts WC, Waller BF. Cardiac amyloidosis causing cardiac dysfunction: analysis of 54 necropsy patients. Am J Cardiol 1983;52:137–147.

Massive Perigraft Aortic Aneurysm Late After Composite Graft Replacement of the Ascending Aorta and Aortic Valve in the Marfan Syndrome

Susanne L. Mautner, MD, Gisela C. Mautner, MD, Charles L. Curry, MD, and William C. Roberts, MD

A major complication of the Marfan syndrome is the development of a fusiform aneurysm of the ascending aorta involving both its sinus and tubular portions. The fusiform aneurysm generally leads to aortic regurgitation, which may become severe, or to aortic rupture, which nearly always is fatal. Treatment of the aneurysm and aortic regurgitation consists of insertion of a composite graft, which involves a substitute aortic valve being sewn into the proximal end of a tube graft. The composite graft is then anastomosed proximally at the aortic valve position and distally to the ascending aorta beyond the aneurysm, and the wall of the aneurysm of the native aorta is wrapped around the composite graft. The coronary arteries are directly anastomosed to small orifices in the tube graft (Bentall operation[1]). This report describes a patient who developed a massive perigraft aortic aneurysm late after operation.

A 30-year-old black man had the Marfan syndrome diagnosed when he was approximately 15 years of age on the basis of ectopia lentis and skeletal features. At the time, the ascending aorta was dilated, and a murmur of aortic regurgitation was audible. Because of progressively worsening aortic regurgitation, the aortic valve and ascending aorta were replaced according to the Bentall operation when he was 23 years old (Figure 1). Within a few months, a mass was observed by echocardiogram surrounding the aortic composite graft, and this mass progressively increased in size to finally reach massive proportions (Figure 2). At age 24 years, retinal detachment occurred that was treated operatively, and also atrial fibrillation appeared. Despite the enlarging periaortic mass, the patient led an active life, including light weight lifting. He weighed 91 kg and was 191 cm in height. A chest radiograph was obtained 7 days before death at a routine follow-up visit (Figure 3). He died suddenly and unexpectedly at home.

Necropsy showed that the large perigraft mass was an aneurysm, the wall of which had been the wall of the previous native aorta (Figure

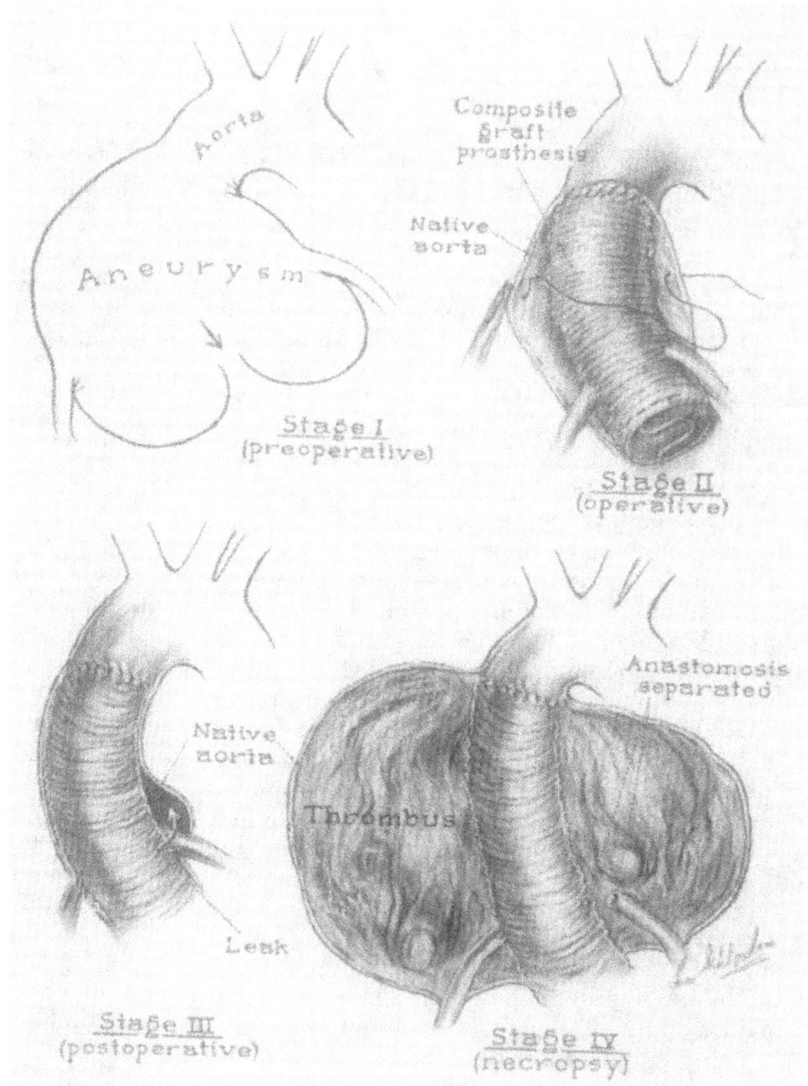

FIGURE 1. Drawing of the mechanism of development of the perigraft aortic aneurysm. Stage I: preoperative aortic regurgitation due to a dilated ascending aorta. Stage II: Bentall procedure with insertion of a composite graft (i.e., graft for the ascending aorta including a prosthesis [Björk-Shiley] in the aortic position). The coronary arteries are implanted into the tube graft and the wall of the native aorta is wrapped around the graft. Stage III: presumed slow leakage at suture line, most likely at the site of the anastomosis of the left main coronary artery to the graft of the ascending aorta (arrow). Stage IV: At necropsy, a massive perigraft aortic aneurysm formed by the wall of the native aorta was present, which was filled with thrombus. The left coronary artery was completely detached from its anastomosis to the composite graft.

From the Pathology Branch, National Heart, Lung, and Blood Institute, National Institutes of Health, Building 10, Room 2N-258, Bethesda, Maryland 20892, and the Department of Medicine, Howard University Medical Center, Washington, D.C. Manuscript received July 9, 1992; revised manuscript received and accepted August 18, 1992.

FIGURE 2. Echocardiogram performed 1 day before death showing the large aortic aneurysm around the graft in the aortic position *(A)*, and the compression of the left and right atria *(B and C)*. *A,* parasternal short-axis view; *B,* parasternal long-axis view; and *C,* 4-chamber view. An = perigraft aortic aneurysm; AV = aortic valve; LA = left atrium; LV = left ventricle; LVFW = left ventricular free wall; MV = mitral valve; RA = right atrium; RV = right ventricle; TV = tricuspid valve; VS = ventricular septum.

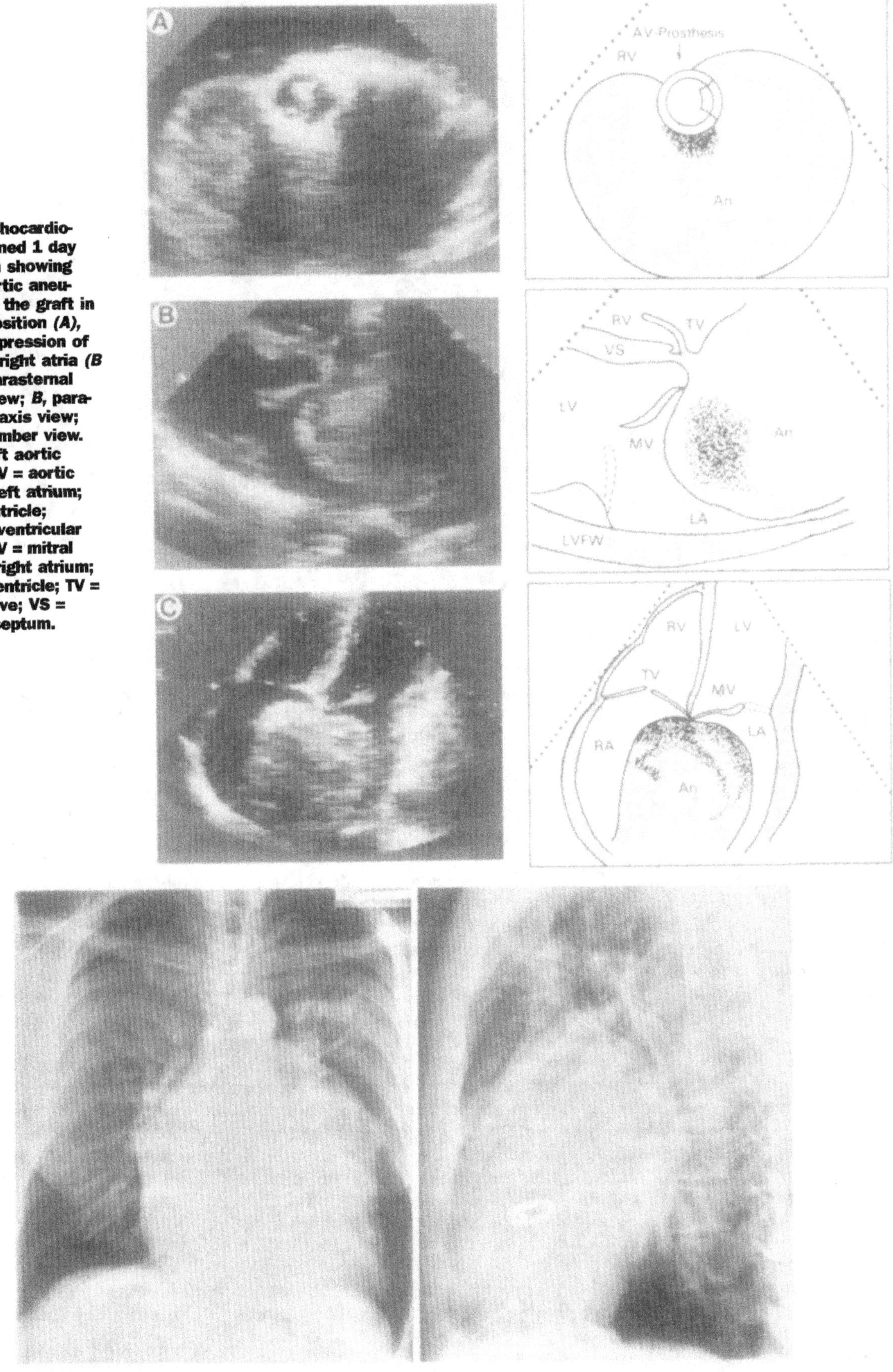

FIGURE 3. Chest radiograph of the patient obtained 7 days before death. *Left,* posteroanterior projection. *Right,* lateral projection. The enlarged heart silhouette is mainly due to the periaortic aneurysm of the ascending aorta.

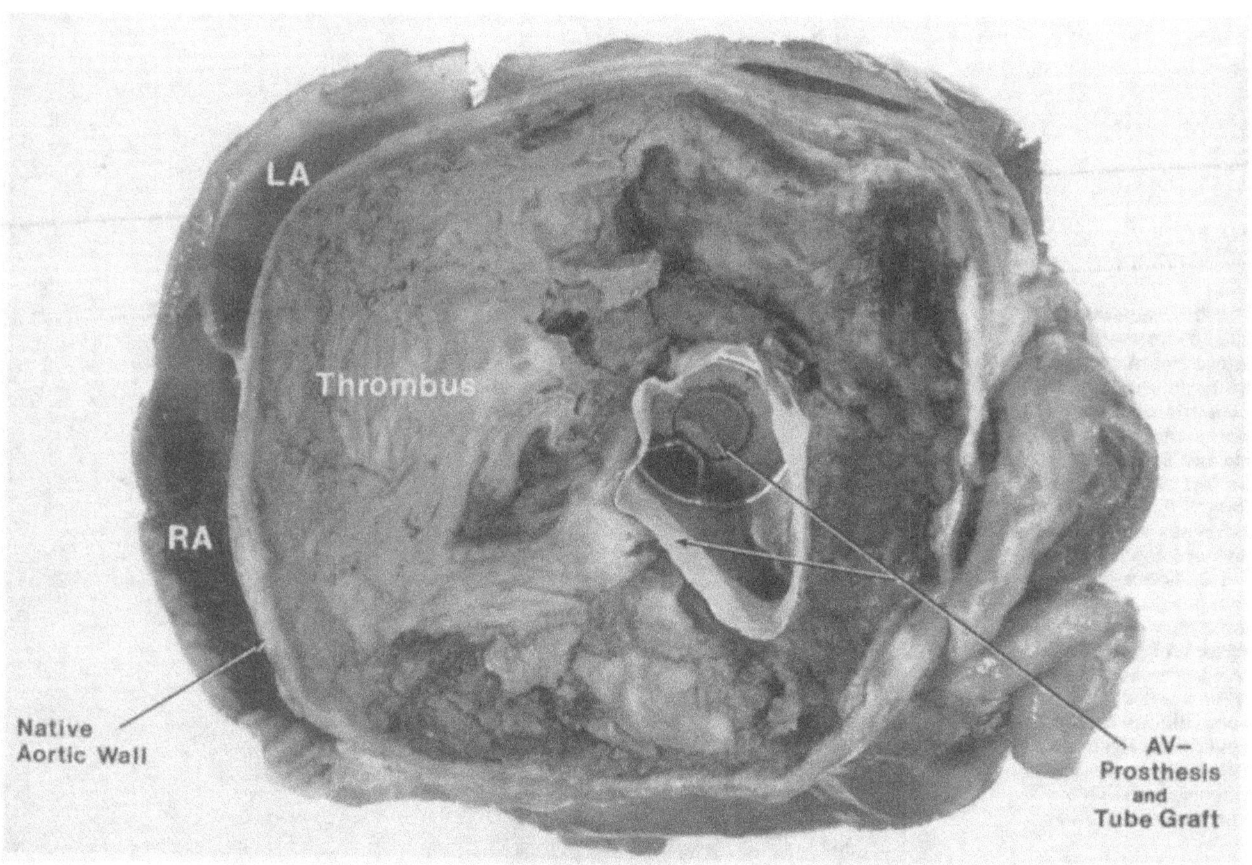

FIGURE 4. Perigraft aortic aneurysm at necropsy. The left and right atria (LA and RA, respectively) are compressed by the massive aneurysm of the ascending aorta. The mechanical valve prosthesis is in the aortic valve (AV) position.

4). The combined weight of the ascending aorta with the aneurysm and the heart was 1,320 g. The aneurysm surrounded the composite graft, did not compress it and contained a large thrombus. The aneurysm was believed to have resulted from a small detachment of the suture line connecting the left main coronary artery to the composite graft. Both atrial cavities were extremely compressed by the aneurysmal mass (Figure 4). The left ventricular wall was free of foci of necrosis and fibrosis, the left ventricular cavity was moderately dilated, and the leaflets of the mitral and tricuspid valves were focally thickened by fibrous tissue. Histology 0sections of the wall of the native aorta disclosed massive loss of elastic fibers.

The patient described in this report developed a huge (12 × 10 × 9 cm) perigraft aneurysm after replacement of most of the ascending aorta with a graft containing a valve prosthesis, and anastomosis of the coronary arteries directly to the Gor-tex graft. Detachment of the left main coronary artery to the composite graft appeared to be the cause of the perigraft aortic hematoma and aneurysm.

Several reports mentioned a peri-composite graft aneurysm after replacement of the ascending aorta with a composite graft with anastomosis of the coronary arteries to the graft.[2–9] At least 3 reports have described aortic graft–coronary arterial disruption after a similar type of operation. Nath et al[10] reported 4 of 15 patients who late after composite graft replacement of the ascending aorta had leakage into the perigraft, intraaortic space at 1 coronary anastomotic site by angiogram. Gott et al[11] described graft dehiscence of the anastomosis of the left main coronary artery in 1 of 50 patients with the Marfan syndrome undergoing composite graft repair. Marvasti et al[12] described 1 of 30 patients undergoing the composite graft operation with aortic wrapping of the graft who had partial disruption of the anastomosis of the right coronary artery to the graft. Two other patients had "pseudoaneurysms" at the site of the right coronary anastomosis to the graft.

The Bentall procedure performed in this patient has had several technical modifications in recent years, and the dramatic complication described herein will hopefully be less frequent with the newer techniques.[13–17] However, regular follow-up including echocardiography is advisable.

In summary, perigraft aortic aneurysm secondary to coronary artery disruption from a composite graft is an infrequent but potentially fatal complication after replacement of the ascending aorta with a composite graft.

Acknowledgment: We thank Michael W. Spencer for his photographic assistance, and Vivian E. Norman for her secretarial support.

REFERENCES

1. Bentall H, De Bono A. A technique for complete replacement of the ascending aorta. *Thorax* 1968; 23:338–339.

2. Nair KK. False aneurysm of the ascending aorta after surgery for Marfan's syndrome. *J Thorac Cardiovasc Surg* 1976;71:765–767.

3. Gallotti R, Ross DN. The Marfan syndrome: surgical technique and follow-up in 50 patients. *Ann Thorac Surg* 1980;29:428–433.

4. Pyeritz RE, Gott VL, McDonald GR, Achuff SC, Brinker JA, Haller JA, Hutchins GM. Surgical repair of the Marfan aorta: technique, indications and complications. *Johns Hopkins Med J* 1982;151:71–82.

5. Probst P, Baur HR, Leupi F, Schüpbach P, Althaus U. Postoperative evaluation of composite aortic grafts: comparison of angiography and CT. *Br J Radiol* 1983;56:797–804.

6. Kitamura S, Onishi K, Nakano S, Kawachi K, Kawashima Y. Early and late results of the Bentall operation for annulo-aortic ectasia. *J Cardiovasc Surg (Torino)* 1983;24:5–12.

7. Kouchoukos NT, Marshall WG Jr, Wedige-Stecher TA. Eleven-year experience with composite graft replacement of the ascending aorta and aortic valve. *J Thorac Cardiovasc Surg* 1986;92:691–705.

8. Josephson RA, Singer I, Levine JH, Maughan L, Pyeritz RE, Gott VL, Weisman HF, Brinker J. Systolic expansion of the aortic root: an echocardiographic and angiographic sign of aortic composite graft dehiscence. *Cathet Cardiovasc Diagn* 1988;14:705–707.

9. Kong B, Ogilby JD, Poynton R. Pseudoaneurysm of a Shiley composite aortic valve and graft prosthesis. *Am Heart J* 1990;120:1002–1004.

10. Nath PH, Zollikofer C, Castaneda-Zuniga WR, Velasquez G, Formanek A, Nicoloff D, Amplatz K. Radiological evaluation of composite aortic grafts. *Radiology* 1979;131:43–51.

11. Gott VL, Pyeritz RE, Magovern GJ Jr, Cameron DE, McKusick VA. Surgical treatment of aneurysms of the ascending aorta in the Marfan syndrome. Results of composite-graft repair in 50 patients. *N Engl J Med* 1986;314:1070–1074.

12. Marvasti MA, Parker FB, Randall PA, Witwer GA. Composite graft replacement of the ascending aorta and aortic valve. Late follow-up with intra-arterial digital subtraction angiography. *J Thorac Cardiovasc Surg* 1988;95:924–928.

13. Cabrol C, Pavie A, Mesnildrey P, Gandjbakhch I, Laughlin L, Bors V, Corcos T. Long-term results with total replacement of the ascending aorta and reimplantation of the coronary arteries. *J Thorac Cardiovasc Surg* 1986;91:17–25.

14. Crawford ES, Svensson LG, Coselli JS, Safi HJ, Hess KR. Surgical treatment of the aneurysm and/or dissection of the ascending aorta, transverse aortic arch, and ascending aorta and transverse aortic arch: factors influencing survival in 717 patients. *J Thorac Cardiovasc Surg* 1989;98:659–674.

15. Belcher P, Ross D. Aortic root replacement — 20 years experience of the use of homografts. *Thorac Cardiovasc Surg* 1991;39:117–122.

16. Kouchoukos NT, Wareing TH, Murphy SF, Perrillo JB. Sixteen-year experience with aortic root replacement. Results of 172 operations. *Ann Surg* 1991;214:308–318.

17. Miyamoto AT. Technique for replacing the ascending aorta and aortic valve with a modified Bentall's operation. *Ann Thorac Surg* 1992;53:1125–1126.

Early descriptions of aortic regurgitation

Steven N. Vaslef, MD, PhD,* and William C. Roberts, MD** *Bethesda, Md.*

Necropsy descriptions. The concept of aortic regurgitation (AR) began to take root in ancient times with the recognition that the function of the aortic valve was to prevent the backflow of "vital spirits" into the left ventricle. Singer[1] reported that an experiment performed around 340 BC in Athens, Greece, was designed to test for valvular competence by determining whether the valve could support a column of water. Doby[2] cited Galen (130-200 AD) who discoursed on valvular function: ". . . the general purpose of the valves is to prevent a reversal of flow of any sort. . . . For nature does not want to tire the heart with unnecessary work, nor commit the error of putting anything at a place from which she intends to take it away again, or lead it away from a place where its presence is necessary." Leonardo da Vinci (1452-1519)[3] depicted how the aortic valve normally functions to prevent AR (Fig. 1).

In 1706 William Cowper (1666-1709),[4] a London surgeon, described necropsy cardiac findings of a man approximately 30 years of age who had aortic valve disease:

> The three semilunar valves of the aorta, which hinder the blood from returning to the heart, after it is expell'd thence by its systole or contraction; these valves . . . were somewhat thicker, and not so plyable as naturally; and did not so adequately apply to each other. . . . Whence it happened sometimes, that the blood of the great artery . . . would recoil. . . . I (also) observed the left ventricle . . . to be a little dilated. . . .

In another patient Cowper described the heart as "larger than that of an ordinary ox," and thus the phrase "cor bovinum" was originated.

In 1715 Raymond Vieussens (1641-1716),[5] a Montpellier physician, described a 35-year-old man who when reclined on his left side had palpitations so vi-

olent that "it seemed to him (the patient) as if one struck on his ribs with a hammer." The pulse was full and strong. Although Vieussens recognized the patient's condition, he was sure that death was imminent, which indeed it was. Necropsy findings disclosed severe left ventricular enlargement. Vieussens noted:

> [T]he semilunar valves are markedly stretched and cut off at their tips: all these cusps . . . were in fact osseous. . . . [A]s they [the cusps] had been cut off the ends could never approach each other closely enough to prevent any opening between them; that is why whenever the aorta contracted, it sent back into the left ventricle a part of the blood which it had just received.

Giovanni Battista Morgagni (1682-1771)[6] described the consequences of AR in a middle-aged woman:

> So that, as some portion of it [the blood] returned into the left ventricle of the heart, when this ventricle ought to receive the blood that was coming in from the lungs, it would necessarily happen that the returning portion, as the portion which had not been extruded just before, must occupy some part of that space, which, from the design of nature, was entirely due to the blood that was coming in from the lungs. Which circumstance, finally, could not but overload both the lungs and heart, and compel the latter to throw out, every now and then, with a great impetus, the blood that stagnated in it.

In another heart observed at autopsy, Morgagni[6] remarked that the cusps of the aortic valve were so "disjoined" that they "admitted a probe betwixt them."

Albrecht von Haller (1708-1777),[7] a Swiss physician, observed "violently throbbing" carotid arteries in a 20-year-old man, determined the prognosis to be poor, and at necropsy recorded that "from the aorta . . . the blood could return between the inexplicably rigid aortic valves into the heart."

Bedford[8] noted that in 1822 Cuming,[9] a Dublin physician, clearly correlated his findings at autopsy of an incompetent aortic valve with the throbbing pulse observed before death. Thomas Hodgkin (1798-1866)[10] reported protrusion of the aortic valve cusps into the left ventricle, "instead of effectually closing the vessel [ventricle] against a reflux of blood."

From the Pathology Branch, National Heart, Lung, and Blood Institute, National Institutes of Health.

*Present address: Department of Surgery, Evanston Hospital.

**Present address: Baylor Cardiovascular Institute Medical Center.

Received for publication Oct. 12, 1992; accepted Nov. 4, 1992.

AM HEART J 1993;125:1475-1483

4/1/44917

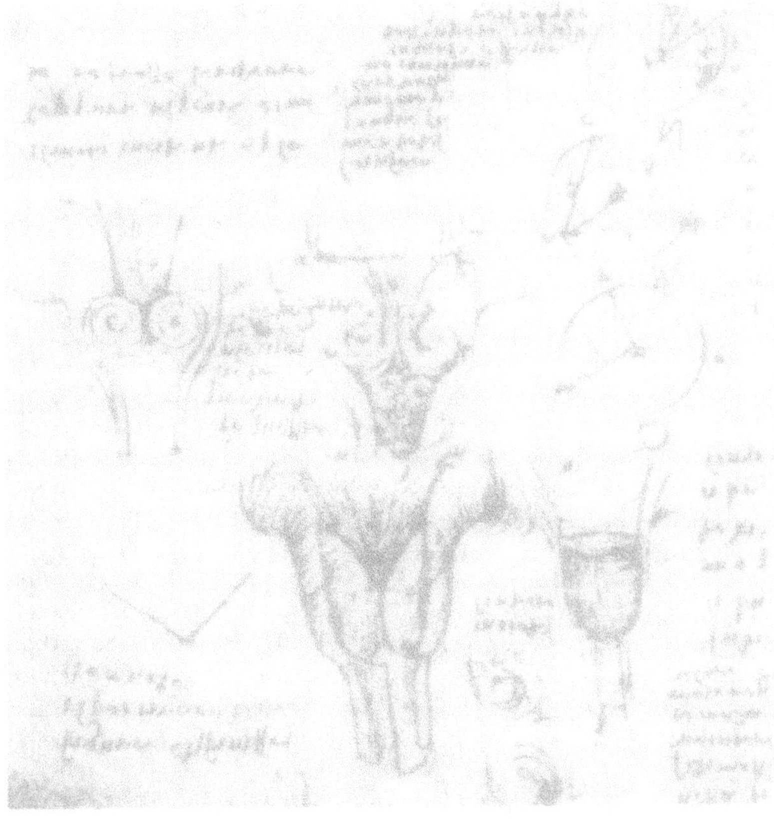

Fig. 1. Leonardo da Vinci's illustrations depicting normal closure of aortic valve. (From O'Malley CD, Saunders JB de CM. Leonardo da Vinci on the human body. New York: Henry Schuman, 1952. Reproduced with permission.)

Etiology. The causes of pure AR may be divided into three categories: (1) those conditions affecting the aortic valve cusps, (2) those affecting the ascending aorta, and (3) those affecting both the aortic valve cusps and ascending aorta.

Diseases involving the aortic valve cusps only. Rheumatic fever, of course, has long been implicated as a cause of AR. Hope[11] in 1832 described a young woman who died 8 years after an attack of "acute rheumatism"; necropsy findings disclosed an incompetent aortic valve. Corrigan[12] in 1832 and Bouillaud[13] in 1835 both described patients in whom AR followed attacks of acute rheumatism.

Infective endocarditis causing fatal AR was described by Billings[14] in 1909. Libman[15] in 1922 stated: "In the course of healing, the lesions of subacute bacterial endocarditis play a role in the development of chronic valvular disease."

Most patients with AR during the first decade of life have congenital abnormalities affecting other cardiovascular structures (for example, ventricular septal defect[16] and aortic isthmic coarctation[17]). It was not until 1981 that Roberts et al.[18] reported 13 patients with pure AR severe enough to warrant aortic valve replacement because of a congenitally bicuspid aortic valve without superimposed infective endocarditis.

Strain or trauma as a cause of AR was first described in 1830 by Plenderleath[19] and later discussed by Howard.[21] Fothergill[21] in 1872 wrote: "... [A]ortic regurgitation is essentially connected with effort. In the iron districts of England this form of disease is unusually frequent."

That rheumatoid arthritis may involve a cardiac valve has been recognized at least since 1944, when Young and Schwedel[22] described the cardiac lesions at autopsy. Goehrs et al.[23] in 1960 noted AR as a cardiac lesion in rheumatoid arthritis. Carpenter et al.[24] in 1967 and Roberts et al.[25] in 1968 observed quadrivalvular cardiac disease, including AR, in patients with rheumatoid arthritis.

Diseases of the aorta. The Marfan syndrome causes AR from dilatation of the proximal portion of ascending aorta. Burch[26] in 1936 and Rados[27] in 1942 stated that incompetence of the valves may occur in this syndrome, but specific evidence of AR was not presented. Baer et al.[28] in 1943 described AR in this syndrome and attributed it to aneurysmal dilatation of the aorta. Weaver et al.[29] in 1959 suggested a forme fruste of the Marfan syndrome as a cause of AR in patients who did not have skeletal or ocular signs of the syndrome.

Syphilis, according to Flaxman,[30] was first mentioned as a cause of AR in 1897 by Broadbent and Broadbent,[31] who stated that AR may be caused by the "syphilitic affection of the valves and the wall of the aorta. . . ." Citron[32] in 1908 first performed the Wasserman test in 16 patients with AR, and results were positive in five of them. Other investigators[33-39] described certain morphologic characteristics of cardiovascular syphilis, and Bulkley and Roberts[40] first delineated morphologic differences between the cardiovascular features of syphilis and ankylosing spondylitis.

Aortic dissection causing peripheral signs of AR was described by Letulle[41] in 1905, Busse[42] in 1906, Börger[43] in 1906, and Resnick and Keefer[44] in 1925. In all four reports the aortic valves appeared normal at necropsy, and regurgitation of blood into the false channel was considered the cause of the signs of AR. Lundberg[45] in 1930 described two patients having healed aortic dissection with AR and attributed the AR to the downward displacement of the aortic valve cusps toward the left ventricle. Gravier[46] 6 years earlier had observed similar displacements of aortic valve cusps. Wood et al.[47] in 1932 attributed the AR to incomplete closure of the valve cusps as a result of distortion of the aortic "ring" by the dissection. Hamman and Apperly,[48] who in 1933 accurately diagnosed AR associated with aortic dissection, considered the aneurysmal sac too small to account for the signs of AR, which they also attributed to distortion of the aortic "ring" by the dissection. Gouley and Anderson[49] in 1940 reported AR in healed aortic dissection.

Systemic hypertension as a cause of AR was described in 1922 by Bergé and Basch.[50] Garvin[51] in 1940 described seven patients with pure AR resulting from hypertension. Waller et al.[52] in 1981 described severe AR caused entirely by hypertension (not associated with aortic dissection), and each of their four patients had aortic valve replacement.

Takayasu's arteritis or "pulseless" disease can cause severe AR, as described initially by Austen and Blennerhassett[53] in 1965.

Although arteriosclerosis has been mentioned as a cause of AR, definite evidence that this mechanism alone could produce AR is lacking.

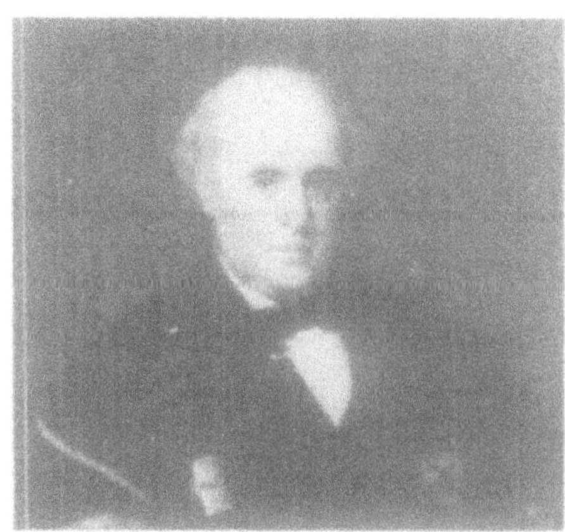

Fig. 2. Sir Dominic John Corrigan (1802-1880) who described collapsing pulse of AR and its cause. (From Major RH. Classic descriptions of disease. 3rd ed. Springfield, IL: Charles C Thomas, 1945. Reproduced with permission.)

Disease of both the aortic valve and aorta. Ankylosing spondylitis as a cause of AR was initially confused with or considered indistinct from rheumatoid arthritis. Bulkley and Roberts[40] in 1973 for the first time described the distinctive cardiovascular morphologic features of ankylosing spondylitis. AR also has been observed in patients with Reiter's syndrome,[40, 54, 55] but the lesion appears to be identical to that found in ankylosing spondylitis.

Diagnosis

Signs and symptoms. In 1832 James Hope (1801-1841)[11] described a prolonged murmur that followed the second heart sound in AR. The murmur, he noted, sounded "like whispering the word 'awe' during inspiration" and was best perceived opposite and above the aortic valve rather than above the apex. Joseph Skoda (1805-1881)[56] in 1839 wrote, "The aortic valves . . . are distended by the blood, but are incapable of performing their office; the blood regurgitates into the left ventricle, and causes a prolonged murmur."

The collapsing pulse in AR was first described in 1715 by Vieussens,[5] who observed that the pulse "struck the ends of my fingers just as a cord would have done which was very tightly drawn and violently shaken." Sir Dominic John Corrigan (1802-1880)[12] (Fig. 2), a Dublin surgeon, was the first to elucidate the cause of the visible pulsation in 1832:

. . . [T]he ascending aorta and arteries from it, pouring back a portion of their contained blood, become- . . . flaccid or lessened in their diameter. While they are in this state, the ventricle again contracts and impels quickly into these vessels a quantity of blood, which suddenly and greatly dilates them [thus producing] the visible pulsation which constitutes one of the signs of the disease.

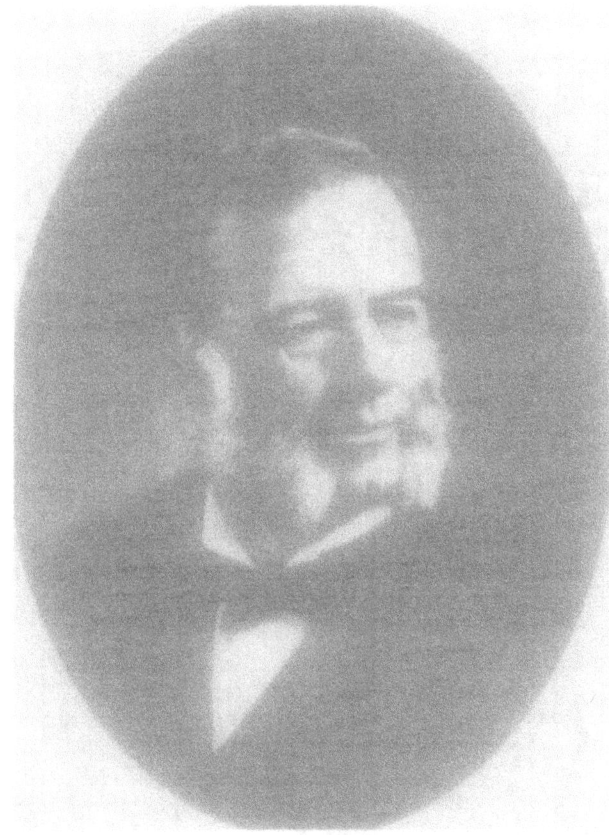

Fig. 3. Austin Flint (1812-1886) who described diastolic mitral rumble in some patients with AR. (From Major RH. Classic descriptions of disease. 3rd ed. Springfield, IL: Charles C Thomas, 1945. Reproduced with permission.)

Corrigan also noted two other signs observed in AR—a *bruit de soufflet* (blowing murmur) heard over the ascending aorta and carotid and subclavian arteries and a fremissement (rushing thrill) over both the carotid and subclavian arteries. Watson[57] in 1843 is credited with likening the pulse to a water-hammer toy.

Paul Louis Duroziez (1826-1897)[58] described an intermittent double murmur over the femoral artery as a sign of AR (Duroziez's sign). The first murmur, resulting from the powerful contraction of the left ventricle, was perceived by pressing the femoral artery 2 cm above the stethoscope; the second murmur (diastolic), believed to be the result of contraction of the arteries in the legs, was heard by pressing the femoral artery 2 cm below the stethoscope. This sign is distinguished from Traube's sign,[59] which is a double tone heard without compressing the femoral artery. The systolic sound, likened to that of a pistol shot, may be due to the sudden distention of the arterial wall.

Austin Flint (1812-1886)[60] (Fig. 3) in 1862 described two patients with AR, each of whom had a diastolic murmur similar to that heard in mitral stenosis. Such a murmur, Flint believed, could be produced without any mitral lesions. The regurgitant stream of blood was thrust into the stream leaving the left atrium, thereby setting the mitral leaflets into vibration, which was responsible for the murmur.

Heinrich Quincke (1842-1922)[61] in 1868 observed an alternating blanching and reddening in the nailbeds in patients with large and rapidly falling arterial pulses. Mueller[62] observed pulsation of the uvula, Sailer[63] noted pulsation of the spleen, and Dennison[64] noted pulsation of the cervix. Delpeuch[65] referred to the synchronous nodding of the head with the heart beat as DeMusset's sign, named after a French poet inflicted with AR. Landolfi[66] described contraction of the pupil in ventricular systole, as a result of hyperemia of the iris, and its dilatation in ventricular diastole. Minervini[67] demonstrated that when the tongue was depressed lightly, the tongue depressor moved up and down because of the strong lingual pulse. Logue[68] observed pulsation of the sternoclavicular joint in a patient with AR resulting from aortic dissection. Hill and Rowlands[69] measured peak systolic pressure gradients between the posterior tibial and radial arteries; they postulated that the greater pressure in the arteries of the legs resulted from their "contraction," thus permitting more blood to go to the brain. Gladstone[70] suggested that this gradient was due to the greater velocity of blood in the leg arteries, which come off of the aorta in a straighter course than in the subclavian arteries. Frank et al.[71] stressed the diagnostic value of measuring the popliteal-brachial peak systolic pressure gradient. Palfrey[72] perceived a pistol-shot sound in the radial artery in AR, and Harvey et al.[73] mentioned excessive sweating, neck pain, abdominal pain, angina pectoris, and a "splashing" sound over the stomach area in patients with AR.

Phonocardiography. Luisada[74] in 1943 described the phonocardiographic features of AR. The murmur was decrescendo like with the vibrations beginning after the second sound and gradually decreasing in intensity (Fig. 4). Wells et al.[75] in 1949 stated that the basal diastolic murmur in AR sometimes had, in addition to the descrescendo phase, a shorter crescendo phase. McKusick[76] in 1958 indicated that the murmur, usually decrescendo, may be crescendo-decrescendo in contour if the murmur sounds "musical." Furthermore, he sometimes noted a gap between the second sound and the murmur and at other times, a long diastolic murmur up to the first sound.

Radiography. Early work in the roentgenologic

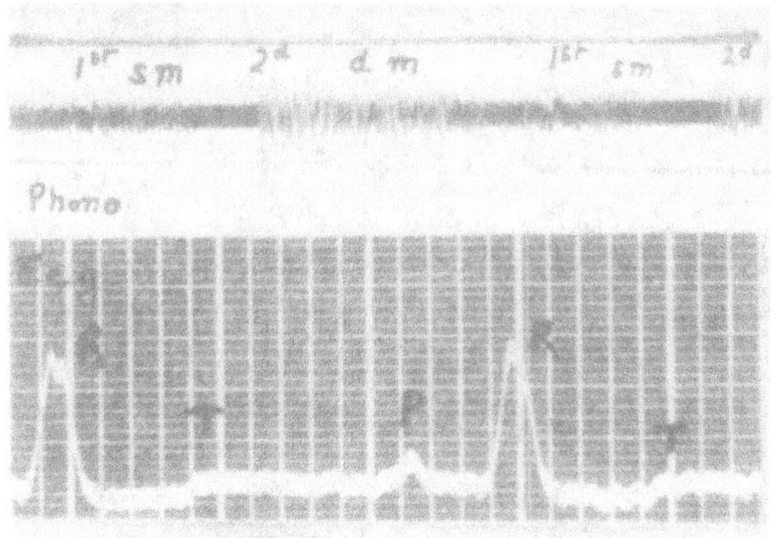

Fig. 4. Early phonocardiographic recording of decrescendo-like murmur of AR. (From Luisada AA. Arch Pediatr 1943;60:498. Reproduced with permission.)

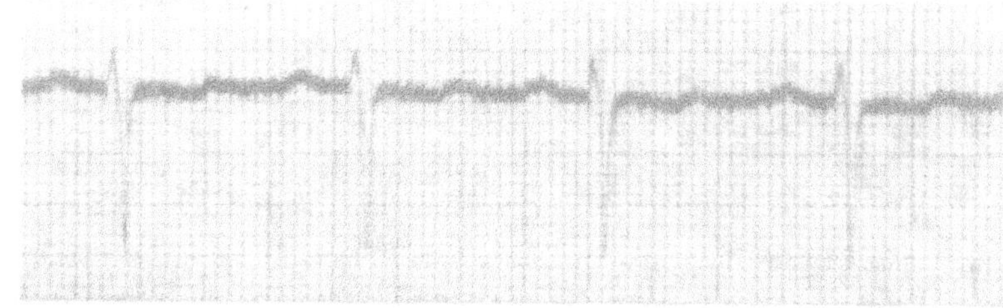

Fig. 5. Electrocardiograph made by Einthoven in 1906 in patient with AR. Recording made from left arm–left leg lead. (From Einthoven W. Arch Int Physiol 1906;4:132-64.)

determination of cardiac shape and size in various cardiac conditions was pioneered by Vaquez and Bordet.[77] In 1913 they observed in AR a lowered, rounded apex and an increased "longitudinal diameter" on the radiograph, findings they attributed to left ventricular hypertrophy. Steel[78] in 1930 differentiated between the radiographic findings in left ventricular hypertrophy and left ventricular dilatation: aortic stenosis was manifested by a change in cardiac shape, and AR by a change in cardiac size. Thus in AR the size of the cardiac silhouette transversely was increased and the apex appeared rounded. Levene and Reid[79] 2 years later emphasized the potential of the roentgenogram in diagnosing cardiac disorders. They observed not only left ventricular dilatation in AR but also left ventricular hypertrophy and an increase in the diameter of the ascending aorta.

Electrocardiography. The first ECG recorded in a patient with AR was by Einthoven[80] in 1906 (Fig. 5).

Although he used only a left arm–left leg lead, Einthoven speculated that the observed downward excursion of the QRS complex was probably due to the left ventricular hypertrophy. Willius[81] in 1920 noted inverted T waves in leads I, II, or III in patients with AR. Lansley[82] in 1921 observed an increased PR interval and a left-sided "preponderance," in addition to T wave inversion in patients with AR. White and Bock[83] in 1918 and White and Burwell[84] in 1924 described left-axis deviation in AR. Willius and Fitzpatrick[85] in 1924 observed "aberrant" QRS complexes, delayed atrioventricular conduction, and rarely atrial fibrillation, in addition to T wave inversion. Singer and Perloff[86] in 1962, in a study of 90 patients with AR, found sinus rhythm in all of them, atrial, nodal, or ventricular premature complexes in 16%, left atrial abnormality in 56%, prolonged PR interval in 37%, complete atrioventricular block in 1%, left-axis deviation in 29%, normal QRS duration in 84%, left bundle branch block in 2%, right bundle

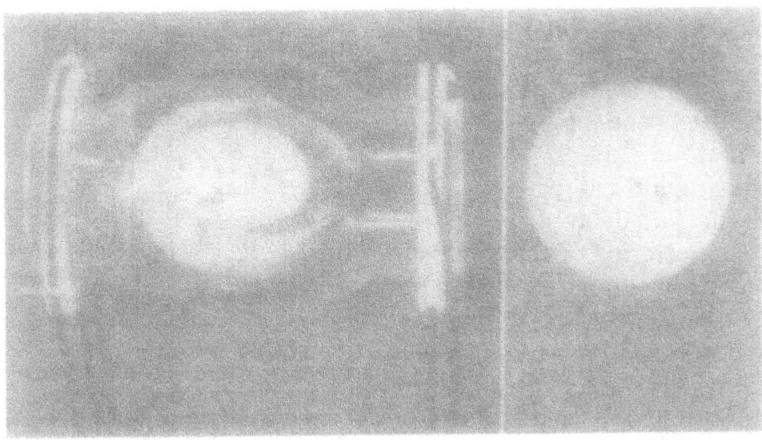

Fig. 6. Hufnagel ball-type valve implanted in 1952 in descending aorta of patient with severe AR. (From Hufnagel CA, Harvey WP, Rabil PJ, McDermott TF. Surgery 1954;35:673. Reproduced with permission.)

branch block in 1%, voltage criteria of left ventricular hypertrophy in 95%, and strain pattern in 69%.

Catheterization and angiocardiography. In 1950 Zimmerman[87] measured left ventricular pressure in 10 patients with AR. The catheter was guided into the left ventricle after being inserted into the radial artery. The left ventricular end-diastolic pressure was increased (average 25 mm Hg) in the seven patients with overt congestive heart failure.

Angiography of the heart and great vessels began in 1929, when Dos Santos et al.[88] injected contrast medium into the abdominal aorta. Ten years later the first countercurrent aortography of the thoracic aorta was performed by Castellanos and Pereiras,[89] who injected contrast medium into what was believed to be the femoral vein but in actuality was the femoral artery. The contrast material was observed in the middescending thoracic aorta. Pérez de los Reyes et al.[90] in 1943 successfully performed retrograde thoracic aortography via the brachial artery, and Radner[91] in 1948 did the same via the radial artery. Bustamente et al.[92] were the first to observe regurgitation of contrast medium into the left ventricle. In 1950 they guided a catheter via the humeral artery to a position 4.5 cm above the aortic valve, at which point the contrast medium was injected and AR observed. Unfortunately the clinical importance of this observation went unnoticed, although these investigators indicated the potential of this technique in other conditions such as patent ductus arteriosus and aortic isthmic coarctation. Castellanos and Garcia[93] in 1953 emphasized the clinical value of retrograde aortography in the diagnosis of AR. Working on both living patients and cadavers, they observed reflux of contrast medium into the left ventricle. Ödman and

Philipson[94] in 1958 found the aortic orifice and the thoracic aorta to be wider than normal in AR. Ross and Criley[95] in 1964 used cineangiocardiography to confirm Flint's postulation that the apical diastolic (Austin Flint) murmur was due to vibration of the anterior mitral leaflet during ventricular diastole.

Echocardiography. The first echocardiograms in a patient with chronic AR demonstrated diastolic vibrations of the anterior mitral leaflet in those patients in whom an Austin Flint murmur was perceptible. Joyner et al.[96] in 1966 observed fluttering of the anterior mitral leaflet by means of ultrasound imaging. Winsberg et al.[97] and Hernberg et al.[98] in 1970 showed fluttering of the anterior mitral leaflet at a frequency of 30 to 40 Hz. Pridie et al.[99] in 1971 used echocardiography to differentiate between organic mitral stenosis and the Austin Flint murmur. Gramiak and Shah[100] in 1970 observed an increase in aortic valve cuspal movement during ventricular systole, and Feizi et al.[101] in 1974 noted the abnormal diastolic separation of aortic valve cuspal echoes in AR. Popp and Harrison[102] in 1970 and Gray and Barritt[103] in 1975 used echocardiography to measure left ventricular diameter from which estimates were made of such parameters as stroke volume.

Several investigators studied AR of recent onset (resulting from infective endocarditis, aortic dissection, or trauma) and found that the echocardiograms differed from those in patients with chronic AR. Pridie et al.[104] in 1970 described premature closure of the mitral valve in AR of acute onset. Nanda et al.[105] recognized diastolic vibration of the anterior mitral leaflet in AR resulting from aortic root dissection. DeMaria et al.[106] in 1975 found acute AR of bacterial endocarditic origin to be associated with premature closure and diastolic vibration of the anterior mitral leaflet; in chronic AR mitral valve preclosure was observed rarely. Thickened aortic valve cusps also were seen in echocardiograms from patients with AR of acute onset. Morganroth et al.[107] in 1977 identified the following echocardiographic characteristics of acute AR: premature closure and delayed opening of the mitral valve, diastolic fluttering of the anterior mitral leaflet (also occurring in chronic AR), normal end-diastolic left ventricular dimensions, normal or decreased septal and free wall motion, and a normal ejection fraction. In chronic AR the echocardiogram revealed increased end-diastolic left ventricular dimensions, increased septal and free wall motion, and an increased ejection fraction. Paoloni et al.[108] in 1977 found left ventricular fractional shortening to be increased in patients with chronic AR who had unimpaired left ventricular function.

Surgical developments. Hufnagel[109, 110] in 1952 successfully implanted a prosthesis in the descending thoracic aorta in a woman with severe AR (Fig. 6). The development of the heart-lung machine[111-113] enabled Harken et al.[114, 115] in 1960 to implant a prosthetic valve in the aortic valve position in a patient with AR.

REFERENCES

1. Singer C. The evolution of anatomy. London: Kegan Pau, Trench, Trubner and Co., Ltd., 1925:17.
2. Doby T. Discoverers of blood circulation. From Aristotle to the times of da Vinci and Harvey. London: Abelard-Schuman, 1963:43.
3. O'Malley CD, Saunders JB de CM. Leonardo da Vinci on the human body. New York: Henry Schuman, 1952:262-71.
4. Cowper W. Of ossifications or petrifactions in the coats of arteries, particularly in the valves of the great artery. Philosophical Transactions of the Royal Society. vol 24. London, 1970-1977:1706.
5. Vieussens R. Traite Nouveau de la structure et des causes du mouvement naturel du coeur. Toulouse, 1715. In: Major RH. Classic descriptions of disease. 3rd ed. Springfield, IL: Charles C Thomas, 1932, 1945:345-6.
6. Morgagni GB. The seats and causes of diseases investigated by anatomy; in five books, containing a great variety of dissections, with remark. To which are added very accurate and copious indexes of the principal things and names therein contained. Translated from Latin by B Alexander in 3 vols. "Facsimile of the London, 1769 edition." vol. I, Book II, Letter XXIII, New York: Hafner Publishing Co., 1960:683, 685.
7. von Haller A. Opuscula pathologica. "Description of calcification of the heart." Lausanne, 1755. In: Willius FA, Keys TE. Cardiac classics. St. Louis: CV Mosby, 1941:170.
8. Bedford DE. An early account of aortic incompetence by Thomas Cuming (1798-1887). Med Hist 1967;11:398-401.
9. Cuming T. A case of diseased heart, with observations. Dublin Hosp Rep 1822;3:319-34.
10. Hodgkin T. On retroversion of the valves of the aorta. London Med Gazette 1829;3:433-43.
11. Hope J. A treatise on the diseases of the heart and great vessels, comprising a new view of the physiology of the heart's action. According to which the physical signs are explained. London: William Kidd, 1832:307-85, 535-8.
12. Corrigan DJ. On permanent patency of the mouth of the aorta, or inadequacy of the aortic valves. Edinburgh Med Surg J 1832;37:225-45.
13. Bouillaud J. Traité clinique des maladies du coeur. vol. 2. Paris: Chez JB Bailliere, 1835; 2nd ed, 1841:265.
14. Billings F. Chronic infectious endocarditis. Arch Intern Med 1909;4:409-31.
15. Libman E. A consideration of the prognosis in subacute bacterial endocarditis. AM HEART J 1922;1:25-40.
16. Taussig HB. Congenital malformations of the heart. New York: The Commonwealth Fund, 1947:19, 401, 433, 482.
17. Campbell M, Baylis JH. The course and prognosis of coarctation of the aorta. Br Heart J 1956;18:475-95.
18. Roberts WC, Morrow AG, McIntosh CL, Jones M, Epstein SE. Congenitally bicuspid aortic valve causing severe, pure aortic regurgitation without superimposed infective endocarditis. Analysis of 13 patients requiring aortic valve replacement. Am J Cardiol 1981;47:206-9.
19. Plenderleath. Rupture of one of the semilunar valves of the aorta. London Med Gazette 1830;7:109-10.
20. Howard CP. Aortic insufficiency due to rupture by strain of a normal aortic valve. Can Med Assoc J 1928;19:12-24.
21. Fothergill JM. The heart and its diseases: With their treatment. London: HK Lewis, 1872:120.
22. Young D, Schwedel JB. The heart in rheumatoid arthritis. A study of thirty-eight autopsy cases. AM HEART J 1944;28:1-23.
23. Goehrs HR, Baggenstoss AH, Slocumb CH. Cardiac lesions in rheumatoid arthritis. Arthritis Rheum 1960;3:298-308.
24. Carpenter DF, Golden A, Roberts WC. Quadrivalvular rheumatoid heart disease associated with left bundle branch block. Am J Med 1967;43:922-9.
25. Roberts WC, Kehoe JA, Carpenter DF, Golden A. Cardiac valvular lesions in rheumatoid arthritis. Arch Intern Med 1968;122:141-6.
26. Burch FE. Association of ectopia lentis with arachnodactyly. Arch Ophthalmol 1936;15:645-76.
27. Rados A. Marfan's syndrome (arachnodactyly coupled with dislocation of the lens). Arch Ophthalmol 1942;27:477-538.
28. Baer RW, Taussig HB, Oppenheimer EH. Congenital aneurysmal dilatation of the aorta associated with arachnodactyly. Bull Johns Hopkins Hosp 1943;72:309-32.
29. Weaver WF, Edwards JE, Brandenburg RO. Idiopathic dilatation of the aorta with aortic valvular insufficiency. A possible forme fruste of Marfan's syndrome. Proc Staff Meeting Mayo Clin 1959;34:518-22.
30. Flaxman N. History of aortic insufficiency. Bull Hist Med 1939;7:192-209.
31. Broadbent WH, Broadbent JFH. Heart disease: With special reference to prognosis and treatment. London: Baillière, Tindall and Cox, 1897:149.
32. Citron J. Ueber Aorteninsufficienz und Lues. Berl Klin Wochenschr 1908;45:2142-6.
33. Lupu N. Untersuchungen über die mikroskopischen Veränderungen der Aortenklappen bei Aortitis syphilitica. Schweiz Med Wochenschr 1920;50:915-8.
34. Scott RW. Syphilitic aortic insufficiency. Arch Intern Med 1924;34:645-57.
35. Clawson BJ, Bell ET. The heart in syphilitic aortitis. Arch Pathol Lab Med 1927;4:922-36.
36. Martland HS. Syphilis of the aorta and heart. AM HEART J 1930;6:1-29.
37. Carr JG. The gross pathology of the heart in cardiovascular syphilis. AM HEART J 1930;6:30-6.
38. Maher CC. Microscopic pathology of cardiac syphilis. AM HEART J 1930;6:36-41.
39. Saphir O, Scott RW. Observations on 107 cases of syphilitic aortic insufficiency, with special reference to the aortic valve area, the myocardium, and branches of the aorta. AM HEART J 1930;6:56-8.
40. Bulkley BH, Roberts WC. Ankylosing spondylitis and aortic regurgitation. Description of the characteristic cardiovascu-

lar lesion from study of eight necropsy patients. Circulation 1973;48:1014-27.

41. Letulle M. Anéurisme disséquant étendu a la totalité de l'aorte et spontanément guéri. Signes d'insuffisance aortique avec intégrité parfaite des valvules sigmoides. Bull Mém Soc Méd Hôp Paris 1905;22:1045-52.

42. Busse O. Ueber Zerreissungen und traumatische Aneurysmen der Aorta. Virchows Arch Pathol Anat Physiol Klin Med 1906;183:440-64.

43. Börger H. Ueber einen Fall von Geheiltem Aneurysma Dissecans der Aorta. Z Klin Med 1906;58:282-95.

44. Resnick WH, Keefer CS. Dissecting aneurysm with signs of aortic insufficiency. Report of a case in which the aortic valves were normal. JAMA 1925;85:422-4.

45. Lundberg A. Three cases of healed aortic rupture. Acta Med Scand 1930;73:19-44.

46. Gravier L. Insuffisance aortique fonctionelle par rupture incomplete de l-'aorte. J Méd Lyon 1924;5:563-6.

47. Wood FC, Pendergrass EP, Ostrum HW. Dissecting aneurysm of the aorta with special reference to its roentgenographic features. Am J Roentgenol Radium Ther 1932;28:437-65.

48. Hamman L, Apperly FL. An instance of spontaneous rupture of the aorta with aortic insufficiency. Int Clin 1933;4:251-72.

49. Gouley BA, Anderson E. Chronic dissecting aneurysm of the aorta, simulating syphilitic cardiovascular diseases. Notes on the associated aortic murmurs. Ann Intern Med 1940;14:978-90.

50. Bergé A, Basch G. Insuffisance aortique par fenestration sigmoidienne réalisée avec l'appoint probable de la dilatation de L'anneau aortique par hypertension. Bull Mém Soc Méd Hôp Paris 1922;46:1700-6.

51. Garvin CF. Functional aortic insufficiency. Ann Intern Med 1940;13:1799-1804.

52. Waller BF, Zoltick JM, Rosen JH, Katz NM, Gomes MN, Fletcher RD, Wallace RB, Roberts WC. Severe aortic regurgitation from systemic hypertension (without aortic dissection) requiring aortic valve replacement. Analysis of four patients. Am J Cardiol 1982;49:473-7.

53. Austen WG, Blennerhassett MB. Giant-cell aortitis causing an aneurysm of the ascending aorta and aortic regurgitation. N Engl J Med 1965;272:80-3.

54. Csonka GW. Litchfield JW, Oates JK, Willcox RR. Cardiac lesions in Reiter's disease. Br Med J 1961;1:243-7.

55. Rodnan GP, Benedek TG, Shaver JA, Fennell RH. Reiter's syndrome and aortic insufficiency. JAMA 1964;189:889-94.

56. Skoda J. Auscultation and percussion. 4th ed. Vienna, 1839. Translated by WO Markham. Philadelphia: Lindsay and Blakiston, 1854:279.

57. Watson T. Lectures on the principles and practice of physic. Delivered at King's College, London. vol. 2. London: John W. Parker, 1843:256.

58. Duroziez PL. Du double souffle intermittent crural, comme signe de l'insuffissance aortique. Arch Gén Méd 1861;107:417-43, 588-605.

59. Traube L. Ueber den Doppleton in der Cruralis Bei Insuffizienz der Aortenklappen. Berl Klin Wochenschr 1872;48:573-4.

60. Flint A. On cardiac murmurs. Am J Med Sci 1862;44:29-54.

61. Quincke H. Beobachtungen ueber Capillar- und Venenpuls. Berl Klin Wochenschr 1868;5:357-8.

62. Mueller F. Zur Pathologie des weichen Gaumens. II. Pulsation des Gaumens bei Aorteninsufficienz. Charité-Annalen 1889;14:251-2.

63. Sailer J. Pulsating spleen in aortic insufficiency. AM HEART J 1928;3:447-53.

64. Dennison AD. Aortic regurgitation; multiple eponyms, physical signs and etiologies. J Ind State Med Assoc 1959;52:1283-9.

65. Delpeuch A. Le signe de musset. Secousses rhythmées de la tete chez les aortiques. Presse Méd 1900;8:237-8.

66. Landolfi M. Un nouveau signe de l'insuffisance aortique. L'hippus circulatoire. Semaine Méd 1909;29:349.

67. Minervini L. Le pouls de la langue dans l'insuffisance aortique. Semaine Méd 1910;30:481-90.

68. Logue RB. A new sign in dissecting aneurysm of aorta. Pulsation of a sternoclavicular joint. JAMA 1952;148:1209-12.

69. Hill L, Rowlands RA. Systolic blood pressure. (1) In change of posture. (2) In cases of aortic regurgitation. Heart 1912;3:219-32.

70. Gladstone S. A few observations on the haemodynamics of the normal circulation; and the changes which occur in aortic insufficiency. Bull Johns Hopkins Hosp 1929;44:83-121.

71. Frank MJ, Casanegra P. Migliori AJ, Levinson GE. The clinical evaluation of aortic regurgitation; with special reference to a neglected sign: the popliteal-brachial pressure gradient. Arch Intern Med 1965;116:357-65.

72. Palfrey FW. Auscultation of the corrigan or water-hammer pulse. N Engl J Med 1952;247:771-2.

73. Harvey WP, Segal JP, Hufnagel CA. Unusual clinical features associated with severe aortic insufficiency. Ann Intern Med 1957;47:27-38.

74. Luisada AA. Clinical applications of phonocardiography. Arch Pediatr 1943;60:498-510.

75. Wells BG, Rappaport MB, Sprague HB. The graphic registration of basal diastolic murmurs. AM HEART J 1949;37:586-611.

76. McKusick VA. Cardiovascular sound in health and disease. Baltimore: Williams & Wilkins Co., 1958:269-85.

77. Vaquez H, Bordet E. Le coeur et l'aorte: Etudes de radiologie clinique. Paris: JB Baillière, 1913:100-10.

78. Steel D. Roentgenological and pathological findings in some of the valvular lesions. Am J Roentgenol Radium Ther 1930;23:384-9.

79. Levene G, Reid WD. The differential diagnosis of organic heart disease by the roentgen ray. Am J Roentgenol Radium Ther 1932;28:466-80.

80. Einthoven W. Le télécardiogramme. Arch Int Physiol 1906;4:132-64.

81. Willius FA. Observations on negativity of the final ventricular T wave of the electrocardiogram. Am Med Sci 1920;160:844-965.

82. Lansley GJ. Aortic incompetence: a clinical study. Lancet 1921;2:1209-12.

83. White PD, Bock AV. Electrocardiographic evidence of abnormal ventricular preponderance and of auricular hypertrophy. Am Med Sci 1918;156:17-9.

84. White PD, Burwell CS. The effect of mitral stenosis, pulmonic stenosis, aortic regurgitation and hypertension on the electrocardiogram. Trans Assoc Am Phys 1924;39:231-4.

85. Willius FA, Fitzpatrick J. Life expectancy with aortic regurgitation. Med J Rec 1924;120:417-21.

86. Singer DH, Perloff JK. Electrocardiogram of free aortic insufficiency [Abstract]. Circulation 1962;26:786-7.

87. Zimmerman HA. Left ventricular pressures in patients with aortic incompetency studied by intracardiac catheterization. J Clin Invest 1950;29:1601-3.

88. Dos Santos R, Lamas, Caldas. L'arteriographie des membres, de l'aorte et de ses branches abdominales. Bull Mém Soc Natl Chir 1929;55:587-601.

89. Castellanos A, Pereiras R. Counter-current aortography. Rev Cubana Cardiol 1939-40;2:187-205.

90. Pérez de los Reyes R, Castellanos A, Pereiras R. Angiocardiography and its value. AM HEART J 1943;25:298-306.

91. Radner S. Thoracal aortography by catheterization from the radial artery. Preliminary report of a new technique. Acta Radiol 1948;29:178-80.

92. Bustamente R, Perez-Stable E, Guerra R, Milanes B. Opacificación de la aorta torácica por el cateterismo de la arteria humeral. Rev Cubana Cardiol 1950;11:96-108.

93. Castellanos A, Garcia O. The diagnosis of aortic insufficiency in the living subject and the cadaver by mean of retrograde aortography. Rev Cubana Pediatr 1953;25:455-70.

94. Ödman P, Philipson J. Aortic valvular diseases studied by percutaneous thoracic aortography. Acta Radiol 1958;suppl:1-172.

95. Ross RS, Criley JM. Cineangiocardiographic studies of the origin of cardiovascular physical signs. Circulation 1964;30:255-61.

96. Joyner CR, Dyrda I, Reid JM. Behavior of the anterior leaflet of the mitral valve in patients with the Austin Flint murmur [Abstract]. Clin Res 1966;14:251.

97. Winsberg F, Gabor GE, Hernberg JG, Weiss B. Fluttering of the mitral valve in aortic insufficiency. Circulation 1970;41:225-9.

98. Hernberg J, Weiss B, Keegan A. The ultrasonic recording of aortic valve motion. Radiology 1970;94:361-8.

99. Pridie RB, Benham R, Oakley CM. Echocardiography of the mitral valve in aortic valve disease. Br Heart J 1971;33:296-304.

100. Gramiak R, Shah PM. Echocardiography of the normal and diseased aortic valve. Radiology 1970;96:1-8.

101. Feizi O, Symons C, Yacoub M. Echocardiography of the aortic valve. I. Studies of normal aortic valve, aortic stenosis, aortic regurgitation and mixed aortic valve disease. Br Heart J 1974;36:341-51.

102. Popp RL, Harrison DC. Ultrasonic cardiac echography for determining stroke volume and valvular regurgitation. Circulation 1970;41:493-502.

103. Gray KE, Barritt DW. Echocardiographic assessment of severity of aortic regurgitation. Br Heart J 1975;37:691-9.

104. Pridie RB, Benham R, Oakley CM. Recognition of aortic regurgitation of recent onset by ultrasound technique [Abstract]. Am J Cardiol 1970;26:654-5.

105. Nanda NC, Gramiak R, Shah PM. Diagnosis of aortic root dissection by electrocardiography. Circulation 1973;48:506-13.

106. DeMaria AN, King JF, Salel AF, Caudill CC, Miller RR, Mason DT. Echography and phonography of acute aortic regurgitation in bacterial endocarditis. Ann Intern Med 1975;82:329-35.

107. Morganroth J, Perloff JK, Zeldis SM, Dunkman B. Acute severe aortic regurgitation. Pathophysiology, clinical recognition, and management. Ann Intern Med 1977;87:223-32.

108. Paoloni HJ, Wilcken DEL, Dado MJ. The role of echocardiography in the assessment of chronic aortic regurgitation. Aust NZ J Med 1977;7:491-6.

109. Hufnagel CA, Harvey WP. The surgical correction of aortic regurgitation: preliminary report. Bull Georgetown Univ Med Center 1953;6:60-1.

110. Hufnagel CA, Harvey WP, Rabil PJ, McDermott TF. Surgical correction of aortic insufficiency. Surgery 1954;35:673-83.

111. Gibbon JH. Artificial maintenance of circulation during experimental occlusion of pulmonary artery. Arch Surg 1937;34:1105-31.

112. Dennis C, Spreng DS, Nelson GE, Karlson KE, Nelson RM, Thomas JV, Eder WP, Varco RL. Development of a pump-oxygenator to replace the heart and lungs; an apparatus applicable to human patients, and application to one case. Ann Surg 1951;134:709-21.

113. Newman MH, Stuckey JH, Levowitz BS, Young LA, Dennis C, Fries C, Gorayeb EJ, Zuhdi M, Karlson KE, Adler S, Gliedman M. Complete and partial perfusion of animal and human subjects with the pump oxygenator; a study of factors yielding consistent survival; successful application to one case. Surgery 1955;38:30-7.

114. Harken DE, Soroff HS, Taylor WJ, Lefemine AA, Gupta SK, Lunzer S. Partial and complete prostheses in aortic insufficiency. J Thorac Cardiovasc Surg 1960;40:744-62.

115. Harken DE, Taylor WJ, Lefemine AA, Lunzer S, Low HBC, Cohen ML, Jacobey JA. Aortic valve replacement with a caged ball valve. Am J Cardiol 1962;9:292-9.

Causes of Pure Aortic Regurgitation in Patients Having Isolated Aortic Valve Replacement at a Single US Tertiary Hospital (1993 to 2005)

William Clifford Roberts, MD; Jong Mi Ko, BA;
Timothy Richard Moore, MD; William Hampton Jones III, MD

Background—The causes of aortic regurgitation (AR) severe enough to warrant aortic valve replacement (AVR) have received little attention in the last 20 years.

Methods and Results—We analyzed the causes of pure AR in 268 patients >20 years of age having isolated AVR at Baylor University Medical Center from 1993 to 2005 that was unassociated with mitral stenosis, mitral valve replacement, or a previous operation involving a cardiac valve or ascending aorta. In 122 patients (46%), the AR resulted from a problem with the aortic valve: congenital malformation unassociated with infective endocarditis, 66 patients (54%); infective endocarditis, 46 patients (38%; 15 with bicuspid valves); probable rheumatic heart disease, 8 patients (6%); and miscellaneous, 2 patients (2%). In the other 146 patients (54%), the AR was the consequence of a condition affecting the ascending aorta: dissection, 28 patients (19%); the Marfan syndrome or its forme fruste variety, 15 patients (10%); aortitis, 12 patients (8%), and in the remaining 91 patients (62%), the cause of the AR was not determined. This latter group was the oldest (mean age 66 years), 83 (91%) had hypertension, 26 (29%) had small calcific deposits in the valve cusps, and 46 (51%) had simultaneous coronary artery bypass grafting.

Conclusions—The causes of pure AR severe enough to warrant isolated AVR are diverse. The most common category in this study was "cause unclear." (***Circulation***. 2006;114:422-429.)

Key Words: bypass ■ calcium ■ coronary disease ■ hypertension ■ regurgitation

---

In contrast to aortic stenosis, which essentially has 3 causes (congenital, atherosclerotic, and rheumatic),[1–3] pure aortic regurgitation (AR; no element of aortic stenosis) has multiple causes, some of which directly affect the aortic valve and others of which are due to problems with the aorta without direct involvement of the aortic valve. Furthermore, unlike aortic stenosis, which essentially is always a slowly progressing chronic condition, AR may develop acutely (acute AR) or over a prolonged period (chronic AR). This report analyzes the causes of pure AR in patients having isolated aortic valve replacement (AVR) at Baylor University Medical Center (Dallas, Texas) from 1993 to 2005.

Clinical Perspective p 429

Methods

Since March 1993, all operatively excised cardiac valves and aortas submitted to the surgical pathology division of the depart-ment of pathology have been examined and described by one of us (W.C.R.). Additionally, the preoperative cardiac catheterization and echocardiographic data, and often pertinent clinical records and operative notes, on most of these patients have been obtained.

The present study was limited to patients who, before AVR, had either no gradient or a negative gradient between peak systolic left ventricular and peak systolic aortic pressures or at least a transvalvular peak systolic pressure gradient of ≤10 mm Hg. Patients with associated mitral valve disease that required mitral replacement or repair or insertion of an annular ring, patients ≤20 years of age at the time of AVR, patients with a previous operation involving the ascending aorta or a cardiac valve, and patients with associated ventricular septal defect or discrete subaortic stenosis or hypertrophic cardiomyopathy were excluded. Mild degrees of mitral regurgitation preoperatively did not exclude patients from inclusion in the present study.

Most operatively excised valves and most operatively excised aortas were weighed (all by W.C.R.) on an Ohaus scale (Ohaus Corporation, Florham Park, NJ) accurate to 2 decimal places. All operatively excised valves and most aortas were photographed. The valves that contained vegetations were sectioned and processed in

---

Received February 27, 2006; revision received May 19, 2006; accepted May 30, 2006.

From the Departments of Pathology and Medicine (Division of Cardiology), Baylor Heart & Vascular Institute (W.C.R., J.M.K.), Baylor University Medical Center, Dallas, Tex; Heart Center, Brownwood Regional Medical Center (T.R.M.), Brownwood, Tex; and Cardiology Association of North Mississippi (W.H.J.), Tupelo, Miss.

Drs Moore and Jones were Cardiology Fellows at Baylor University Medical Center, Dallas, Tex, at the time of this study.

Correspondence to William C. Roberts, MD, Baylor Heart & Vascular Institute, Baylor University Medical Center, 3500 Gaston Ave, Dallas, TX 75246. E-mail wc.roberts@baylorhealth.edu

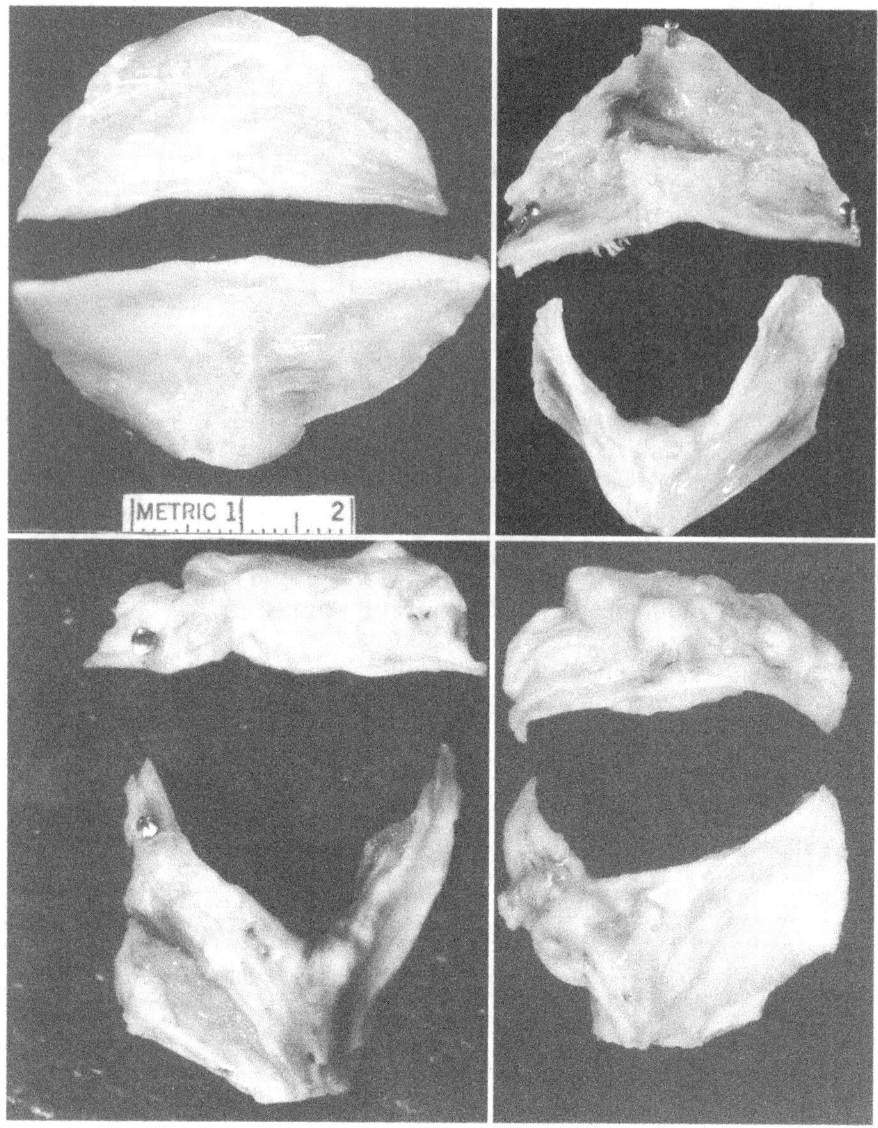

Figure 1. Congenitally bicuspid aortic valves unassociated with infective endocarditis in 4 men. Upper left, Age 53 years. The valve was devoid of calcific deposits and weighed 1.69 g. Upper right, Age 56 years. The valve weighed 1.65 g. Lower left, Age 66 years. The valve weighed 1.05 g. Lower right, Age 71 years. The valve weighed 2.43 g. The last 3 valves had calcific deposits on both cusps, mainly in their raphe.

alcohols and xylene, and sections were cut and stained, one with hematoxylin-eosin and another with the Gram method. All aortas were also processed for histological study and, after they were cut, were stained, one with hematoxylin-eosin and another by the Movat method.

The study protocol was approved by the Institutional Review Board of Baylor University Medical Center.

The authors had full access to the data and take full responsibility for its integrity. All authors have read and agree to the manuscript as written.

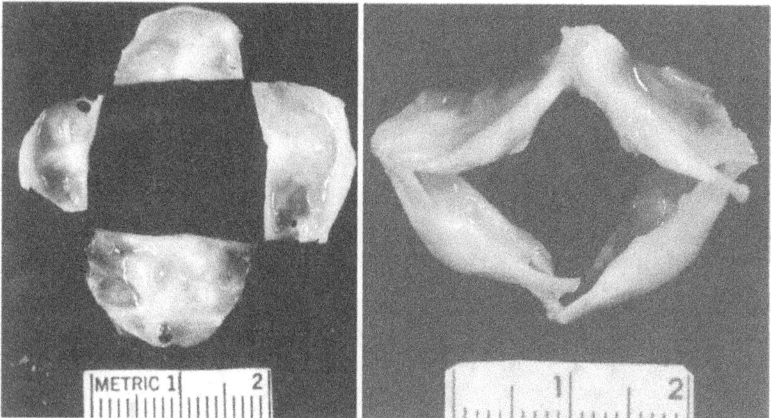

Figure 2. Congenitally quadricuspid aortic valves in 2 women. Left, Age 79 years. The valve weighed 0.57 g. Right, Age 53 years. The valve weighed 1.13 g.

TABLE 1. Causes of AR in Patients Having Isolated AVR at Baylor University Medical Center (1993–2005)

Cause of AR	Total	Ages at Operation, Range (Mean), y	M	F	Acute	Chronic	SH	Coronary Artery Bypass Grafting	Portions of Ascending Aorta		
									Excised	Examined Histologically	CMN (3+, 4+)
Valve (122 [46%])											
Congenital malformation without Infective endocarditis											
Bicuspid	59 (22%)	22–77 (55)	49	10	0	59	39 (66%)	18 (31%)	22	22	11
Quadricuspid	2 (1%)	53–79 (66)	0	2	0	2	0	1 (50%)	0	0	0
Tricuspid	5 (2%)	33–48 (40)	3	2	0	5	2 (40%)	0	1	1	0
Infective endocarditis	46 (17%)	21–82 (45)	31	15	27	19	29 (63%)	7 (15%)	6	4	0
Rheumatic?	8 (3%)	25–63 (47)	6	2	0	8	6 (75%)	2 (25%)	0	0	0
Miscellaneous	2 (1%)	24–42 (33)	1	1	0	2	2 (100%)	1 (50%)	0	0	0
Nonvalve (146 [54%])											
Aortic dissection	28 (10%)	25–78 (58)	20	8	21	7	22 (79%)	5* (17%)	28	20	5
Marfan or forme fruste	15 (6%)	21–71 (47)	9	6	0	15	10 (67%)	1† (7%)	15	13	13
Aortitis	12 (4%)	35–82 (66)	5	7	0	12	10 (83%)	5 (42%)	12	12	12
Cause unclear	91 (34%)	50–84 (66)	58	33	0	91	83 (91%)	46 (51%)	7	7	0
Total	268 (100%)	21–84 (57)	182 (68%)	86 (32%)	48 (18%)	220 (82%)	203 (76%)	86 (32%)	91 (34%)	76	41

SH indicates systemic hypertension; M, male; F, female; CMN, cystic medial necrosis; and BAV, bicuspid aortic valve.

Cystic medial necrosis is used here to refer to the magnitude of loss of elastic fibers in the aorta's media.

*Four other patients had CABG due to extension of the aortic dissection into a coronary artery.

†One additional patient had CABG due to extension of the aortic dissection into a coronary artery.

‡No. of cases with aortic valve weight.

Results

The study included all patients having AVR for pure AR who met the above criteria and had AVR from March 24, 1993, to March 31, 2005. A total of 268 patients aged 21 to 84 years (mean 57 years) met the above criteria, and the findings in these patients are summarized in Table 1. The 268 patients were divided into 2 major groups: those in whom the AR was secondary to a problem with the valve (n=122, 46%) and those in whom the AR was secondary to a problem with the ascending aorta (nonvalve; n=146, 54%). Of the 268 patients, 48 (18%) had acute AR, which in 27 was due to active infective endocarditis and in 21 to acute aortic dissection; the remaining 220 patients had chronic AR.

Hemodynamic or echocardiographic data were available in 235 (88%) of the 268 patients: One hundred thirty-seven patients had both cardiac catheterization data and echocardiographic data available; 40 other patients had only cardiac catheterization data available, and 58 others had only echocardiographic data available. Of the 177 patients with hemodynamic data from cardiac catheterization, 67 (38%) had transvalvular peak systolic pressure gradients that varied from 1 to 10 mm Hg.

Of the 268 operatively excised aortic valves, the valve was weighed in 226 patients, and its weight ranged from 0.48 to 2.99 g (mean 1.22 g) in the men and from 0.31 to 2.50 g (mean 0.81 g) in the women. Of the 91 patients in whom portions of ascending aorta were resected, the resected specimens were weighed on the same scales in 63 (69%) and ranged from 0.40 to 60 g (median 13 g) in the men and from 0.40 to 37 g (median 13 g) in the women. Whether the ascending aorta was resected was determined by its size, by its appearance, and by the operator. Of the latter 63 patients, the aorta weighed ≤4 g in 13 patients and >4 g in 50 patients.

Valve Problem

Congenital Malformation of the Aortic Valve Unassociated With Infective Endocarditis

This group included 59 patients with congenitally bicuspid aortic valves (Figure 1), 2 with quadricuspid valves (Figure 2), and 5 with tricuspid valves (Figure 3). At operation in each of the latter 5 patients, 1 or 2 of the 3 aortic valve cusps was described as being prolapsed such that the free margins of the cusps did not coapt with each other at the same cephalad level. Examination of the operatively excised valves in these 5 patients did not disclose cuspal inequality but indeed similar-sized cusps. In other words, examination of the operatively excised valves in these 5 patients did not allow us to determine or predict which cusps had prolapsed. In 19 (32%) of the 59 patients with congenitally bicuspid aortic valves, the ascending aorta was dilated, and a large portion (>4 g) of it was resected. Histological study of the

TABLE 1. Continued

BAV	Calcium Deposits on AV Cusps	Aortic Valve Weight (g), Range (Mean)	
		Men	Women
59	31	0.52–2.99 (1.42)	0.68–1.80 (1.24)
0	0	...	0.57–1.13 (0.85)
0	0	1.11–1.40 (1.23)	0.34–0.66 (0.50)
15	8	0.77–2.31 (1.53)	0.44–2.50 (0.98)
0	3	1.10–2.45 (1.81)	1.31–1.83 (1.57)
0	0	0.55	...
3	4	0.51–1.19 (0.81)	0.37–0.90 (0.59)
0	2	0.73–1.01 (0.94)	0.35–0.85 (0.66)
0	2	0.63–0.79 (0.70)	0.35–0.70 (0.54)
0	26	0.48–2.13 (1.08)	0.31–1.74 (0.73)
77 (29%)	76/263 (29%)	0.48–2.99 (1.22) 151‡	0.31–2.50 (0.81) 75‡

resected aorta showed severe loss of medial elastic fibers in 11 cases (58%).

Infective Endocarditis

In 46 patients, the cause of the pure AR was infective endocarditis (Figure 4), which was active in 27 patients (59%) and healed in 19 (41%). Each of the 27 patients with active infective endocarditis had an acute onset of AR, whereas each of the 19 patients with healed infective endocarditis had chronic AR. Of these 46 patients, 15 (33%) had the infection superimposed on a 2-cuspid aortic valve, and in the other 31 patients (67%), the infection involved a 3-cuspid aortic valve.

Probable Rheumatic Heart Disease

In 8 patients, the pure AR was attributed to rheumatic heart disease (Figure 5). Each of the 3 cusps in each of these 8 patients was quite thickened, mainly by fibrous tissue, but in 3 of the 8 patients, the cusps also contained small calcific deposits. Cardiac catheterization in 5 of these 8 patients disclosed small (2 to 9 mm Hg) peak systolic pressure gradients between left ventricle and aorta. None of these 8 patients had hemodynamic or echocardiographic evidence of mitral stenosis, although mild mitral regurgitation was present in several of them.

Miscellaneous

Two patients had 3-cuspid aortic valves that were mildly and focally thickened by fibrous tissue. No abnormalities of the aorta were described. One patient, a 24-year-old woman, had the Behçet syndrome with multiple noncardiovascular problems. The other patient, a 42-year-old obese woman, took phentermine-fenfluramine, and the AR was believed to be related to that medication. Histologically, however, no features of the phentermine-fenfluramine (carcinoid) valve lesion were evident.

Aortic (Nonvalve) Problem

Aortic Dissection With Tear in Ascending Aorta

In 28 patients, the AR was secondary to aortic dissection, acute in 21 (75%) and healed in 7 (25%; Figure 6). Portions of ascending aorta were excised in all 21 cases with acute dissection and were weighed in 10 cases; the resected aorta weighed from 0.40 to 51 g (median 13 g). Histologically, the number of patients with a clear loss of medial elastic fibers was 3. In 7 with healed dissection, the 6 resected aortas weighed from 11 to 60 g (mean 38 g); histologically, the media contained a normal number of elastic fibers in 5 and were severely deficient in elastic fibers in 2 patients.

The Marfan Syndrome and Forme Fruste Varieties of It

Pure AR was attributed to the Marfan syndrome in 15 patients. The resected ascending aorta weighed from 6 to 24 g (mean 13 g); portions of the resected aortas in 13 cases submitted for histological study showed massive loss of medial elastic fibers with normal intima and adventitia, which resulted in an aortic wall that was thinner than normal, and each of them had intima-media tears, without dissection in 14 and with dissection in 1.

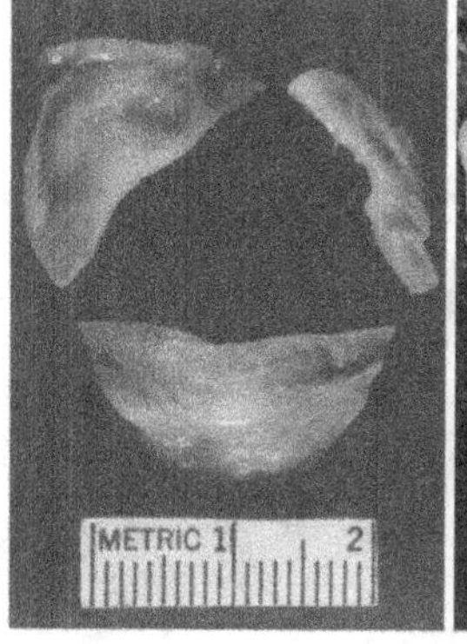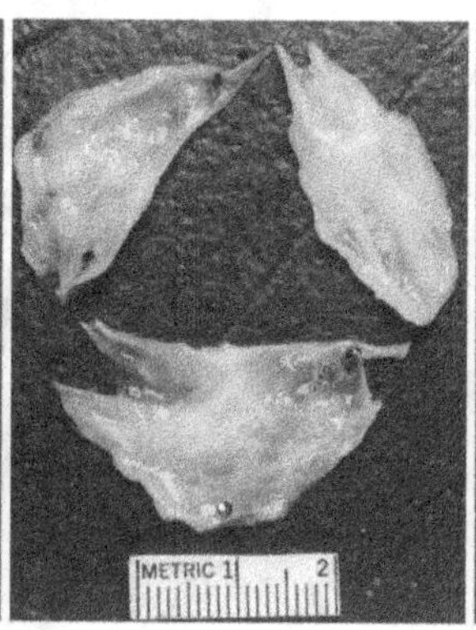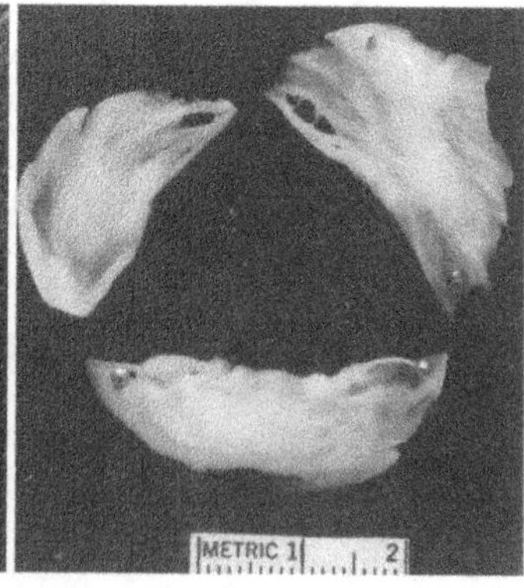

Figure 3. Congenitally malformed tricuspid aortic valves. Left, In a 33-year-old woman, the valve weighed 0.34 g. Middle, In a 44-year-old man, the valve weighed 1.11 g. Right, In a 33-year-old man, the valve weighed 1.19 g. Which of these cusps were attached more caudally than normal was not discernible after the cusps had been excised.

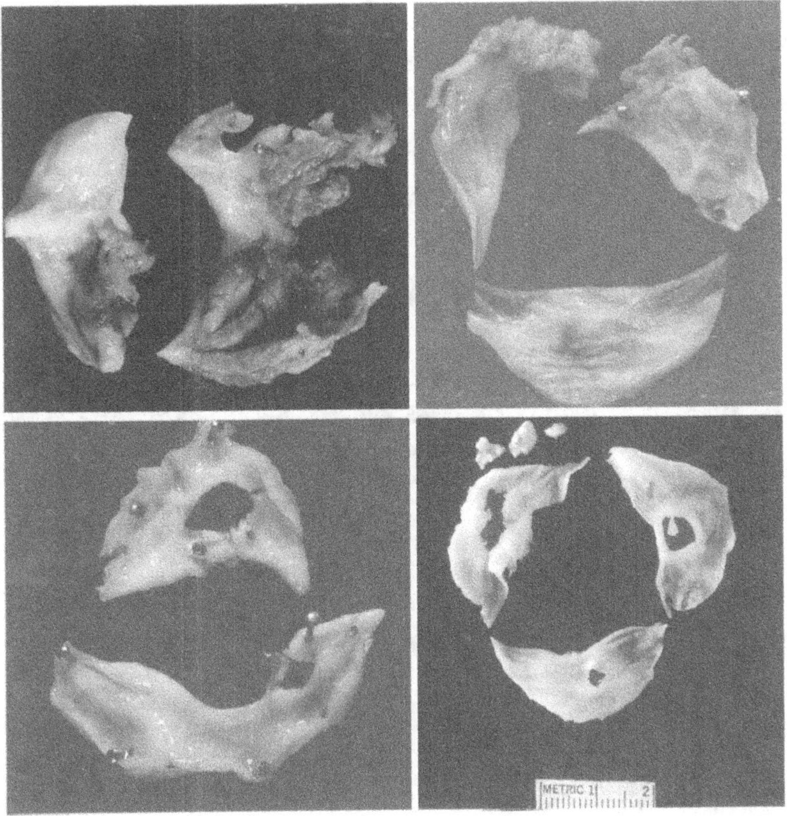

Figure 4. Infective endocarditis. Upper left, Acute infection in a bicuspid valve in a 41-year-old man. Upper right, Acute infection in a tricuspid valve in a 40-year-old man. The valve weighed 1 g. Lower left, Healed infection with cuspal perforations in a bicuspid valve in a 27-year-old man. The valve weighed 0.86 g. Lower right, Healed infection with cuspal perforations in a tricuspid valve in a 69-year-old man. The valve weighed 0.96 g.

Diffuse Aortitis

The AR was secondary to diffuse aortitis of the ascending aorta in 12 patients (Figure 7): granulomatous in 3 and nongranulomatous in 9. Eight (aged 42 to 82 years [mean 67 years]) of the latter 9 patients had typical histological features of syphilis; the ninth, aged 35 years, was believed to have Takayasu arteritis. In the 3 patients with granulomatous aortitis, its cause was not determined. The only difference between these 2 types of aortitis was the presence of multinucleated giant cells in 1 group and their absence in the other group. In both groups, both the intima and the adventitia were considerably thickened, mainly by fibrous tissue. The resected ascending aorta weighed from 0.40 to 25 g (median 18 g). Of these 12 patients, 8 were ≥65 years of age.

Cause Unclear

Each patient in this group had 3-cuspid aortic valves (Figure 8). Seven, aged from 51 to 81 years (mean 67 years), had a portion of the ascending aorta excised (weight 1 to 31 g [median 12 g]), but 3 were small biopsies. In all 7, the aorta histologically was normal. Most of them had mildly dilated aortas, probably the result of aging alone. Of these 91 patients, 83 (91%) had either a history of systemic hypertension or a directly or indirectly measured peak systolic systemic pressure >140 mm Hg. Of these 91 patients, 46 (51%) also had coronary artery bypass grafting at the time of AVR.

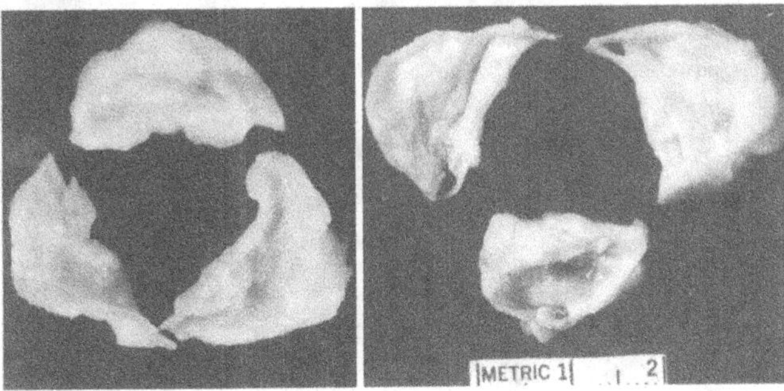

Figure 5. Probable rheumatic heart disease. Left, Tricuspid valve in a 60-year-old man. The valve weighed 2.06 g. Right, Tricuspid valve in a 55-year-old man. The valve weighed 1.52 g. The cusps in both patients are thickened by fibrous tissue.

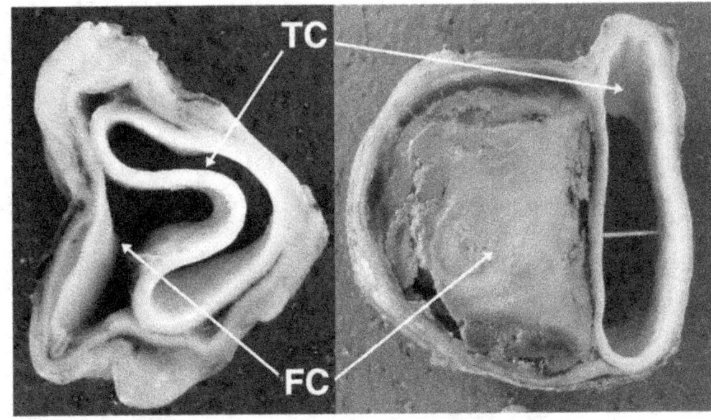

Figure 6. Aortic dissection. Left, Cross section of a portion of ascending aorta in an acute dissection in a 42-year-old man. The partition between the false channel (FC) and the true channel (TC) buckled into the lumen of the TC. Right, Cross section of a portion of ascending aorta in a healed dissection in a 79-year-old man. The FC is filled with a thrombus and is larger than the TC.

Discussion

The present study describes causes of pure (no element of stenosis) AR in 268 patients having isolated AVR unassociated with mitral stenosis or mitral valve replacement. The patients were divided into 2 groups: those in whom the cause of the AR was a problem with the valve (46%) and those in whom the cause was a problem with the aorta (54%). Hemodynamic or echocardiographic data were available in 235 patients (88%). All excised valves and ascending aortas were examined by the same physician (W.C.R.), who has been examining operatively excised aortic valves for 45 years.

Several findings in the present study were surprising to the authors, the main one being the high frequency with which we were unable to determine the cause of the AR, an occurrence in 91 patients (34% of the total or 62% of the 146 patients in whom the AR was considered the consequence of a problem with the aorta). The ages of these 91 patients were among the oldest of any of the groups, namely, 50 to 84 years (mean 66 years), and all 91 had tricuspid aortic valves. Although probably all had some degree of dilatation of the ascending aorta, mainly due to aging,[4] only 4 had significant portions of the ascending aorta resected, and in each of them, it was histologically normal. Of these 91 patients, at least 83 (91%) had either a transvalvular peak systolic aortic pressure >140 mm Hg, an end-diastolic aortic pressure >90 mm Hg, or both. It appears reasonable to believe that the systemic hypertension in some way caused or at least contributed to the AR in these patients. The operatively excised aortic valve cusps contained small calcific deposits in 26 (29%) of these 91 patients, but the valve weights were relatively small- (mean 0.73 g in women and 1.08 g in men). Almost certainly, some of these 91 patients had a cardiac operation primarily because of severe coronary artery disease; 46 (51%) of these 91 patients had CABG. Nevertheless, the degree of AR appears to have been similar in the patients with versus those without simultaneous coronary bypass. In 79 of these 91 patients, the degree of AR was classified by either aortic angiography or echocardiography; the AR was severe in 67 (85%) and mild to moderate in 12 (15%).

That systemic hypertension can cause AR severe enough to warrant AVR has been debated. Waller and colleagues[5] in 1982 described 4 patients with severe AR from systemic hypertension (without aortic dissection) who underwent AVR, and they reviewed previously reported patients with systemic hypertension and pure AR. Of their 4 patients, the systemic arterial pressures ≈1 month postoperatively remained elevated in 2 of the 3 survivors. Among previous reports describing precordial murmurs consistent with AR in patients with systemic hypertension, Waller and colleagues found 7 studies that analyzed 79 patients with AR associated with systemic hypertension, and 17 had severe AR with evidence of considerable heart failure. In 11 of the 17 patients, systemic hypertension appeared to be the only reasonable cause of the AR. Barlow and Kincaid-Smith[6] studied 100 patients with systemic hypertension and peak systolic pressures >180 mm Hg; 9 had diastolic blowing murmurs consistent with AR. Their report and reports of others pointed out that among hypertensive

patients, the higher the systemic arterial pressure, the greater the chance that AR would develop. Among patients with similar levels of systemic arterial pressure, older patients had a higher frequency of AR than did younger patients. Of patients of similar age and with similar blood pressures, those with systemic hypertension of longer duration had a higher frequency of AR than did those with hypertension of shorter duration. Among the few patients with severe AR due to systemic hypertension, arterial diastolic pressure is usually >60 mm Hg; nevertheless, the pulse pressure is high (often >100 mm Hg).

Another finding, not unexpected, was the high frequency of a congenitally bicuspid aortic valve, which occurred in 77 (29%) of the 268 patients, including 74 (61%) of the 122 patients in whom the AR was a consequence of a valve problem and 3 (2%) of the 146 patients in whom the AR appeared to be the consequence of a problem with the aorta. All 3 of the latter patients were among the 28 patients with aortic dissection. Thus, 11% of the patients in whom the AR resulted from aortic dissection had a congenitally bicuspid aortic valve. Of the 74 patients with a congenitally bicuspid aortic valve, the AR in 59 (80%) was in patients who had never had a clinical event compatible with active or healed infective endocarditis and 15 (33%) were in the 46 patients in whom the AR appeared to result from active or healed infective endocarditis superimposed on a congenitally bicuspid aortic valve. Small calcific deposits were present in 34 (44%) of the 77 congenitally bicuspid aortic valves. The calcific deposits usually were localized to the raphe. Although its high frequency in patients with aortic valve stenosis is well appreciated, the bicuspid aortic valve as a cause of pure AR—at least, when unassociated with infective endocarditis—is less well appreciated. Indeed, that a bicuspid aortic valve could cause AR severe enough to warrant AVR in the absence of active or healed infective endocarditis was not described initially until 1981.[7]

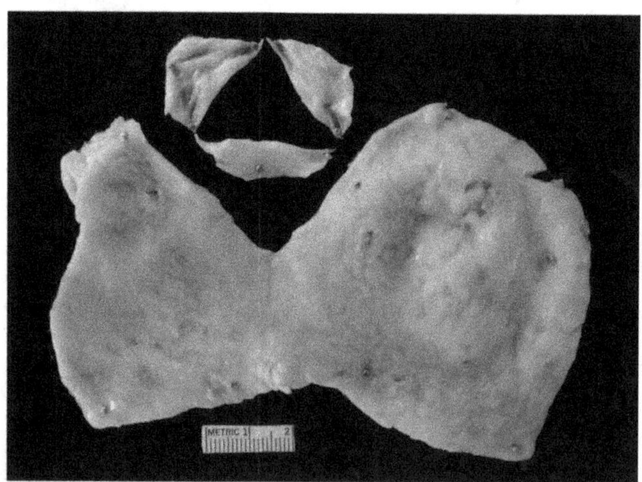

Figure 7. Diffuse aortitis. Valve and a portion of an ascending aorta in a 69-year-old man with syphilis. The aortic wall is thickened, and the intimal surface is 100% involved by the process. The tricuspid aortic valve is essentially normal and weighed 0.63 g.

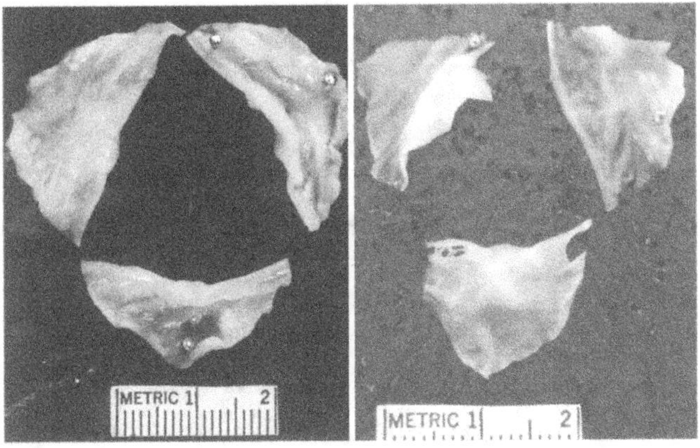

Figure 8. Cause of AR unclear. Left, Valve in a 74-year-old man. The valve weighed 1.08 g. Right, Valve in a 56-year-old woman. The valve weighed 0.31 g. The cusps are focally but minimally thickened.

In addition to the findings of a congenitally bicuspid aortic valve in 77 patients, 7 other patients had congenitally malformed aortic valves. Two had quadricuspid valves, and 5 had tricuspid aortic valves. In each of the latter 5 patients, 1 or 2 of the 3 cusps was attached more caudally than usual such that the free margins of these cusps did not coapt with the normally attached cusp(s), which resulted in prolapse. The prolapsed cusp, however, was usually similar in size to the nonprolapsed cusps, just attached more caudally. That a tricuspid aortic valve can be congenitally malformed or malpositioned is not a well-recognized cause of AR.

Portions of the ascending aorta were resected in 91 (34%) of the 268 patients, and in 63 of them, the excised portion of aorta was weighed (range 0.40 to 60 g [median 13 g] in men and 0.40 to 37 g [median 13 g] in women); in 13 patients (21%), the excised portion of aorta weighed ≤4 g, and in the other 50 patients, it weighed >4 g. Ascending aortas having features of the Marfan syndrome, aortitis (usually syphilis), and acute or healed dissection were excised. Patients having AR secondary to congenitally bicuspid aortic valves unassociated with infective endocarditis often (22 [37%] of 59 patients) had portions of the aorta excised, and the aortas histologically usually had evidence of loss of medial elastic fibers.

There are few reported studies to which the present data can be compared. Roberts and colleagues[7] in 1981 briefly described causes of pure AR in 177 patients, aged 18 to 70 years, having AVR at the National Heart, Lung, and Blood Institute from 1963 to 1979. Of the 177 patients fulfilling the same criteria as in the present study, these authors attributed the AR to rheumatic heart disease in 94 patients (53%); to infective endocarditis in 41 (23%; bicuspid aortic valve in 7 and tricuspid valve in 34); to the Marfan syndrome or its forme fruste variety in 15 (8%); to a congenitally bicuspid aortic valve unassociated with infective endocarditis in 13 (7%)[7]; to syphilis in 9 (5%); to aortic dissection in 2 (1%); and to trauma in 1 (<1%). Thus, there were no patients in whom the AR was attributed to an unclear cause.

Olson and colleagues[8] in 1984 described 221 patients with "clinically pure aortic insufficiency" having AVR at the Mayo Clinic during the 4 years of 1965, 1970, 1975, and 1980. In contrast to the present study, however, these authors included patients who also had simultaneous mitral valve replacement (80 patients [36%]) or who were aged <20 years (8 patients), and none had the presence of pure AR confirmed by hemodynamic data, angiography, or echocardiography. Rheumatic heart disease was the most frequent cause of "clinically pure" AR in their patient population (100 [45%] of 221 patients). The second most common cause was "idiopathic aortic dilatation" (43/221 [19%]). We suspect that their group of "idiopathic aortic dilatation" would have been similar to our group classified as "cause unclear." The Mayo clinic study did not provide information on blood pressure, and therefore, the frequency of hypertension in this group is not known. Their third most common cause of AR was congenitally bicuspid aortic valve unassociated with either infective endocarditis or aortic dissection (42/221 [19%]). Infective endocarditis was next (21/221 [10%], 9 of whom had a bicuspid aortic valve). Other causes included the Marfan syndrome (4 patients), aortic dissection (3 patients, each of whom had a bicuspid aortic valve), ankylosing spondylitis (3 patients), indeterminate (2 patients), and syphilis (1 patient). Their study did not include any information regarding coronary artery bypass grafting or resection of the ascending aorta, and there was no information regarding preoperative echocardiographic or hemodynamic data.

No previous studies have weighed operatively excised purely regurgitant aortic valves. Table 2 shows the range and mean weights of the purely regurgitant aortic valves in the present study and the weights for comparative

TABLE 2. Comparison of Aortic Valve Weight (g) in Patients Having Isolated AVR for Pure AR Versus Aortic Stenosis (With or Without Associated AR)*

	Bicuspid		Tricuspid	
	Men	Women	Men	Women
AR	0.52–2.99 (1.39)	0.68–1.80 (1.24)	0.48–2.45 (1.06)	0.31–1.83 (0.70)
No. of cases with aortic valve weight	45	9	86	55
AS†	0.89–11.30 (3.57)	0.73–4.97 (2.30)	1.03–6.60 (2.40)	0.45–4.81 (1.56)
No. of cases with aortic valve weight	237	104	181	152

*Patients with infective endocarditis were excluded.
†Data from Roberts et al.[3]

purposes of operatively excised stenotic aortic valves-
(with or without associated AR).[3] In both groups, the
mean weights were heavier in the men than in the women. The mean weights of the purely regurgitant valves
ranged from 39% to 54% of the mean weights of the
stenotic valves. The normal aortic valve in adults weighs
≈ 0.5 g.[9]

Disclosures

None.

References

1. Roberts WC, Ko JM. Weights of operatively-excised stenotic unicuspid,
   bicuspid, and tricuspid aortic valves and their relation to age, sex, body
   mass index, and presence or absence of concomitant coronary artery
   bypass grafting. *Am J Cardiol.* 2003;92:1057–1065.
2. Roberts WC, Ko JM. Frequency by decades of unicuspid, bicuspid, and tricuspid
   aortic valves in adults having isolated aortic valve replacement for aortic stenosis,
   with or without associated aortic regurgitation. *Circulation.* 2005;111:920–925.
3. Roberts WC, Ko JM, Hamilton C. Comparison of valve structure, valve
   weight, and severity of the valve obstruction in 1849 patients having
   isolated aortic valve replacement for aortic valve stenosis (with or without
   associated aortic regurgitation) studied at 3 different medical centers in 2
   different time periods. *Circulation.* 2005;112:3919–3929.
4. Roberts WC. Morphological features of the elderly heart. In: Tresch D,
   Aronow WS. 2nd ed. *Cardiovascular Disease in the Elderly Patient.* New
   York, NY: Marcel Dekker; 1999:17–42.
5. Waller BF, Zoltick JM, Rosen JH, Katz NM, Gomes MN, Fletcher RD,
   Wallace RB, Roberts WC. Severe aortic regurgitation from systemic
   hypertension (without aortic dissection) requiring aortic valve
   replacement. *Am J Cardiol.* 1982;49:473–477.
6. Barlow J, Kincaid-Smith P. The auscultatory findings in hypertension. *Br
   Heart J.* 1960;22:505–514.
7. Roberts WC, Morrow AG, McIntosh CL, Jones M, Epstein SE. Congenitally bicuspid aortic valve causing severe, pure aortic regurgitation
   without superimposed infective endocarditis. *Am J Cardiol.* 1981;47:
   206–209.
8. Olson LJ, Subramanian R, Edwards WD. Surgical pathology of pure aortic
   insufficiency: a study of 225 cases. *Mayo Clin Proc.* 1984;59:835–841.
9. Silver MA, Roberts WC. Detailed anatomy of the normally functioning
   aortic valve in hearts of normal and increased weight. *Am J Cardiol.*
   1985;55:454–461.

CLINICAL PERSPECTIVE

In the first 30 years of aortic valve replacement (AVR) for pure aortic regurgitation (AR), the cause of the AR was usually
readily apparent. We reviewed causes of pure AR among 268 patients having AVR from 1993 to 2005. To our surprise,
despite examining the operatively excised valves and occasionally portions of ascending aorta and the medical records, the
cause of the AR was clear in 177 patients (66%) and unclear in 91 (34%). The frequency of simultaneous coronary bypass
was much less in the clear-cause group than in the unclear-cause group (40/177 [23%] versus 46/91 [51%]).

Natural History of Syphilitic Aortitis

William Clifford Roberts, MD[a,b,*], Jong Mi Ko, BA[a], and Travis James Vowels[a,c]

No large studies of cardiovascular syphilis at necropsy have been reported since 1964. We examined at necropsy 90 patients who had characteristic morphologic findings of syphilitic aortitis. None had ever undergone cardiovascular surgery. With the exception of 2 cases seen more recently, the hearts and aortas of the 90 patients were examined and categorized by one of us (W.C.R.) from 1966 to 1990. All 90 had extensive involvement of the tubular portion of the ascending aorta by the syphilitic process, which spared the sinuses of Valsalva in all but 4 patients. The aortic arch was also involved in 49 (91%) of 54 patients and the descending thoracic aorta in 47 (90%) of 52 patients. Syphilis was the cause of death in 23 (26%) of the 90 patients. It was secondary to rupture of the ascending or descending thoracic aorta in 12, severe aortic regurgitation leading to heart failure in 10, and severe narrowing of the aortic ostium of the right coronary artery in 1 patient. Of the 40 patients who had undergone serologic testing for syphilis, 28 (70%) had a positive (reactive) finding. Those patients with a negative or nonreactive test or who did not undergo a serologic test for syphilis had morphologic and histologic findings in the aorta at necropsy similar to the findings of those patients who had had a positive serologic test for syphilis. In conclusion, cardiovascular syphilis has not disappeared. In patients with dilated ascending aortas, with or without aortic regurgitation, a serologic test for syphilis is recommended. If the findings are positive or if characteristic morphologic features of cardiovascular syphilis are suspected, irrespective of the results of the serologic tests, antibiotic therapy appears desirable.   © 2009 Elsevier Inc. All rights reserved. (Am J Cardiol 2009;104:1578–1587)

Syphilis was so common in the nineteenth century—estimated to affect 15% of United States adults during that period—that an entire specialty (syphilology) focused on it. Although relatively few with primary syphilis subsequently develop tertiary syphilis, the cardiovascular manifestations of late syphilis are at least life-threatening, if not fatal. The cause of the cardiovascular features of syphilis are unclear, because the spirochete *Treponema pallidum* has never convincingly been demonstrated in histologic sections of the aorta in patients with this complication of syphilis, and *T. pallidum* cannot be cultured. Because of its decreased frequency in the past several decades and because serologic tests for syphilis are now infrequently performed, it seemed appropriate to review a large number of cases of cardiovascular syphilis studied at necropsy by a single investigator during an approximately 50-year period to learn more about the morphologic features of the cardiovascular consequences. Only patients who had never undergone cardiovascular surgery were included.

Methods

The autopsy files of the Pathology Branch of the National Heart, Lung, and Blood Institute, National Institutes of Health (Bethesda, Maryland; where W.C.R. was chief for 29 years) were searched for cases coded as "cardiovascular syphilis." Except for 2 cases seen subsequently, all hearts and aortas were studied by W.C.R. from 1966 through 1990. None of the 90 patients had ever undergone cardiovascular surgery. Of the 90 cases studied, 77 were submitted from Washington, DC area hospitals or institutions (Washington DC Medical Examiners Office, n = 17; Georgetown University Medical Center, n = 17; Washington DC Veterans Affairs Hospital, n = 11; Washington DC General Hospital, n = 12; Howard University Hospital, n = 6; George Washington University Hospital, n = 4; Sibley Memorial Hospital, n = 3; National Institutes of Health, n = 2; Suburban Hospital, n = 2; Franklin Square Hospital, n = 2; National Naval Medical Center, n = 1, and non-Washington, DC area hospitals, n = 13). Patients for whom a serologic test for syphilis was positive (reactive) but in whom the aorta was not involved by the syphilitic process were not included in the present study.

Each heart and aorta was examined initially and later by W.C.R. All hearts had extensive involvement of the tubular portion of the ascending aorta by a process typical of cardiovascular syphilis (to be described subsequently). Many of the hearts and aortas were photographed, and several were drawn by a professional artist (Leon Schlossberg).

Partial or complete clinical records for each case were provided by the submitting institution. Most cases were seen initially by W.C.R. at the submitting institution at a teaching conference. He examined the specimen there and discussed the findings and then brought the heart and aorta back to the National Institutes of Health for additional study. Histologic sections of the aorta and heart were pre-

[a]Baylor Heart and Vascular Institute, Baylor University Medical Center, Dallas, Texas; and [b]Pathology Branch, National Heart, Lung, and Blood Institute, National Institutes of Health, Bethesda, Maryland; [c]University of Texas at Austin, Austin, Texas. Manuscript received July 6, 2009; revised manuscript received and accepted July 6, 2009.

*Corresponding author: Tel: (214) 820-7911; fax: (214) 820-7533.

E-mail address: wc.roberts@baylorhealth.edu (W.C. Roberts).

Table 1

Necropsy cases of syphilitic aortitis without operative intervention

Variable	Total (n = 90)	Men (n = 59)	Women (n = 31)
Age (years)			
Range	19–91	19–88 (66 ± 13)	32–91 (70 ± 14)
Mean ± SD	67 ± 14		
Race			
African American	60	44	16
European American	20	12	8
Unclear	10	3	7
Serologic test for syphilis (positive/No. done)	28/40 (70%)	20/27 (74%)	8/13 (62%)
Aortic regurgitation	23 (26%)	14 (24%)	9 (29%)
Systemic hypertension	41/72 (57%)	28/48 (58%)	13/24 (54%)
Heart failure	26/84 (31%)	23/56 (41%)	3/28 (11%)
Cause of death			
Syphilis			
Aortic rupture	12 (13%)	5 (8%)	7 (23%)
Aortic regurgitation → heart failure	10 (11%)	8 (14%)	2 (6%)
Ostial narrowing, right coronary artery	1 (1%)	0	1 (3%)
Coronary artery disease	17 (19%)	14 (24%)	3 (10%)
Stroke	5 (6%)	2 (3%)	3 (10%)
Noncardiac, nonvascular	38 (42%)	27 (46%)	11 (35%)
Unclear	7 (8%)	3 (5%)	4 (13%)
Heart weight (g)			
Range	215–850	260–850	215–750
Mean ± SD	486 ± 135	507 ± 135	443 ± 127
Coronary artery narrowing >75% of cross-sectional area	46/71 (65%)	35/48 (73%)	11/23 (48%)
Left ventricular infarct			
Acute	5 (6%)	4 (7%)	1 (3%)
Healed	28 (31%)	24 (41%)	4 (13%)
Both	1 (1%)	0	1 (3%)
Coronary ostial narrowing			
Right	13 (14%)	9 (15%)	4 (13%)
Left main	2 (2%)	1 (2%)	1 (3%)

pared at the National Institutes of Health in the Pathology Branch for each case and were examined by W.C.R.

Results

The pertinent findings for the 59 men and 31 women are listed in Table 1. The men ranged in age from 19 to 88 years (mean 66 ± 13), and the women from 32 to 91 years (mean 70 ± 14). The race was known for 80 patients: 60 (75%) were African American and 20 (25%) were European American. At least 23 patients had some degree of aortic regurgitation; 3 others had evidence of aortic valve stenosis (a nonsyphilitic process) at necropsy. All 90 patients had 3-cuspid aortic valves. At least 41 (57%) of the 72 patients in whom it was noted had a history of systemic hypertension or had had a peak systolic pressure >140 mm Hg or an end-diastolic pressure >90 mm Hg, or both. At least 26 (31%) of the 84 patients in whom it was noted had had clinical evidence of heart failure. At least 40 patients had undergone a serologic test for syphilis (either the Venereal Disease Research Laboratory or fluorescent treponemal antibody), and in ≥28 (70%), 1 or both test results were positive (reactive).

The cause of death in the 90 patients was as follows: cardiovascular syphilis from rupture of the ascending or descending thoracic aorta in 12 patients, severe aortic regurgitation producing heart failure in 10 patients, or severe narrowing of the ostium of the right coronary artery in 1 patient (total 23 patients [26%]); coronary heart disease in 17 patients; stroke in 5 patients; cancer in 14 patients; renal failure in 3 patients; and a noncardiac, nonvascular, and noncancer cause in 28 patients, including chronic obstructive pulmonary disease in 4, amyloidosis in 2, and unclear in 7.

At necropsy, the hearts of the 46 men weighed 260 to 850 g (mean 507 ± 135, median 505). In 33 (72%) of these 46 patients, the heart weighed >400 g (upper limit of normal for men). The hearts of the 23 women weighed 215 to 750 g (mean 443 ± 127, median 420). In ≥18 (78%) of these 23 women, the heart weighed >350 g (upper limit of normal for women).

In all 90 patients, the tubular portion of the ascending aorta was extensively involved by the syphilitic process (Figures 1 to 9). In only 4 of the 90 patients did the process extend into the wall of aorta behind the sinuses of Valsalva. In the other 86 patients, the process began at the sinotubular junction. The aortic arch was available for examination in 54 of the 90 patients. Of the 54 patients, the aortic arch was also involved by the syphilitic process in 49 (91%). The descending thoracic aorta was available for examination in 52 of the 90 patients, and in 47 (90%) the process also involved this portion of the aorta. The abdominal portion of aorta was available for examination in 47 patients, and in 39

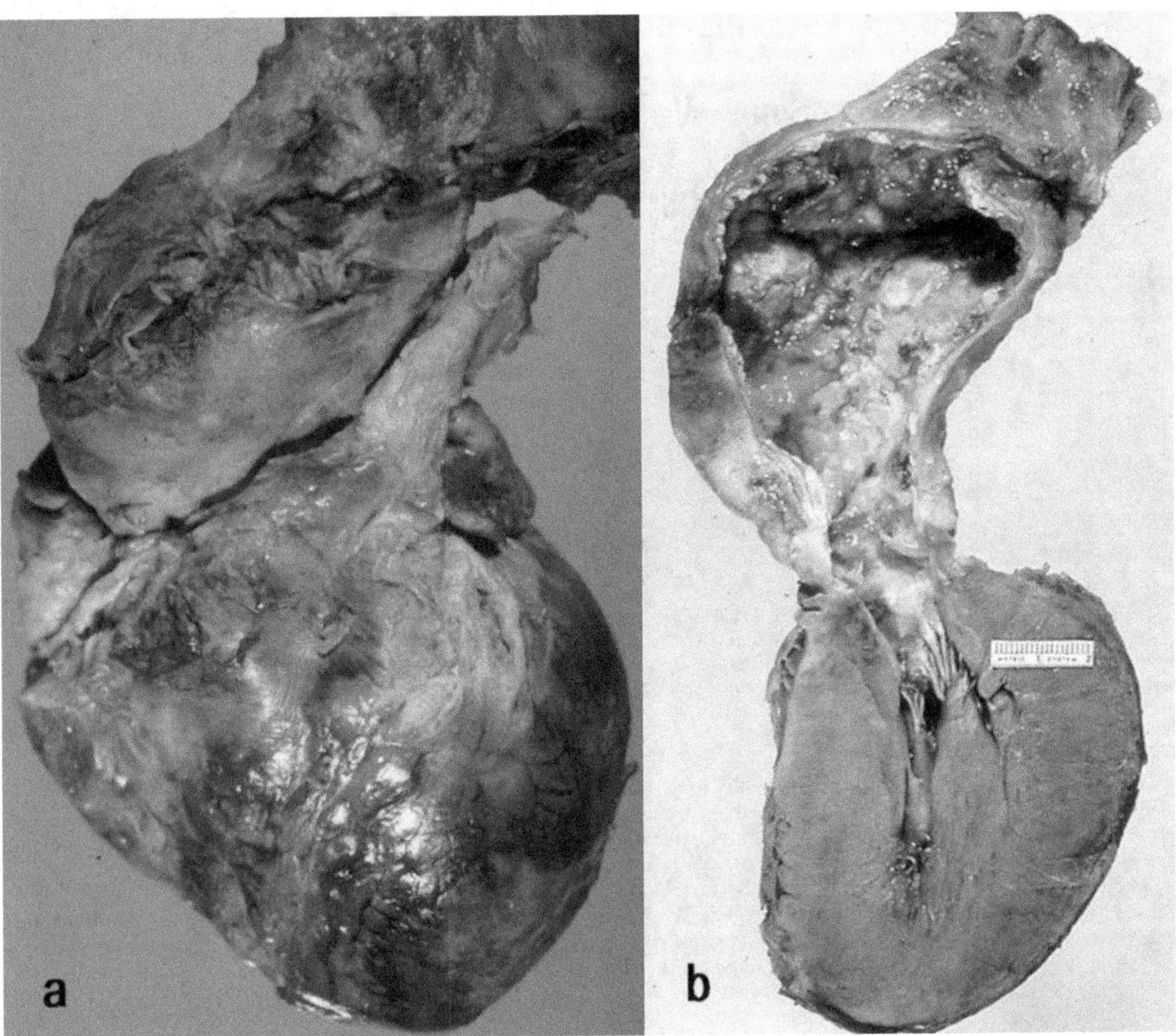

Figure 1. Heart and aorta in 67-year-old European-American woman with positive Venereal Disease Research Laboratory and fluorescent treponemal antibody serologic test results for syphilis with huge fusiform aneurysm of ascending aorta. (*a*) Anterior view of heart and aorta. Huge aortic aneurysm compresses adjacent pulmonary trunk. (*b*) Opened aorta showing severe involvement of tubular portion by syphilitic process with sparing of sinus portion. Right ventricle and atria have been excised from remaining left ventricle. The lack of dilation of the left ventricular cavity strongly suggests the lack of aortic regurgitation, of which no evidence was seen during her life.

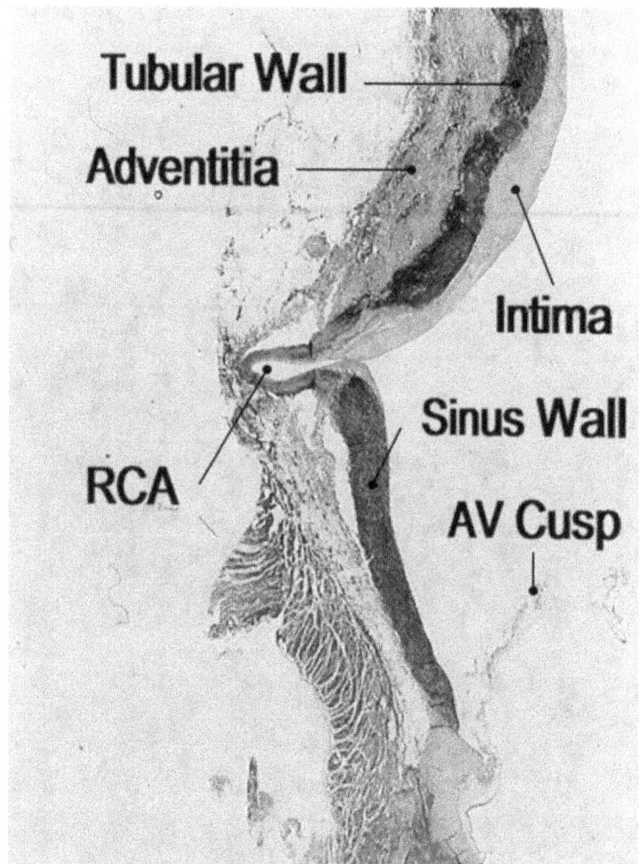

Figure 2. Histologic section of sinus and proximal tubular portion of ascending aorta in 32-year-old African-American woman who was killed in an automotive crash. Ascending aorta had a maximal diameter of 6 cm. Media *(black stained)* of sinus wall was normal, and no intimal or adventitial thickening seen. Wall of tubular portion was 4 times thicker than that of sinus portion. Thickening resulted from severe thickening of both intima and adventitia by fibrous tissue. Transverse scars replaced medial elastic tissue in 3 different areas. Ostium of right coronary artery severely narrowed by intimal fibrous tissue. Movat stain, original magnification ×5. RCA = right coronary artery; AV = aortic valve.

(83%), this portion of the aorta contained atherosclerotic plaques. However, the process was quite different from that involving the more proximal portions of the aorta in that the process involved only the intima and spared the adventitia.

The syphilitic process involving the thoracic aorta caused aneurismal dilation of the involved segment in some patients but not in others. The aneurismal process involved the entire wall of aorta (fusiform) in all patients, and in 10 of them, one or more saccular aneurysms were present within the fusiform dilated portion. (Only a portion of the aortic wall was involved in the saccular aneurysm.)

Histologically, the wall of the thoracic aorta was much thicker than normal, the result of fibrous thickening of the adventitia and fibrous and/or fibrocalcific thickening of the intima (Figures 2 and 8). Within the adventitial fibrous tissue were focal collections of plasmacytes and lymphocytes, often surrounding the vasa vasora, the walls of which were usually quite thickened and their lumens quite narrowed. The media of the aorta was not thickened but its elastic fibers, as demonstrated by Movat stain, were focally interrupted such that in some areas of media no elastic fibers

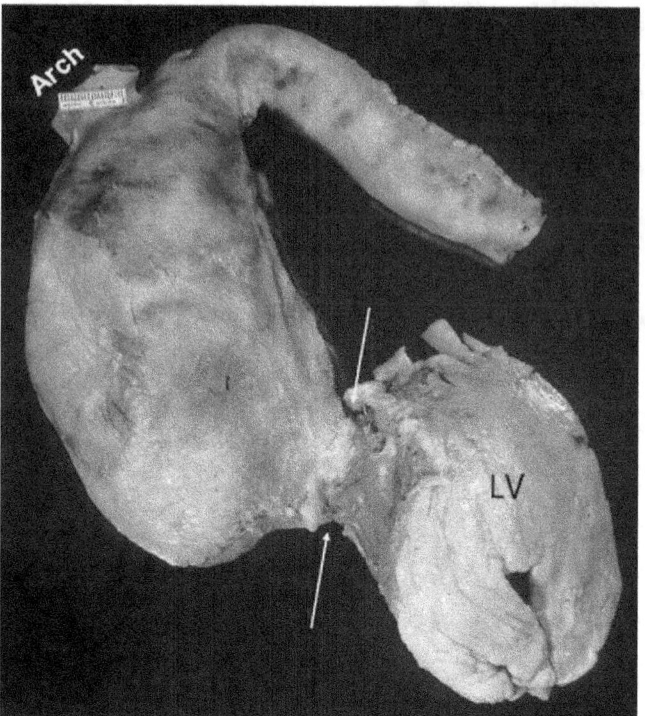

Figure 3. Thoracic aorta and left ventricle from 79-year-old woman who died from cancer. Maximal transverse diameter of ascending aorta was 8.7 cm. Dilation began just above sinus portion *(between arrows)*, which was not dilated. Entire arch and descending thoracic aorta were also diffusely involved by syphilitic process. Both Venereal Disease Research Laboratory and fluorescent treponemal antibody serologic test results for syphilis were negative. LV = left ventricle.

were present and fibrous scars had replaced the medial elastic fibers and smooth muscle cells. The intimal process appeared to be typical atherosclerotic plaque.

At least 46 (65%) of the 71 patients in whom the arteries were carefully examined had >75% narrowing in the cross-sectional area of one or more major (right, left main, left anterior descending, left circumflex) epicardial coronary arteries. Of the 85 patients in whom the ostia of the 2 coronary arteries in the aorta were carefully examined, 13 (15%) had definite narrowing of the ostium of the right coronary artery and 2 (2%) had definite narrowing of the ostium of the left main coronary artery.

Grossly visible myocardial infarcts were observed at necropsy in 34 (38%) of 89 patients: acute infarcts only in 5 patients (6%), healed infarcts only in 28 patients (31%), and both acute and healed infarcts in 1 patient (1%).

Discussion

The present study has described the cardiovascular findings at necropsy in 90 patients with characteristic morphologic findings in the ascending aorta of tertiary syphilis. Each heart and aorta was examined and categorized by the same investigator (W.C.R.). No patient had ever undergone cardiovascular surgery. Although it was positive (reactive) for only 70% of the patients who had a serologic test for syphilis, the changes in ascending aorta were similar in the patients with reactive and nonreactive findings for syphilis

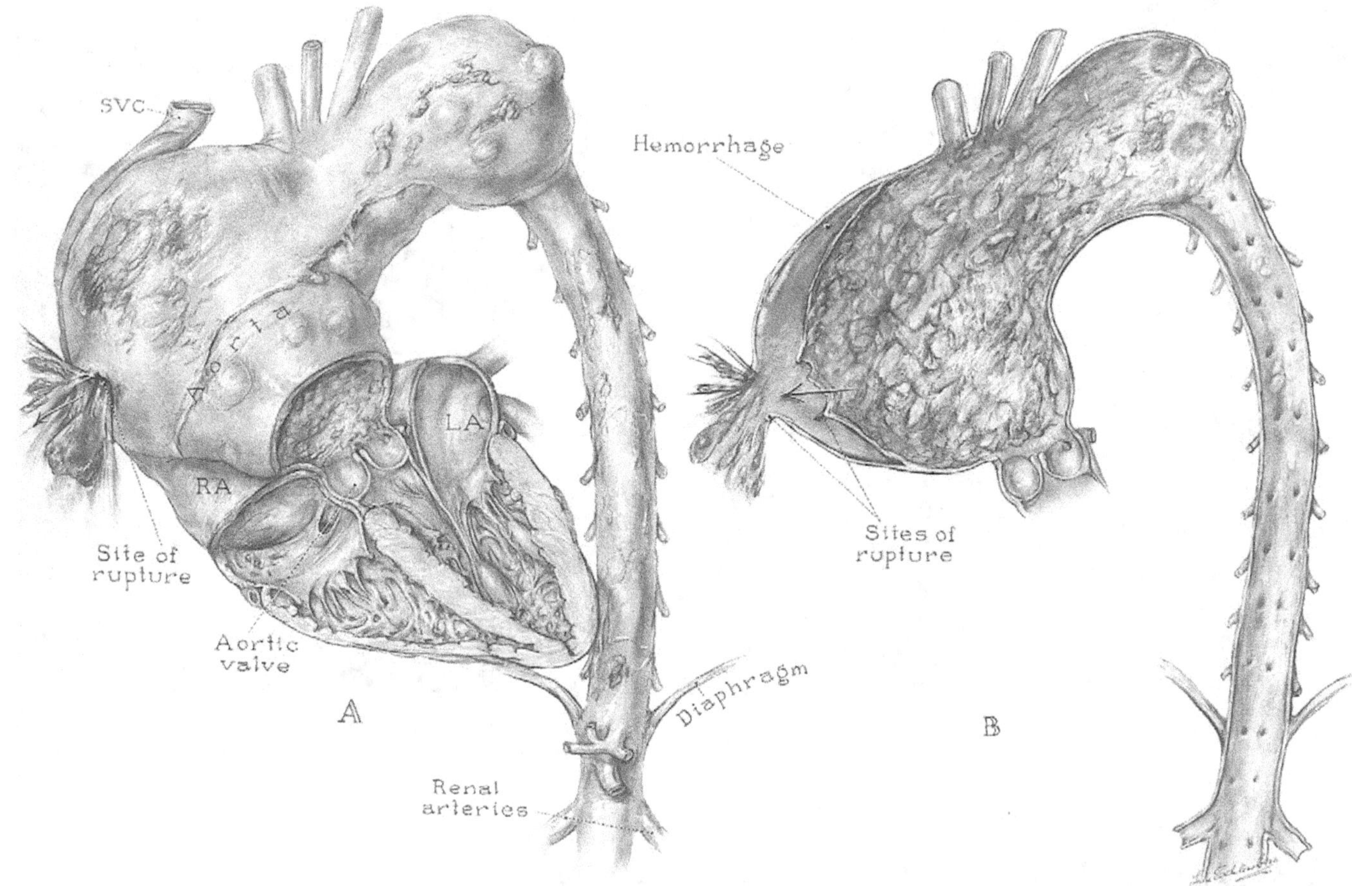

Figure 4. Drawing of thoracic aorta, which ruptured in 60-year-old European-American woman. She had died suddenly at home in the bathroom. Largest transverse diameter of ascending aorta was 9.5 cm. Sinus portion of aorta was normal. The rupture was into the pericardial sac. SVC = Superior vena cava.

and in the patients who did not have a serologic test for syphilis recorded. Of the 90 patients studied, men outnumbered women nearly 2 to 1 and African Americans outnumbered European Americans nearly 3 to 1. Evidence of aortic regurgitation was present clinically in only 1/4 of the patients, and systemic systolic blood pressure >140/90 mm Hg was present in virtually 60% of the patients. Evidence of heart failure was recorded clinically in nearly 1/3 of the patients. The causes of death varied. Syphilis was the cause in only 1/4 of the patients, with nonsyphilitic causes responsible in 3/4. Nearly 70% had one or more major (right, left main, left anterior descending, left circumflex) coronary arteries narrowed >75% in cross-sectional area by atherosclerotic plaques (nonsyphilitic), and nearly 40% of the patients had acute or healed myocardial infarct, or both. The ostium of the right coronary artery was very narrow in 15% of the patients.

Examination of our necropsy patients supports the view that cardiovascular syphilis is essentially limited to the thoracic aorta with occasional involvement of the arch arteries. The involvement when present always included the ascending aorta, but any portion of the thoracic aorta can be affected by the syphilitic process. Although some of our patients had severe atherosclerotic involvement of the abdominal aorta, with or without fusiform aneurysm, the process was clearly different from that involving the thoracic aorta in that it spared the adventitia and only indirectly involved the media (presumably from pressure from the overlying heavy atherosclerotic plaques). Similarly, although the coronary ostia can be narrowed by the syphilitic process in the aorta, the coronary arterial involvement is clearly not a part of the syphilitic process. The narrowing of the coronary arteries themselves resulted from typical atherosclerosis, a process involving the intima only, except for focal thinning of the media, again presumably the result of the overlying heavy atherosclerotic plaques. The adventitia of the coronary arteries was spared (i.e., not thickened).

The syphilitic process appears to involve only arteries in which the vasa vasora are present or at least easily identified histologically. The vasa vasora are either absent from the coronary arteries or difficult to identify. The vasa vasora are present in the entire thoracic aorta but are absent from the abdominal aorta and their absence from this portion of the aorta appears to be the explanation for the absence of syphilitic involvement of the abdominal aorta.

The major consequence of syphilitic involvement of the aorta is thickening of its wall (Figure 10). The thickening results from dense scarring of the adventitia and from less dense fibrous tissue with or without calcium in the intima. The media is not thickened and might be thinner than normal. The media contains many foci of fibrosis, and these scars are usually oriented transversely. In these scarred areas, the elastic fibrils and smooth muscle cells may have vanished completely, and, even in the nonscarred areas of

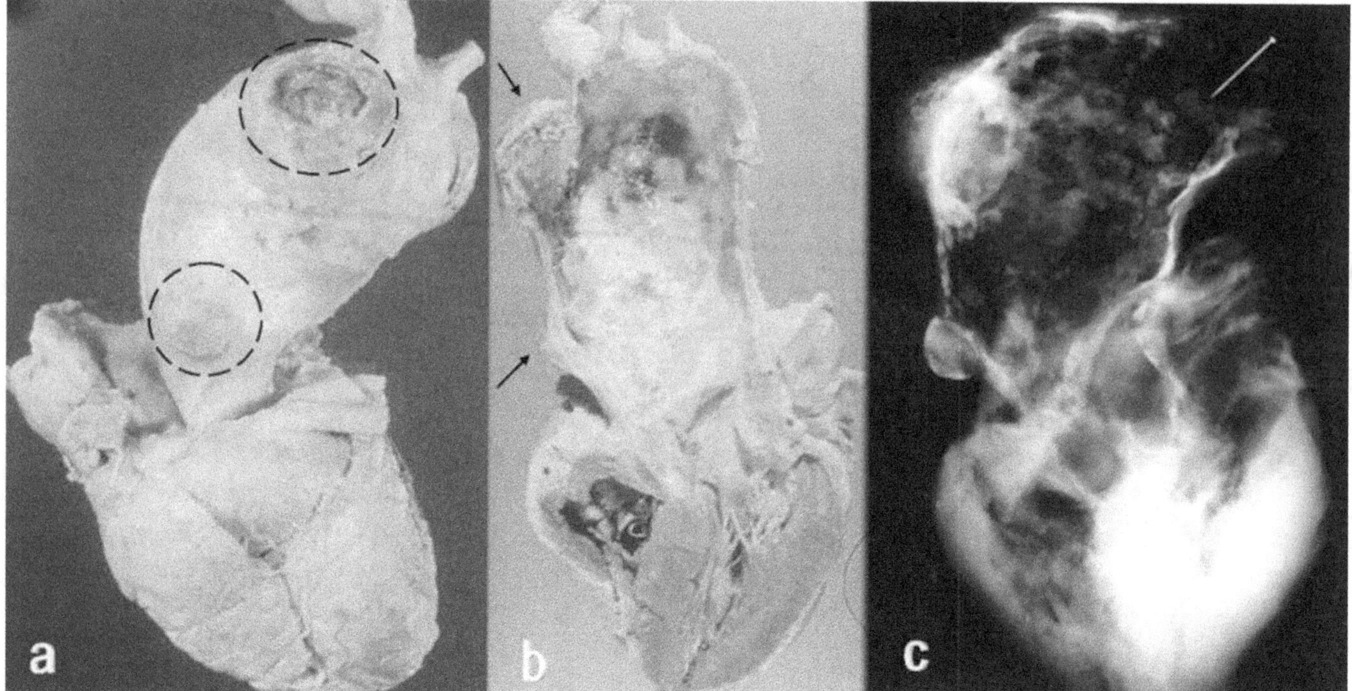

Figure 5. Fusiform and saccular aneurysm of ascending aorta in 81-year-old African-American man who died from a diabetic coma. (*a,b*) One of 2 saccular aneurysms *(arrows and circles)* within fusiform aneurysm had burrowed into the sternum. Thrombus was present in both saccular aneurysms. Sinus portion of aorta was normal. Heart size was normal. (*c*) Calcific deposits present in aortic wall.

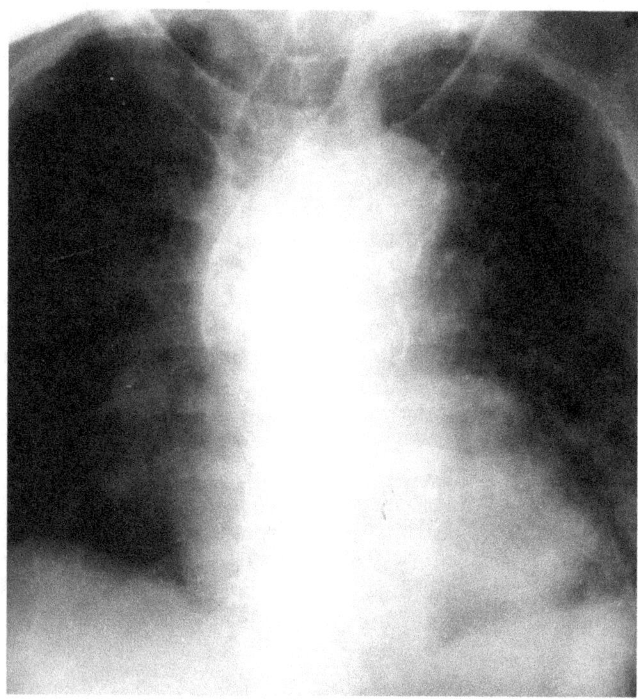

Figure 6. Radiograph of chest in patient described in Figure 5. Linear calcific deposits present in tubular portion of ascending aorta. Calcific deposits present only in intima of aorta.

the media, the elastic fibers are often disrupted. Despite the thickening, the involved arterial wall is weaker than normal because of the disruption of the elastic fibrils and smooth muscle cells of the media. Because the strength of a vessel is dependent on the integrity of its media, which is disrupted, the involved portion of the aorta usually dilates. Where the media has been totally disrupted, the dilation will be particularly severe, resulting in an increase in focal saccular aneurysms.

Accurately reported information on patients in whom cardiovascular syphilis was found at necropsy is relatively limited, primarily because the data obtained was from autopsy protocols and not from examination by the same investigator of a large number of cases or from re-examination by one or more investigators. Clawson and Bell[1] in 1927 reported the findings from necropsy protocols of 126 patients with syphilitic aortitis: 104 (83%) were men and 22 (17%) were women (the ratio of men to women in their total autopsy cases, however, was 2:1). Aortic regurgitation had been evident in 46 patients (37%), rupture of aortic aneurysm occurred in 35 (28%), and myocardial gummas were found in 3 (2%). Sudden death from coronary ostial narrowing occurred in 25 (20%) and the cause of death was nonsyphilitic for 17 (13%).

Martland,[2] in 1930, described necropsy findings from autopsy protocols in 101 patients with morphologic evidence of cardiovascular syphilis: 28 (28%) had ascending aortic aneurysms, 36 (36%) had aortic regurgitation, and 15 (15%) had narrowing of one or more coronary arteries.

Carr,[3] in 1930, briefly described the autopsy findings in 119 patients with morphologic features of cardiovascular syphilis: 13 (11%) had aneurismal dilation of the ascending aorta and 24 (20%) had morphologic evidence of aortic regurgitation; ≥49 patients (41%) had atherosclerotic coronary artery disease.

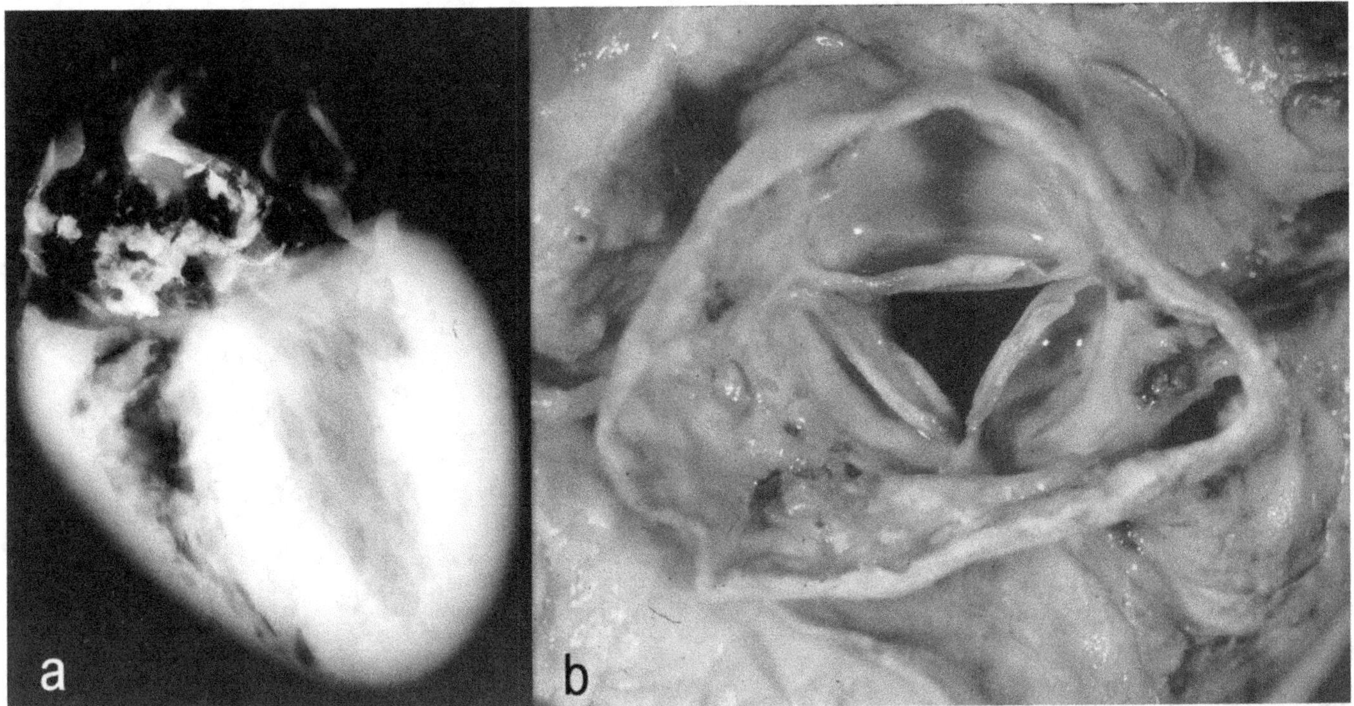

Figure 7. Radiograph of heart and proximal aorta (*a*) at necropsy and of aortic valve and proximal aorta from above (*b*) in 68-year-old African-American woman who had clinical evidence of aortic regurgitation and died from heart failure. Radiograph shows heavy calcific deposits in proximal aorta (*a*). Aortic valve orifice was triangular owing to dilation of ascending aorta. Tubular portion of aorta is diffusely involved by syphilitic process. Venereal Disease Research Laboratory serologic test result for syphilis was nonreactive.

Heggtveit,[4] in 1964, summarized findings from necropsy reports in 100 patients with syphilitic aortitis studied at Kings County Hospital Center (Brooklyn, New York). A clinical diagnosis of syphilis was established in only 17 of the patients. The patients' age range was 30 to 92 years (mean 63): 57 were European American and 43 were African American. Only 23 had ever been treated for syphilis. The blood serology findings (Venereal Disease Research Laboratory and Kolmer) was positive in 40, negative in 28, and not done in 32 patients. Of the 100 patients, 36 had "uncomplicated" aortitis, 40 had aortic aneurysm, 29 had evidence of aortic regurgitation, and 26 had coronary ostial stenosis. In 14 (35%) of the 40 patients with thoracic aortic aneurysms, fatal rupture occurred. In 43 of the 73 men, the heart weighed >400 g and in 18 of the 27 women, the heart weighed >350 g. No large studies of cardiovascular syphilis at necropsy have been reported subsequently.

The frequency of cardiovascular involvement among patients with untreated syphilis has been derived primarily from 2 large studies: the Oslo study and the controversial (i.e., unethical) Tuskegee, Alabama, study, both of which yielded numerous publications in medical journals. The Oslo study[5] analyzed native Oslo patients initially hospitalized with primary syphilis from 1890 to 1910 and followed thereafter for 40 to 60 years. Cardiovascular syphilis (with or without "saccular" thoracic aortic aneurysm, aortic regurgitation or coronary ostial stenosis) was diagnosed in 45 (15%) of the 303 men and in 47 (8%) of the 584 women. Of the patients who were studied at necropsy, 9% of the men had uncomplicated aortitis and 25% had complicated (aneurysm, aortic regurgitation,

coronary ostial stenosis) aortitis, and 11% of the women had "uncomplicated" and 10% had "complicated" disease of the aorta.

The Tuskegee study involved 408 African-American men hospitalized with primary syphilis initially in 1932 and followed through 1972.[6-9] None were treated with penicillin, which had become available in the United States in 1943. By 1952, about 1/3 of the patients had died, and necropsy findings were available for 89. "Fusiform aneurysm of the thoracic aorta" was present in 40 patients (45%), "saccular aneurysm of the thoracic aorta" in 7 (8%), and "aortitis" (by histologic examination) in 41 patients (46%). Of the 89 patients studied at necropsy, 60 (67%) had had positive blood serologic test findings for syphilis when last tested, 3 had "doubtful" test results, and 24 had negative results. Of the 69 hearts (those with weights available), 48 (70%) weighed >400 g. A clinical diagnosis of cardiovascular syphilis corresponded with the necropsy diagnosis in 88% of the patients.

The present study had many limitations. First, we had virtually no information on the presence or absence of primary syphilis in the distant past. Second, the results of the serologic tests for syphilis for most patients were not available to us. Third, the entire aorta of many patients was unavailable for examination by us. Fourth, whether syphilitic cardiovascular disease had been diagnosed clinically was not known for most patients. Finally, the number of patients who had ever received antibiotic therapy for syphilis was unknown to us. Nevertheless, the morphologic data were collected and studied extensively by a single investi-

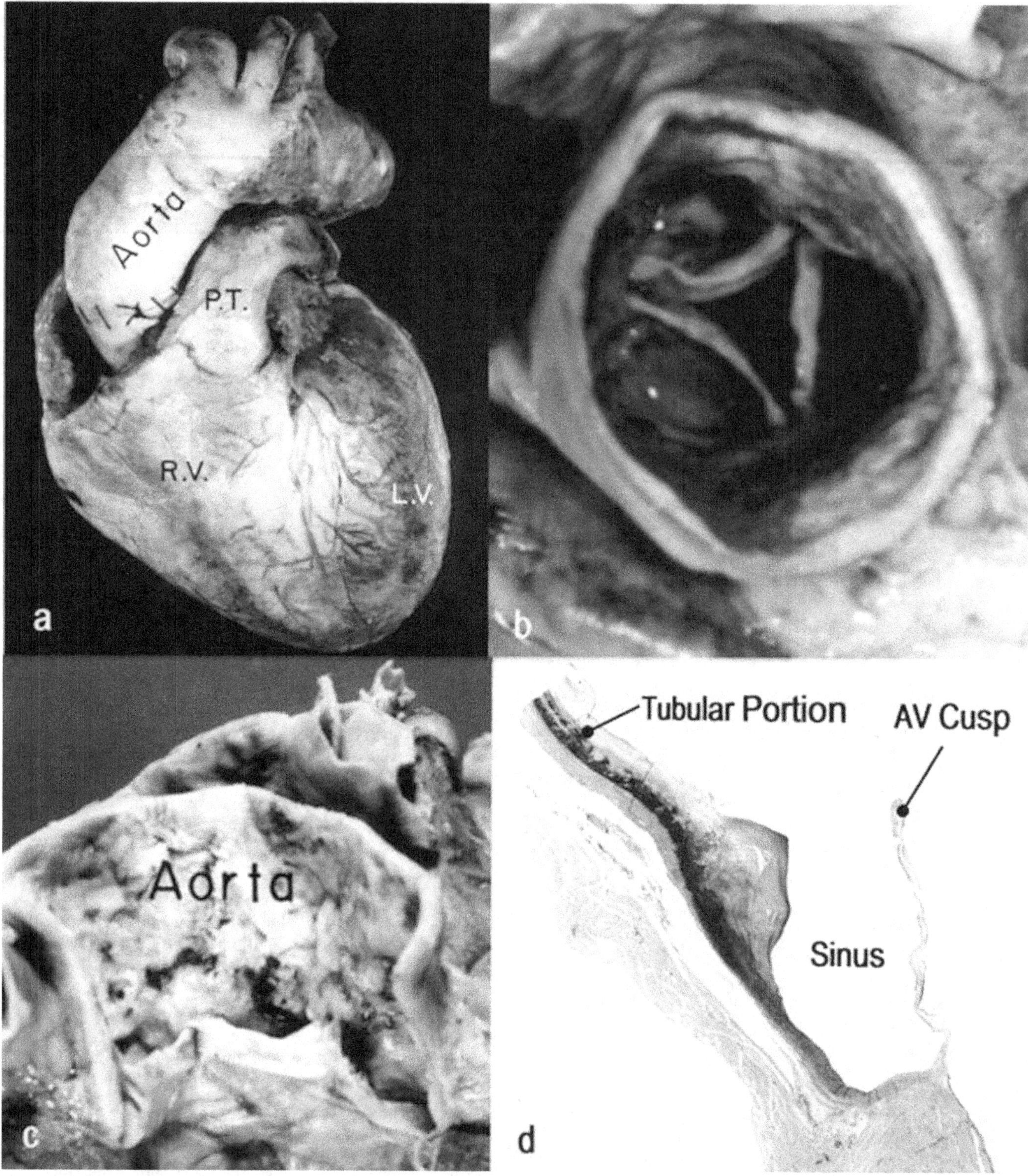

Figure 8. Heart and aorta from 69-year-old African-American man who died from heart failure secondary to severe aortic regurgitation (systemic blood pressure 170/50 mm Hg). Venereal Disease Research Laboratory serologic test result for syphilis was positive (reactive). (*a*) Heart, which weighed 640 g, and dilated ascending aorta. L.V. = left ventricle; P.T. = pulmonary trunk; R.V. = right ventricle. (*b*) Aortic valve from above with eccentric triangular orifice. Wall of aorta was very thick. (*c*) Opened aortic valve and aorta showing diffuse syphilitic involvement of tubular portion. (*d*) Photomicrograph of aortic valve cusp and proximal aorta. Wall behind sinus portion was normal, and wall in tubular portion was about 3 times thicker than aortic wall behind sinus. Elastic van Gieson stain, original magnification ×5.

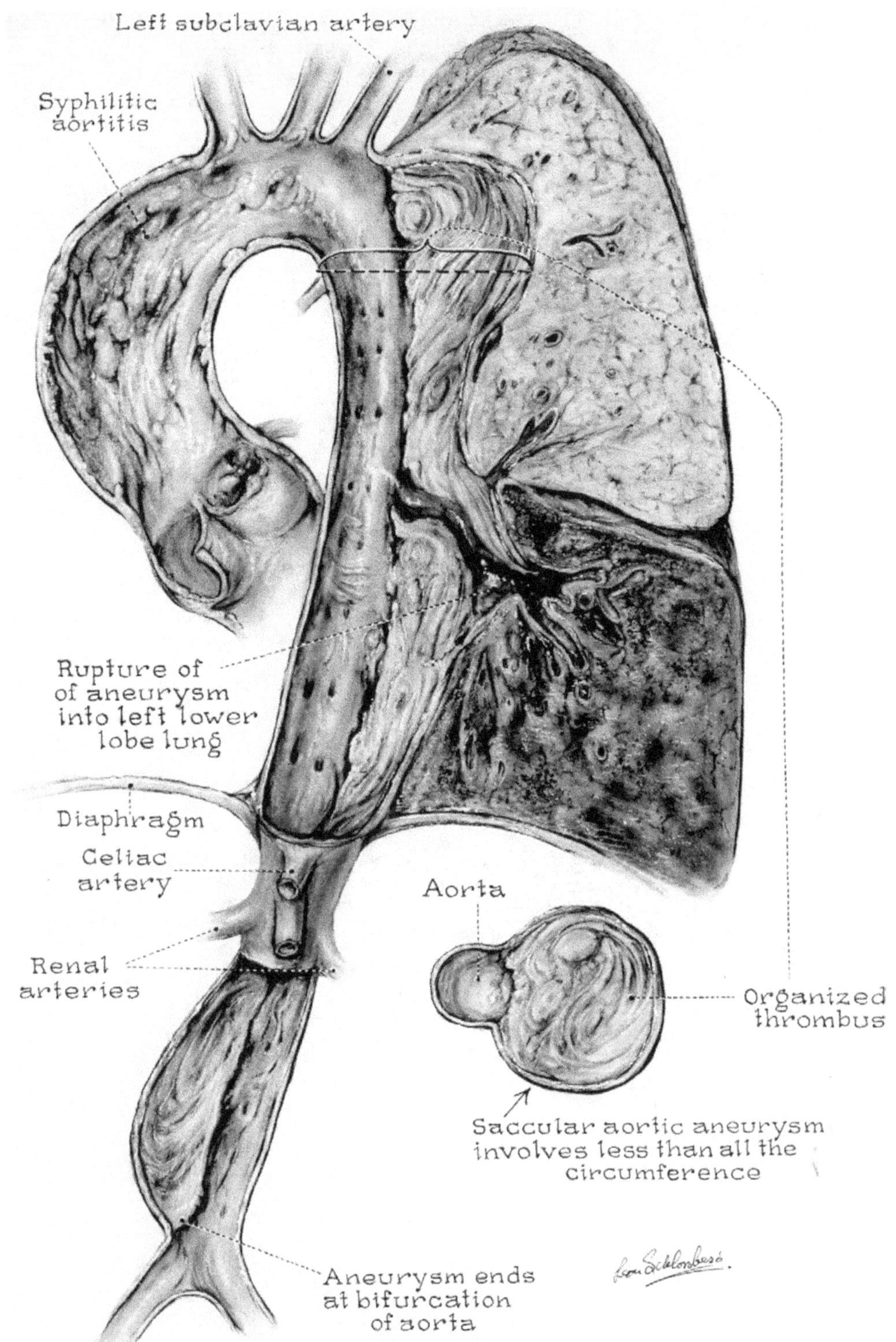

Figure 9. Drawing of aorta and portion of lung from 44-year-old African-American man who died from rupture of descending thoracic aneurysm into his left lung. Ascending aorta was typical of syphilitic aortitis. Wall of aorta behind sinuses was normal. Heart weighed 350 g.

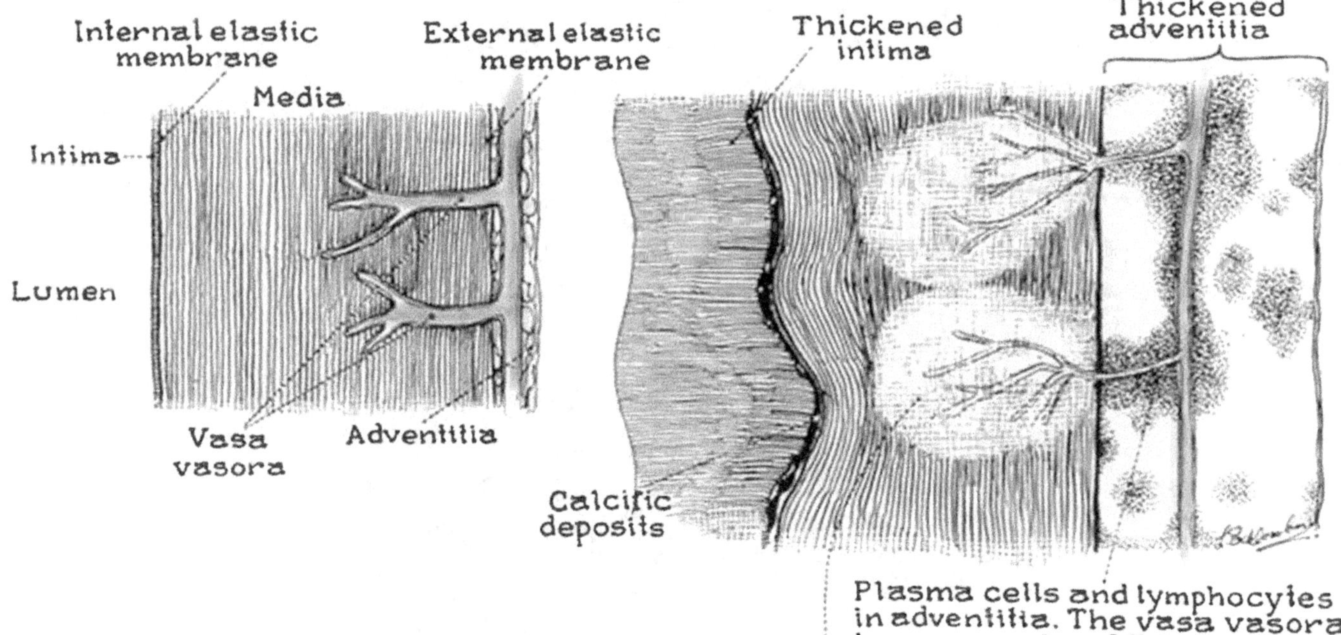

Figure 10. Diagram showing normal aorta *(Left)* and syphilitic aorta *(Right)*.

gator, an occurrence made possible only by not discarding the specimens soon after necropsy.

1. Clawson BJ, Bell ET. The heart in syphilitic aortitis. *Arch Pathol Lab Med* 1927;4:922–936.
2. Martland HS. Symposium on cardiovascular syphilis: syphilis of the aorta and heart. *Am Heart J* 1930;6:1–29.
3. Carr JG. The gross pathology of the heart in cardiovascular syphilis. *Am Heart J* 1930;6:30–36.
4. Heggtveit HA. Syphilitic aortitis: a clinicopathologic autopsy study of 100 cases, 1950 to 1960. *Circulation* 1964;29:346–355.
5. Clark EG, Danbolt N. The Oslo study of the natural history of untreated syphilis: an epidemiologic investigation based on a rest-udy of the Boeck-Brussgaard material. *J Chronic Dis* 1955;2:311–344.
6. Peters JJ, Peers JH, Olansky S, Cutler JC, Gleeson GA. Untreated syphilis in the male Negro: pathologic findings in syphilitic and non-syphilitic patients. *J Chronic Dis* 1955;1:127–148.
7. Rockwell DH, Yobs AR, Moore MB Jr. The Tuskegee study of untreated syphilis: the 30th year of observation. *Arch Intern Med* 1964;114:792–798.
8. Caldwell JG, Price EV. Schroeter AL, Fletcher GF. Aortic regurgitation in Tuskegee study of untreated syphilis. *J Chronic Dis* 1973;26:187–194.
9. White RM. Unraveling the Tuskegee study of untreated syphilis. *Arch Intern Med* 2000;160:585–598.

Combined congenitally bicuspid aortic valve and mitral valve prolapse causing pure regurgitation

William C. Roberts, MD, Saleha Zafar, MD, Jong Mi Ko, Melissa M. Carry, MD, and Robert F. Hebeler, MD

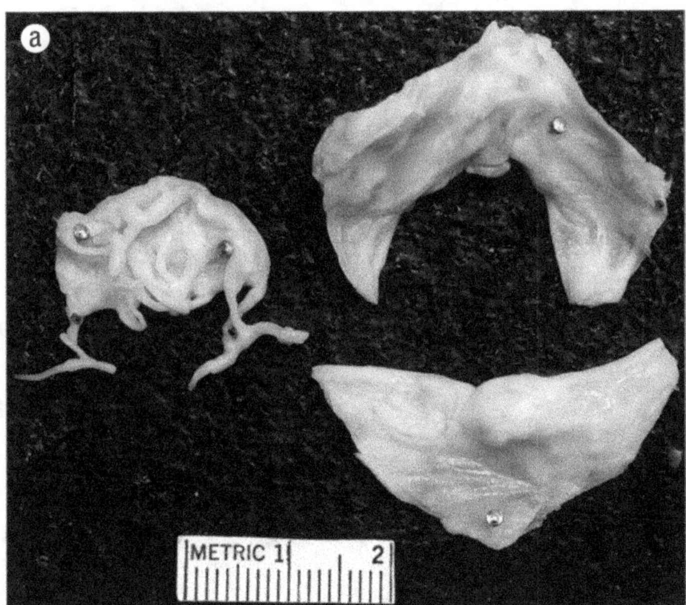
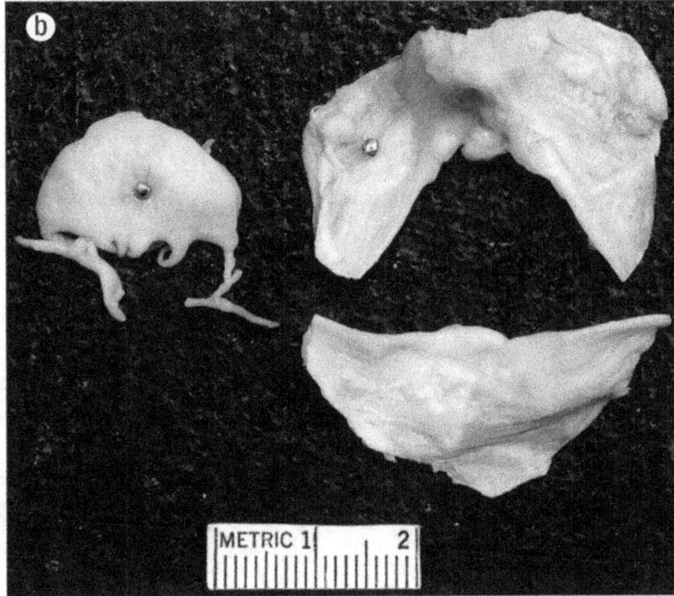

Figure 1. Mitral and aortic valves of the patient described. **(a)** Ventricular aspect of the resected portion of the posterior mitral leaflet and of the congenitally bicuspid aortic valve. Several chordae are missing, indicating that they had ruptured in the past and later became incorporated in the superimposed fibrous tissue on the ventricular aspect of the leaflet (see Figure 2). **(b)** Atrial aspect of the mitral leaflet and aortic aspect of a congenitally bicuspid aortic valve.

Described herein is a patient with a purely regurgitant congenitally bicuspid aortic valve and a purely regurgitant prolapsing mitral valve. Although it is well established that the bicuspid aortic valve is a congenital anomaly, it is less well appreciated that mitral valve prolapse is almost certainly also a congenital anomaly. The two occurring in the same patient provides support that mitral valve prolapse is also a congenital anomaly.

I t is well appreciated that the bicuspid aortic valve (BAV) is usually of congenital origin. It is less well appreciated that mitral valve prolapse (MVP) is usually of congenital origin. Most patients with a congenitally BAV (unless complicated by superimposed infective endocarditis) have a structurally normal mitral valve. It is most unusual for a patient with a congenitally BAV, particularly one that is purely regurgitant, to have associated MVP. Such was the case, however, in the patient described herein.

CASE DESCRIPTION

A 64-year-old white man with a doctorate, who was born in June 1947, had been well until November 2011, when he had the first of several episodes of syncope. During hospitalization for acute appendicitis, an electrocardiogram disclosed the presence of atrial fibrillation. Another syncopal episode and the appearance of exertional and nocturnal dyspnea in 2012 prompted a visit to a cardiologist. His body mass index was 30 kg/m^2. A grade 2/6 basal precordial systolic murmur and a grade 4/6 blowing apical systolic murmur with radiation into the left axilla were heard. The initial electrocardiogram showed supraventricular tachycardia with a ventricular rate of

From the Divison of Cardiology, Department of Internal Medicine (Roberts, Zafar, Ko, Carry), and Department of Cardiothoracic Surgery (Hebeler), Baylor Heart and Vascular Hospital and Baylor University Medical Center at Dallas.

Corresponding author: William C. Roberts, MD, Baylor Heart and Vascular Institute, 621 North Hall Street, Dallas, TX 75226 (e-mail: wc.roberts@baylor-health.edu).

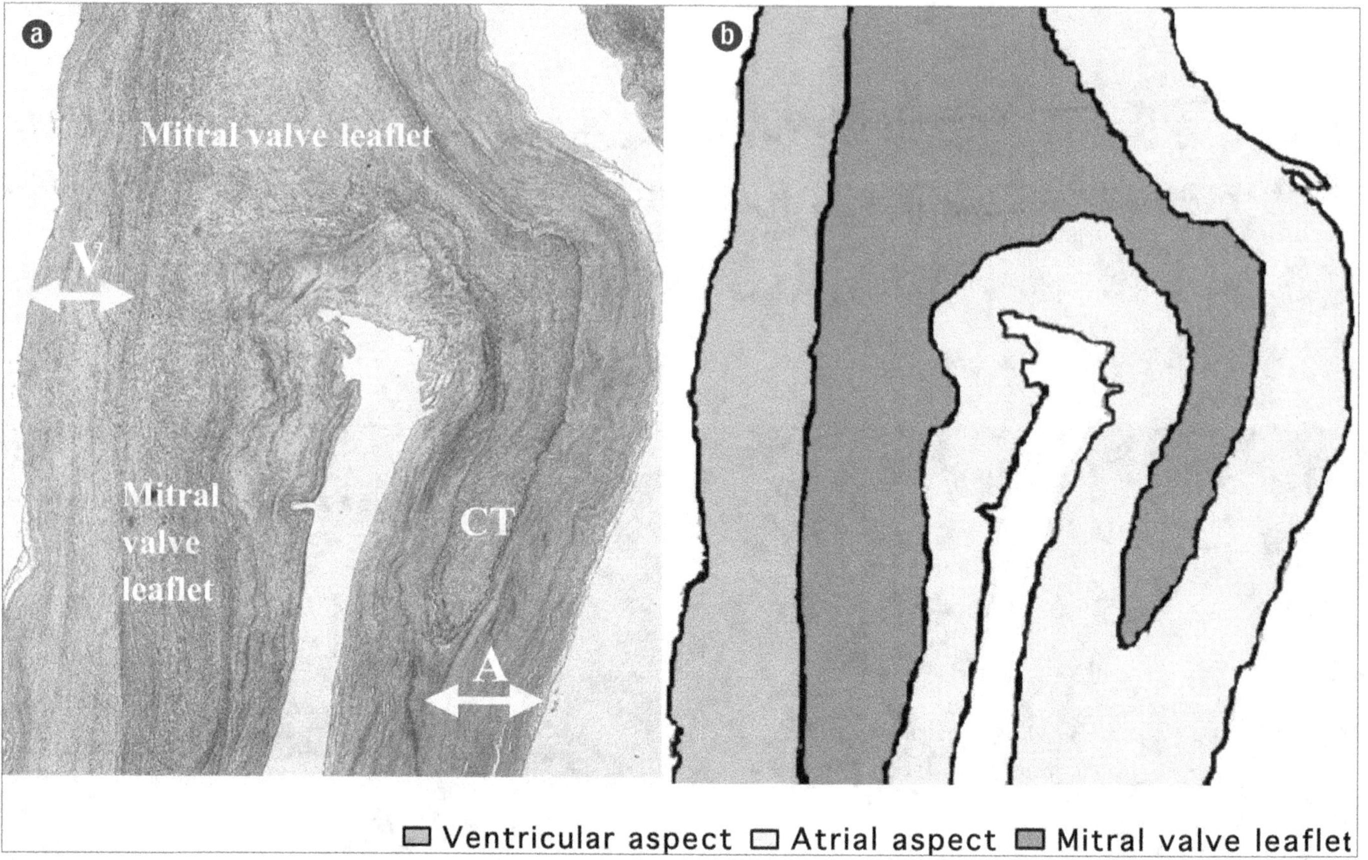

Figure 2. (a) Photomicrograph of a portion of the posterior mitral valve leaflet and attached chordae tendineae (CT). The leaflet and chordal thickening is the result of superimposed fibrous tissue on both atrial (A) and ventricular (V) aspects of the leaflet and surrounding the chordae. The leaflet itself consists primarily of the fibrosa element; the spongiosa element is minimal. These histological features are characteristic of mitral valve prolapse. Elastic von Gieson stain, ×40. **(b)** A color-coded replica with green representing the ventricular aspect, yellow representing the atrial aspect, and red representing the mitral valve leaflet.

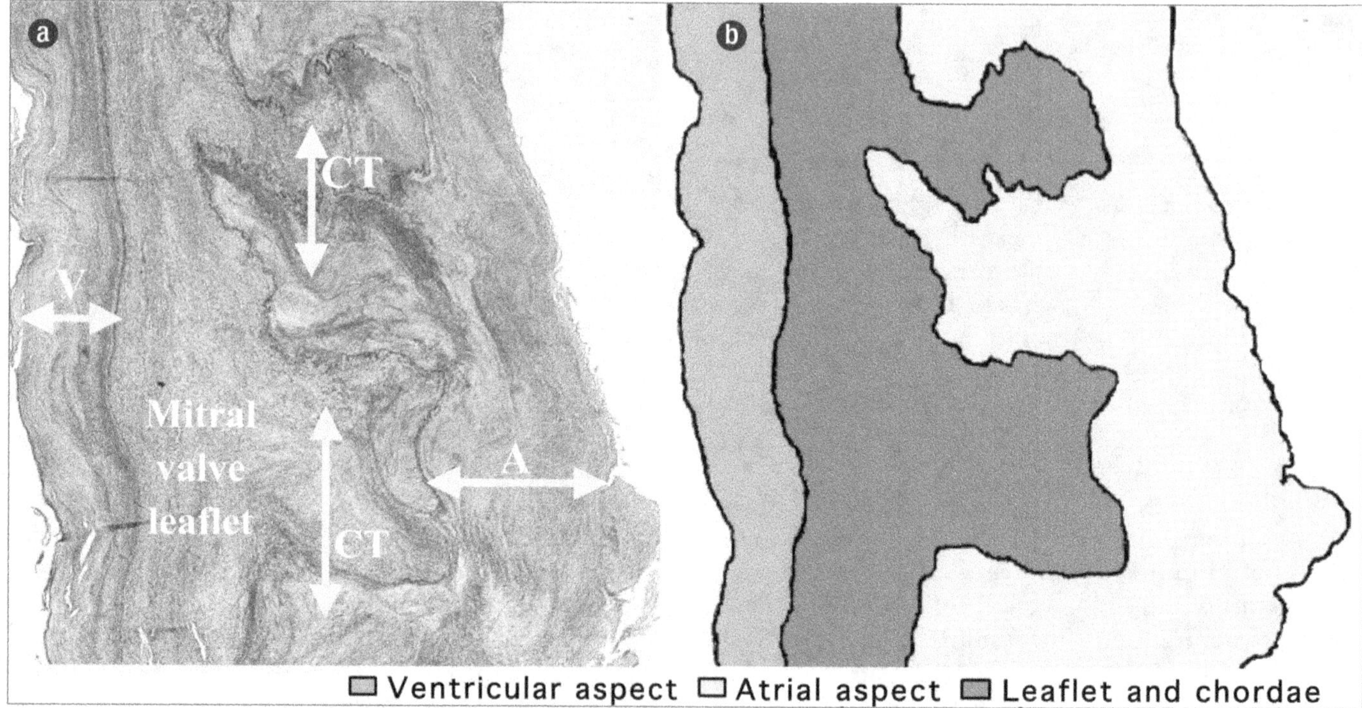

Figure 3. (a) Photomicrograph of a portion of the mitral leaflet and chordae tendineae (CT) with superimposed fibrous tissue on the atrial (A) aspect and on the ventricular (V) aspect. The underlying normal leaflet and chordae tendineae are outlined by a black-staining elastic membrane. It is likely that the chordae had ruptured in the distant past and later the portion closest to the leaflet was covered by fibrous tissue. Elastic von Gieson stain, ×40. **(b)** A color-coded replica with green representing the ventricular aspect, yellow representing the atrial aspect, and red representing the leaflet and chordae.

Table. Previously reported patients having simultaneous aortic and mitral valve operations for a dysfunctioning congenitally bicuspid aortic valve and a dysfunctioning mitral valve*

Valve dysfunction	Patients (n)	Ages, years: Range (mean)	Etiology of MR				
			IE	IC	RHD	MVP	Unknown
AS + MS	6	46–74 (59)	0	0	4	0	2
AS + MR	13	52–84 (66)	2	2	0	4	5
AR + MS	0	0	0	0	0	0	0
AR + MR	9	24–66 (46)	7	0	0	1	1
Totals	28	24–84 (56)	9	2	4	5	8

*From Fernicola and Roberts, 1994 (3) and Roberts et al, 2012 (4).
AR indicates aortic regurgitation; AS, aortic stenosis; IC, ischemic cardiomyopathy; IE, infective endocarditis; MR, mitral regurgitation; MS, mitral stenosis; MVP, mitral valve prolapse; RHD, rheumatic heart disease.

140 beats a minute. An echocardiogram showed MVP with a flail P_2 portion of the posterior leaflet and severe mitral regurgitation. The aortic valve was bicuspid, and moderate aortic regurgitation was present. The left ventricular cavity was of normal size, and its ejection fraction was 60%. Cardiac catheterization disclosed the following pressures in mm Hg: left ventricle, 136/33; aorta, 139/70; pulmonary artery wedge, a wave 23, v 38, mean 11; pulmonary artery, 34/13; right ventricle, 39/14; and right atrium, a wave 14, v wave 13, mean 11. The cardiac index was 2.9 L/min/m². Coronary angiogram disclosed no luminal narrowing; the right coronary was the dominant artery. Left ventricular cavity size and contractility were normal. The aortic regurgitation was graded 2+/4+.

Five days later the purely regurgitant aortic valve was replaced with a #29 Mosaic porcine xenograft. The mitral valve was repaired by resecting P_2, replacing two chordae, and inserting a #37 ATS annuloplasty ring *(Figures 1–3)*. Additionally, a Maze procedure was performed. Seven days postoperatively, because of the development of complete atrioventricular disassociation, a dual-chamber pacemaker was inserted. Electrocardiogram in July 2012 disclosed sinus rhythm (75 beats a minute) and complete left bundle branch block. When seen on September 11, 2012, 3 months after the valve operation, the patient was asymptomatic and "feeling great."

DISCUSSION

The occurrence of both a congenitally BAV and MVP in the same patient suggests that both conditions are of congenital origin. That the BAV is a congenital anomaly is well accepted, but that MVP is also likely a congenital anomaly—at least some of the leaflet and chordal tissue is congenitally deficient—is less well appreciated.

Iqbal and colleagues (1) in 1980 appear to have been the first to report MVP associated with a congenital BAV. They described two patients, one a 39-year-old man who underwent mitral and aortic valve replacement for combined mitral and aortic regurgitation and the other, a 23-year-old man with mitral regurgitation and a normally functioning congenitally BAV.

Chisholm (2) in 1981 found a congenitally BAV in 8 of 257 black patients with MVP. None of his 8 patients had either mitral or aortic dysfunction severe enough to warrant operative intervention. All 8 patients had evidence of trace aortic regurgitation, and none had evidence of aortic stenosis. None apparently had significant mitral regurgitation. The cardiac size in all 8 patients was normal.

In 1994 Fernicola and Roberts (3) described 11 patients who underwent aortic valve replacement for a dysfunctioning congenitally BAV and mitral replacement for a purely regurgitant mitral valve. In 2012 Roberts and colleagues (4) described another 16 patients at another institution who had aortic valve replacement for a dysfunctioning congenitally BAV and simultaneous mitral valve operation for a dysfunctioning mitral valve. The *Table* summarizes the findings in the combined studies by Fernicola and Roberts (3) and by Roberts et al (4). Of their 28 patients, the BAV was stenotic in 19 (68%) and purely regurgitant in 9 (32%); the mitral valve was stenotic in 6 (21%) and purely regurgitant in 22 (79%). Of the 19 patients with stenotic BAVs, at least 4 (21%) had MVP; of the 9 patients with a purely regurgitant BAV, only 1 (11%) had MVP, as did the patient described herein.

1. Iqbal MZ, Eybel CE, Messer JV. Mitral valve prolapse associated with bicuspid aortic valve. *Cardiovasc Rev Rep* 1980;1:465–468.
2. Chisholm JC. Mitral valve prolapse syndrome associated with congenital bicuspid aortic valve. *J Natl Med Assoc* 1981;73(10):921–923.
3. Fernicola DJ, Roberts WC. Pure mitral regurgitation associated with a malfunctioning congenitally bicuspid aortic valve necessitating combined mitral and aortic valve replacement. *Am J Cardiol* 1994;74(6):619–624.
4. Roberts WC, Janning KG, Vowels TJ, Ko JM, Hamman BL, Hebeler RF Jr. Presence of a congenitally bicuspid aortic valve among patients having combined mitral and aortic valve replacement. *Am J Cardiol* 2012;109(2):263–271.

Anomalous Cord From the Raphe of a Congenitally Bicuspid Aortic Valve to the Aortic Wall Producing Either Acute or Chronic Aortic Regurgitation

Travis J. Vowels, BBA,* Gonzalo V. Gonzalez-Stawinski, MD,† Jong M. Ko, BA,*
Gregory D. Trachiotis, MD,‡ Brad J. Roberts, BS, RCS,* Charles S. Roberts, MD,§
William C. Roberts, MD*‖¶

Dallas, Texas; Washington, DC; and Charleston, South Carolina

Objectives	This report calls attention to an unappreciated cause of both acute and chronic aortic regurgitation (AR).
Background	Although stenosis develops in most patients with a congenitally bicuspid aortic valve (BAV), in others with this anomaly, pure AR (no element of stenosis) develops, some in the absence of infection or other clear etiology.
Methods	We describe 5 men who underwent aortic valve replacement for pure AR associated with a BAV containing an anomalous cord attaching the raphe of the conjoined cusp near its free margin to the wall of the ascending aorta cephalad to the sinotubular junction.
Results	Three of these 5 patients had a history of progressive dyspnea, and the anomalous cord, which was intact at operation, appeared to cause chronic AR by preventing proper coaptation of the 2 aortic valve cusps. The other 2 patients heard a "pop" during physical exertion and immediately became dyspneic, and at operation, the anomalous cord was found to have ruptured. Prolapse of the conjoined aortic valve cusp toward the left ventricular cavity resulted in severe acute AR.
Conclusions	This variant of the purely regurgitant BAV may cause either chronic AR (when the anomalous cord does not rupture) or acute severe AR (when the cord ruptures). (J Am Coll Cardiol 2014;63:153–7) © 2014 by the American College of Cardiology Foundation

The congenitally bicuspid aortic valve (BAV) occurs in an estimated 1% of the population, such that in the United States, an estimated 3 million individuals have this malformation (1). Although in some individuals the BAV functions normally for an entire lifetime, stenosis develops in most, superimposed infection (infective endocarditis)

develops in some, and pure aortic regurgitation (AR) unassociated with infective endocarditis or its consequences develops in some (2). A subgroup of those with pure AR unassociated with infection have an anomalous cord extending from the raphe of 1 of the 2 cusps to the wall of the aorta, and the cord serves to keep the raphe cusp from prolapsing toward the left ventricle (Table 1). During a 50-year period, we examined 5 operatively excised purely regurgitant BAVs with an anomalous cord from the raphe to the wall of the aorta. A brief description of these 5 cases is the purpose of this report.

Methods

During a nearly 50-year period, we examined 5 operatively excised aortic valves that were congenitally bicuspid and had a cord attached from the margin of the raphe cusp to the wall of the aorta. The clinical records in all 5 patients were subsequently examined, and all 5 valves were photographed.

From the *Baylor Heart and Vascular Institute, Baylor University Medical Center, Dallas, Texas; †Department of Cardiothoracic Surgery, Baylor University Medical Center, Dallas, Texas; ‡Division of Cardiothoracic Surgery, The George Washington University Medical Center and Veterans Affairs Medical Center, Washington, DC; §Palmetto Cardiovascular and Thoracic Associates, Trident Medical Center, Charleston, South Carolina; ‖Department of Internal Medicine (Division of Cardiology), Baylor University Medical Center, Dallas, Texas; and the ¶Department of Pathology, Baylor University Medical Center, Dallas, Texas. The study was funded by the Baylor Health Care System Foundation, Dallas, Texas. Mr. Vowels is a second-year medical student at the University of Texas Medical School at Houston. The authors have reported that they have no relationships relevant to the contents of this paper to disclose.

Manuscript received July 27, 2013; revised manuscript received August 30, 2013, accepted September 10, 2013.

Abbreviations and Acronyms

AR = aortic regurgitation

BAV = bicuspid aortic valve

Results

Pertinent findings in the 5 patients are summarized in Table 2; all patients were men. Three (Patients #1, #2, and #5) had chronic AR and 2 had acute AR. The latter 2 were asymptomatic until 1 or 2 days before aortic valve replacement: both heard a popping noise in his chest, 1 patient while working in his yard and 1 while working on his car beneath the hood. Both became suddenly dyspneic, and the dyspnea progressed rather rapidly, prompting pulmonary edema and hospitalization. A median sternotomy was emergently performed in each for severe AR. The cord extending from the raphe to the wall of the aorta had ruptured, causing the raphe cusp to prolapse toward the left ventricular cavity (Fig. 1). Each of the other 3 patients had chronic AR, and in none of them had the anomalous cord ruptured.

Photographs of the operatively excised BAVs are shown in Figures 2 to 5.

Discussion

This report describes 5 men with a BAV and pure AR with an anomalous cord extending from the raphe of the conjoined cusp to the wall of the ascending aorta cephalad to the sinotubular junction. In the 3 patients who presented with chronic AR, the cord appeared to prevent complete coaptation of the 2 aortic valve cusps by pinning the raphe of the conjoined cusp to the aortic wall. In the 2 patients who presented with acute AR, the cord had ruptured, resulting in the conjoined cusp prolapsing toward the left ventricular cavity and the acute onset of symptoms.

This variant of the BAV has been previously described (Table 1), and its association with AR has been well documented (1,3–13). Of the 33 previously published cases, 25

Table 1 — Previous Publications of Patients Having an Anomalous Cord Extending From the Raphe of a Congenitally BAV to the Wall of the Aorta Causing Either Acute or Chronic Pure Aortic Regurgitation

Year of Publication	First Author (Ref. #)	No. of Patients With a BAV Containing an Anomalous Cord	No. With Cord Rupture	Mean Age, yrs (Range)	No. of Men	Severity of AR (No. of Patients) 1+	2+	3+	4+
1970	Roberts (1)	1*	0	27	1	0	0	0	1
1971	Carter et al. (3)	1	1	59	1	NA	NA	NA	NA
1977	Becker and Düren (4)	1	1	45	1	0	0	0	1
1984	Olson et al. (5)	11†	1	NA	NA	NA	NA	NA	NA
1986	Yamagishi et al. (6)	1	0	32	1	0	0	0	1
1990	Waller et al. (7)	2	0	53	2	0	0	0	2
1990	Arikawa et al. (8)	2	NA	NA	NA	NA	NA	NA	NA
1992	Hamada et al. (9)	2	1	53	NA	NA	NA	1	NA
1993	Misawa et al. (10)	1	NA	NA	NA	NA	NA	NA	NA
1994	Walley et al. (11)	9	2	61 (46–73)	7	1	1	1	6
2000	Akiyama et al. (12)	1	1	57	1	0	0	1	0
2011	Journigan and Clements (13)	1	1	48	1	0	0	0	1
Total		33	8 (24%)		15/17 (88%)				12/16 (75%)

*Patient is included in the present study (Patient #1). †The author described the bicuspid aortic valves as containing "either a fenestrated raphe or a raphal cord."

BAV = bicuspid aortic valve; NA = not available.

Table 2 — Clinical Data for 6 Men Having AVR for a Purely Regurgitant (4+/4+) Congenitally Bicuspid Aortic Valve With an Anomalous Cord Extending From the Raphe of One Cusp to the Wall of the Aorta

Patient #	Age, yrs	Age, yrs — Precordial Murmur First Heard	Age, yrs — S/S of Heart Failure First Appeared	SH	LVEF, %*	Rupture of Anomalous Cord	AVR (yr)	Type of Valve Implanted
1†‡	27	17	25	0	NA	−	1966	Mechanical
2	45	NA	NA	+	50	−	2013	Mechanical
3	49	49	49	0	55	+§	2012	Bioprosthesis
4	55	55	55	0	NA	+§	2012	Bioprosthesis
5	71	70	70	+	50	−	2012	Bioprosthesis

*LVEF was measured by echocardiography in Patients #2 and #3 and by cardiac catheterization in patient 5. †Patient was previously reported by Roberts (1) in 1970. ‡Patient's aorta coursed over his right main bronchus (right aortic arch). §Producing acute aortic regurgitation.

AVR = aortic valve replacement; LVEF = left ventricular ejection fraction; NA = not available; SH = systemic hypertension; S/S = signs and symptoms; + = positive or present; − = negative or absent.

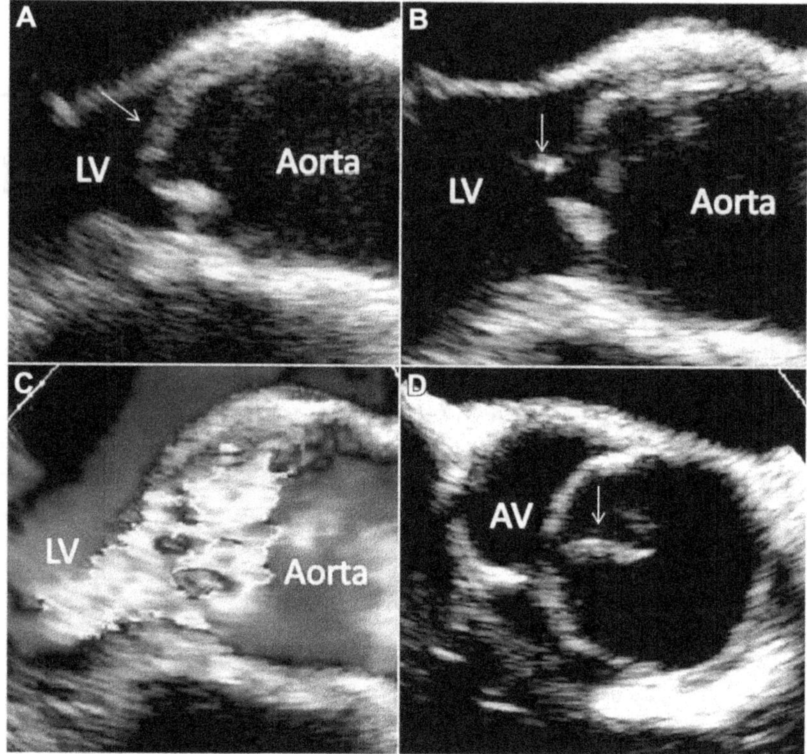

Figure 1   Patient #3: Pre-Operative Transesophageal Echocardiogram Showing a Congenitally Bicuspid Aortic Valve

(A) Long-axis view showing the conjoined cusp **(arrow)** prolapsing toward the left ventricular cavity during diastole. **(B)** Long-axis view showing the anomalous cord **(arrow)** prolapsing toward the left ventricular cavity during diastole. **(C)** Long-axis color Doppler view showing aortic regurgitation. **(D)** Short-axis view showing the flail cord **(arrow)**. AV = aortic valve; LV = left ventricle.

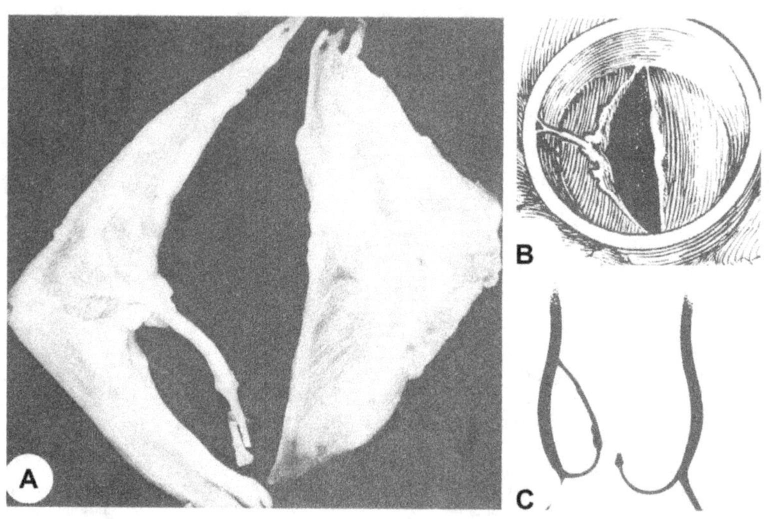

Figure 2   Patient #1

(A) A congenitally bicuspid aortic valve devoid of calcific deposits containing an anomalous cord attached to the conjoined cusp in a 27-year-old man who was found to have a murmur consistent with aortic regurgitation at age 17 years. He remained asymptomatic until age 25 years when exertional dyspnea appeared. On pre-operative cardiac catheterization, the left ventricular pressure was 125/35 mm Hg, the brachial arterial pressure was 125/55 mm Hg, and the cardiac index (Fick method) was 2.2 l/min/m². The patient underwent aortic valve replacement with a mechanical aortic valve prosthesis for chronic aortic regurgitation and died 13 months later. His heart weighed 800 g. **(B)** Diagram of a short-axis view of the aortic aspect of the bicuspid aortic valve before aortic valve replacement showing the attachment of the anomalous cord from the raphe to the wall of the aorta. **(C)** Diagram of a long-axis view of the same valve. Reproduced with permission from Roberts (1).

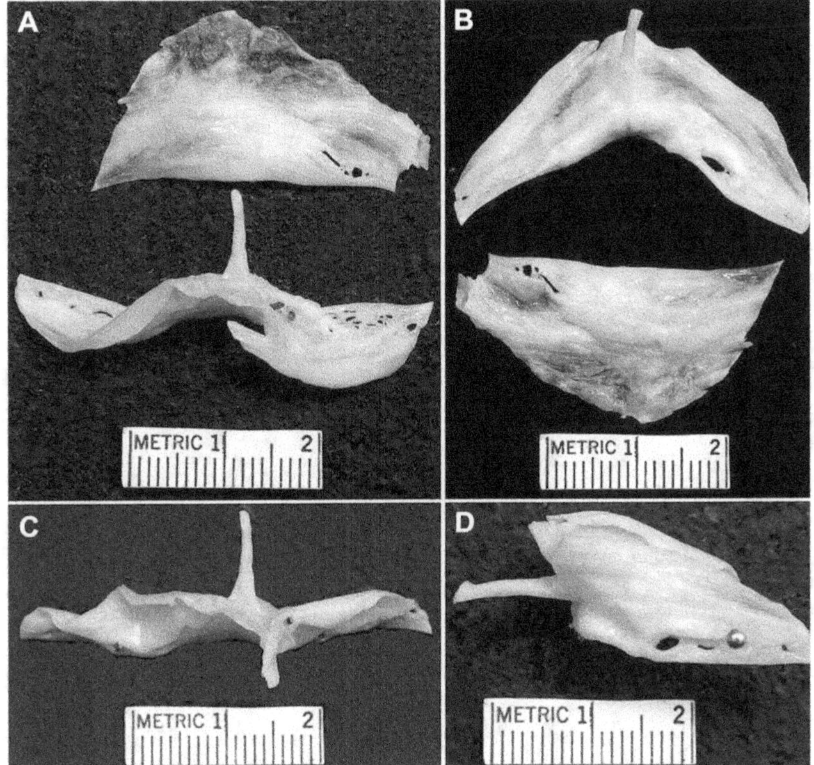

Figure 3   Patient #2

A congenitally bicuspid aortic valve with an anomalous cord extending from the raphe of the conjoined right and left coronary cusps in a 45-year-old man with a history of dyspnea. Pre-operative echocardiogram revealed 4+/4+ aortic regurgitation and a 50% left ventricular ejection fraction. He underwent successful aortic valve replacement with a 27 mm St. Jude Medical Regent mechanical aortic valve (St. Jude Medical Inc., St. Paul, Minnesota). **(A)** View of valve from ventricular aspect. **(B)** View from aortic aspect. **(C)** Lateral view showing the length of the anomalous cord. **(D)** Similar to **C**.

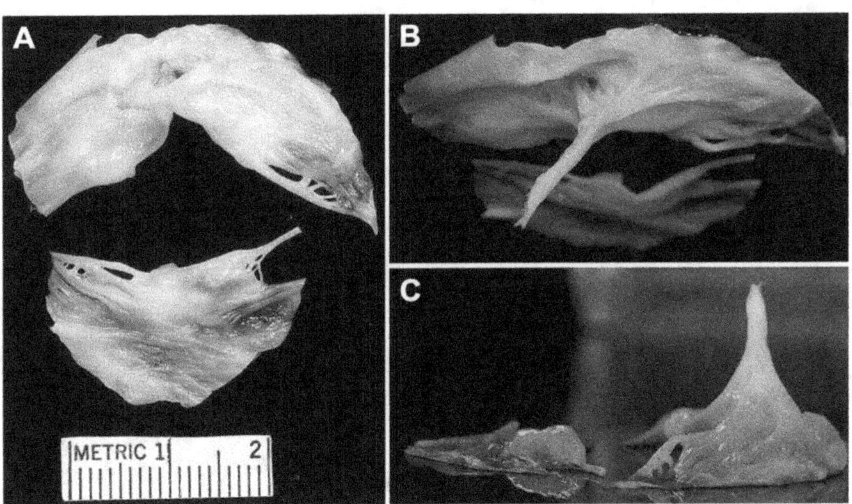

Figure 4   Patient #3

(A) The aortic aspect of a congenitally bicuspid aortic valve with an anomalous cord extending from the raphe in a 49-year-old man who heard a loud "pop" while working in his yard with subsequent chest pain and dyspnea. Two days later, he presented to the emergency department with severe dyspnea, and a chest radiograph revealed bilateral pulmonary edema. A precordial murmur was later heard, and echocardiography revealed a "flail" aortic valve cusp causing severe aortic regurgitation. The left ventricular ejection fraction was 55%. Aortotomy disclosed an anomalous cord attached to his bicuspid aortic valve, and it had ruptured. The valve was replaced with a 23-mm Carpentier-Edwards PERIMOUNT pericardial bioprosthesis (Edward Lifesciences Inc., Irvine, California). **(B)** The torn edge of the anomalous cord. **(C)** From the side of the same valve.

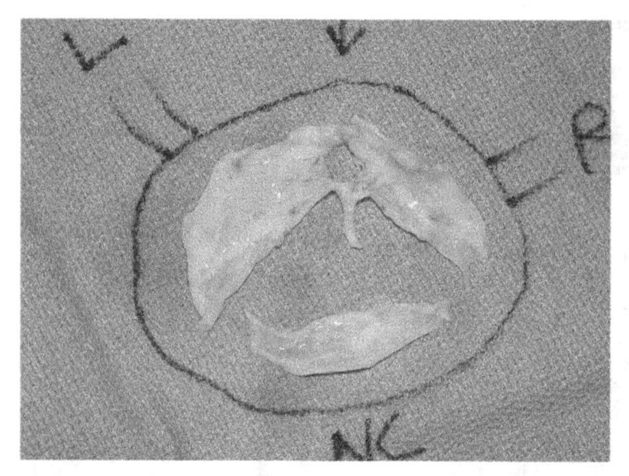

Figure 5 | Patient #4

A congenitally bicuspid aortic valve with an anomalous cord attached at 1 end to the raphe near the free margin in a 55-year-old man who heard a loud "pop" while working on his car and suddenly became dyspneic. He underwent emergent aortic valve replacement with a bioprosthesis for severe acute aortic regurgitation caused by rupture of the anomalous cord where it attached to the wall of the aorta.

(76%) had evidence of chronic AR as a result of having an intact anomalous cord, and 8 (24%) patients presented with acute AR due to rupture of the anomalous cord. Waller et al. (14) in 1973 described 2 other patients, not included in Table 2, with similar BAVs: 1 was an 8-year-old boy with coarctation of the aorta, and 1 was an 81-year-old man with no other associated congenital anomalies. There was no mention of function of the BAV in these 2 patients. In 1994, Walley et al. (11) described 8 patients with this anomalous cord attached to a stenotic BAV in addition to the 9 patients with a purely regurgitant BAV included in Table 1. The presence of an anomalous cord extending to the wall of the aorta from the raphe of a BAV thus may be associated with stenosis but far more commonly with pure AR.

In none of the 5 men included in the present study was the diagnosis of this variant of the purely regurgitant BAV made pre-operatively. Most symptomatic patients with this congenital anomaly present with chronic AR and slowly progressing symptoms. Rupture of an anomalous cord should be considered as a possible etiology of pure acute AR

when infection, aortic dissection, and trauma have been ruled out.

Reprint requests and correspondence: Dr. William C. Roberts, Baylor Heart and Vascular Institute, Baylor University Medical Center at Dallas, 3500 Gaston Avenue, Dallas, Texas 75246. E-mail: wc.roberts@baylorhealth.edu.

REFERENCES

1. Roberts WC. The congenitally bicuspid aortic valve. A study of 85 autopsy cases. Am J Cardiol 1970;26:72–83.
2. Roberts WC, Vowels TJ, Ko JM. Natural history of adults with congenitally malformed aortic valves (unicuspid and bicuspid). Medicine 2012;91:287–308.
3. Carter JB, Sethi S, Lee GB, Edwards JE. Prolapse of semilunar cusps as causes of aortic insufficiency. Circulation 1971;43:922–32.
4. Becker AE, Düren DR. Spontaneous rupture of bicuspid aortic valve. An unusual cause of aortic insufficiency. Chest 1977;72:361–2.
5. Olson LJ, Subramanian R, Edwards WD. Surgical pathology of pure aortic insufficiency: a study of 225 cases. Mayo Clin Proc 1984;59: 835–41.
6. Yamagishi M, Anzai N, Yamada M. An exceptional form of congenitally bicuspid aortic valve resulting in pure aortic regurgitation. Jpn Heart J 1986;27:267–71.
7. Waller BF, Taliercio CP, Dickos DK, Howard J, Adlam JH, Jolly W. Rare or unusual causes of chronic, isolated, pure aortic regurgitation. Clin Cardiol 1990;13:577–81.
8. Arikawa K, Chosa N, Kinjoh T, et al. Pure aortic valve regurgitation due to congenital bicuspid valve. Analysis of 7 cases and a report of 2 rare cases. Nihon Kyobu Geka Gakkai Zasshi 1990;38:2401–3.
9. Hamada Y, Iijima T, Yoshida I, et al. Bicuspid aortic valve with sudden onset of aortic insufficiency due to rare causes: report of two cases. Kyobugeka 1992;45:519–21.
10. Misawa Y, Hasegawa T, Oyama H, Sudo H, Hasegawa N, Kamisawa O. Congenital bicuspid aortic valve with regurgitation. A rare case showing a fibrous band between the conjoined cusp and the ascending aorta. Nihon Kyobu Geka Gakkai Zasshi 1993;41:2156–9.
11. Walley VM, Antecol DH, Kyrollos AG, Chan KL. Congenitally bicuspid aortic valves: study of a variant with fenestrated raphe. Can J Cardiol 1994;10:535–42.
12. Akiyama K, Taniyasu N, Iba Y, Hirota J, Asano S. Sudden deterioration of aortic regurgitation due to rupture of a raphal cord on the conjoined cusp. Jpn Circ J 2000;64:477–80.
13. Journigan JG, Clements SD Jr. Case study: acute aortic regurgitation due to spontaneous rupture of a congenitally malformed bicuspid valve. J Med Assoc Ga 2011;100:26–7.
14. Waller BF, Carter JB, Williams HJ Jr., Wang K, Edwards JE. Bicuspid aortic valve: comparison of congenital and acquired types. Circulation 1973;48:1140–50.

Key Words: aortic regurgitation ▪ bicuspid aortic valve ▪ congenital heart disease.

Characteristics of Adults Having Aortic Valve Replacement for Pure Aortic Regurgitation Involving a Congenitally Bicuspid Aortic Valve Unaffected by Infective Endocarditis or Aortic Dissection

William C. Roberts, MD[a,b,*], Sean P. McCullough[c], and Anupama Vasudevan, BDS, MPH, PhD[d]

Few reports have appeared describing patients with a purely regurgitant congenitally bicuspid aortic valve (BAV) unassociated with active or healed infective endocarditis or with acute or healed aortic dissection. This report describes a large group of such patients who had replacement of the purely regurgitant BAV with or without concomitant resection of the ascending aorta. Operatively excised purely regurgitant BAVs were examined and then their clinical records were examined to confirm that the valves indeed were purely regurgitant. The patients were aged 21 to 86 years (median 50). Of the 133 patients, 114 (86%) were men. The degree of aortic regurgitation (AR) ranged from 1+ to 4+/4+. Of the 133 patients, 52 (39%) had simultaneous resection of the ascending aorta, its frequency varying inversely with the degree of AR. Histologic study of sections of the operatively excised aortas disclosed that 28 (54%) had a normal or nearly normal aorta (0-1+ loss of medial elastic fibers) and that 24 (46%) had an abnormal loss (grade 2+ -4+/4+). In conclusion, the congenitally BAV, unassociated with either infective endocarditis or aortic dissection, is a common cause of pure AR in adults in the Western World undergoing AVR for AR. About half the patients had a dilated ascending aorta and those resected were histologically abnormal half the time. Why one BAV becomes stenotic, another purely regurgitant, another the site of infective endocarditis, and another functions normally for an entire lifetime remains unclear. © 2018 Elsevier Inc. All rights reserved. (Am J Cardiol 2018;122:2104−2111)

Many studies have described real and potential consequences of the congenitally bicuspid aortic valve (BAV).[1−21] A few patients live a full lifetime with a BAV without its developing any complications. Most, however, are not so lucky. The most common complication is aortic stenosis. Infective endocarditis (IE),[10] as pointed out by William Osler, is a well-recognized complication. Often, the tubular portion of the aorta is dilated in patients with a normally functioning BAV as well as in those with aortic stenosis or pure aortic regurgitation (AR) involving a BAV.[11−17] Both aortic isthmic coarctation and coronary arterial anomalies are also more common in patients with bicuspid than in patients with tricuspid aortic valves.[18−20] Patients with congenitally BAVs also have higher frequencies of developing aortic dissection than persons of similar age and sex with tricuspid aortic valves.[21] Although minimal degrees of AR are common in patients with BAVs, the occurrence of pure AR (with or without associated dilatation of the ascending aorta) severe enough to warrant aortic valve replacement (AVR) unassociated with IE or aortic dissection is believed to be relatively uncommon. A description of a group of such patients seen over a 50-year period is the purpose of this report.

Method

Since March 1993, one of us (W.C.R.) has examined and described all cardiac specimens submitted by cardiac surgeons to the department of pathology of Baylor University Medical Center at Dallas. From March 1993 through July 2017, a period of just under 25 years, a total of 112 congenitally BAVs, later confirmed to be purely regurgitant, were received. Each valve was weighed by the same individual (W.C.R.) on a scale accurate to 0.01 g. Before weighing the cusps any formaldehyde/water was removed by patting the cusps with paper towels. After describing the excised cusps, the valves were photographed, and the clinical records were reviewed to confirm that pure AR indeed had been present. Additionally, clinical, echocardiographic, and hemodynamic findings and the operative reports were examined. Also included, in addition to these 112 cases, were 13 patients previously studied at the National Institutes of Health by W.C.R. and reported[22]; 2 other cases came from each of 2 different non-Dallas hospitals and they too were previously reported,[23] and 2 more came from another Dallas hospital. Thus, a total of 133 cases were included in this study.

The ascending aorta was resected at the time of the AVR in 52 (39%) of the 133 patients. The resected portions of

[a]Baylor Scott & White Heart and Vascular Institute, Dallas, Texas; [b]Department(s) of Internal Medicine and Pathology, Baylor University Medical Center, Dallas, Texas; [c]Baylor University, Waco, Texas; and [d]Baylor Scott & White Research Institute, Dallas, Texas. Manuscript received August 29, 2018; revised manuscript received and accepted August 31, 2018.

Funding: No outside funding was provided for this manuscript.

See page 2110 for disclosure information.

*Corresponding author: Tel: (214) 820-7911; fax: (214) 820-7533.

E-mail address: william.roberts1@BSWHealth.org (W.C. Roberts).

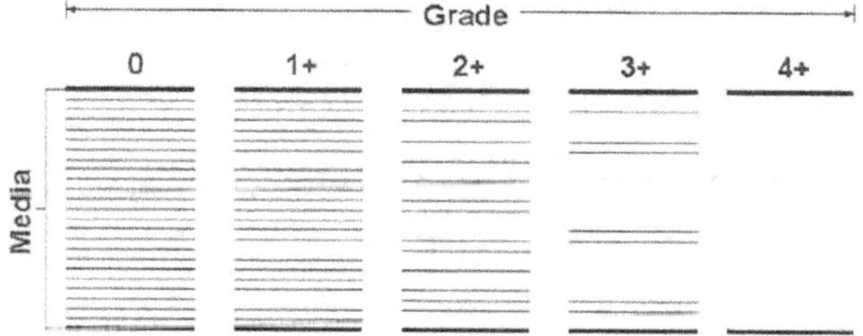

Figure 1. This figure represents a grading system for loss of medial elastic fibers in the aorta. Grade 1 represents no loss. Generally, there are 56 elastic fibers in the aortic media. Grade 1+ represents a minor loss which occurs normally with aging. Grades 2+, 3+, and 4+ represent abnormal loss of medial elastic fibers. Grade 2+ is considerably more than 1+, grade 3+ shows severe loss of medial elastic fibers and grade 4+ shows that at one or more sites no elastic fibers are present between the internal and external elastic membranes.

aorta were weighed and sectioned for histologic study. The sections were stained by the Movat method. At least 20 cm of Movat-stained sections were examined histologically in each patient (With this stain the medial elastic fibers are well-defined). The loss of medial elastic fibers was graded 0 to 4+ as illustrated in Figure 1.

Statistical analyses were done using STATA 14.2. Categorical variables were presented as proportions and continuous variables as mean (SD) or median (range) as applicable. Chi-square/Fisher exact tests were conducted to compare proportions and Student t-test Test/Wilcoxon rank sum test were conducted to compare continuous variables as appropriate. Trend tests (np-trend) were conducted for ordinal variables such as grades of aortic regurgitation and age groups.

Results

The findings are summarized in Table 1. The ages of the 133 patients ranged from 21 to 86 years (mean 50);

114 (86%) were men and 19 (14%) were women. The degree of AR was graded 1+ to 4+ with 1+ being minimal; 2+ mild; 3+ moderately severe and 4+ severe. In 63 patients, left ventricular and systemic arterial pressures were available from cardiac catheterization: all had peak transvalvular gradients ≤ 10 mm Hg; most were 0.

The ascending aortas were resected in 52 patients (39%); the diameter of the ascending aorta preoperatively ranged from 37 to 60 mm (mean 52). Of these 52 patients, 28 (59%) had no loss or minimal loss of medial elastic fibers (graded as 0 to 1+ [considered normal for age]); 24 (46%) had 2+ to 4+ loss of medial elastic fibers (considered abnormal). The frequency of excision of the ascending aorta at the time of AVR was significantly higher in the 20 patients with 1+ or 2+ AR than in the 89 patients with 3+ or 4+ AR (75% vs 30%) (Figure 2). No relation was found between the degree of AR and the frequency of concomitant coronary artery bypass grafting, which occurred in 19 patients (14%). The frequency of resection of the aorta by age decade is shown in Figure 3 and by year decade in Figure 4.

The operatively excised aortic valves, weighed in 119 patients (89%), ranged from 0.42 to 2.9 g (mean 1.27), and the mean weights were significantly larger in the men than in the women. The operatively excised ascending aortas, weighed in 49 patients (94%), ranged from 5.2 to 51.0 g (mean 15.7). Three other patients had biopsies of the ascending aorta and they disclosed either 0 or 1+ loss of medial elastic fibers. (These 3 cases were not included in Table 1.) Several operatively excised aortic valves with or without ascending aortas are shown in Figures 5–7.

Discussion

This study describes findings in 133 patients undergoing AVR for pure AR (no element of stenosis) associated with a congenitally BAV but unassociated with IE

Table 1

Clinical and morphological characteristics of patients with congenitally bicuspid aortic valves having aortic valve replacement for pure chronic aortic regurgitation without infective endocarditis or aortic dissection (n = 133)

Variable	Total (n = 133)	Men (n = 114)	Women (n = 19)	p value
Age (years) at aortic valve replacement (mean ± SD)	50.3 ± 13.1	49.6 ± 12.8	54.3 ± 14.5	0.15
Coronary artery bypass grafting	19 (14%)	18 (16%)	1 (5%)	0.69
Aortic regurgitation grade				0.97
1+	9 (8%)	8 (9%)	1 (7%)	
2+	11 (10%)	10 (11%)	1 (7%)	
3+	26 (24%)	23 (24%)	3 (20%)	
4+	63 (58%)	53 (56%)	10 (67%)	
Aortic valve weight (g) (n = 119)				
Mean ± SD	1.26 ± 0.46	1.30 ± 0.46	1.05 ± 0.41	
Median (range)	1.2 (0.42–2.90)	1.32 (0.42–2.90)	1.05 (0.42–1.80)	0.03
Ascending aorta excised	52 (39%)	41 (36%)	11 (58%)	0.07
Number with ascending aorta weight	49 (94%)	39 (95%)	10 (91%)	
Ascending aorta weight (g) mean ± SD	15.64 ± 7.42	14.66 ± 4.61	19.49 ± 13.57	
Ascending aorta weight (g) median (range)	15.1 (5.17–51.0)	15.07 (5.17–23.10)	14.87 (9.58–51.0)	0.74
Number with ascending aortic diameter	39 (75%)	32 (78%)	7 (64%)	
Aortic diameter (mm) mean ± SD	51.87 ± 5.21	51.90 ± 5.46	51.71 ± 4.23	
Aortic diameter (mm) median (range)	53 (37–60)	53 (37–60)	53 (43–55)	0.84
Loss of medial elastic fibers (0-4+) (grade)				0.16
0 − 1+	28 (54%)	20 (49%)	8 (73%)	
2+ − 4+	24 (46%)	21 (51%)	3 (27%)	

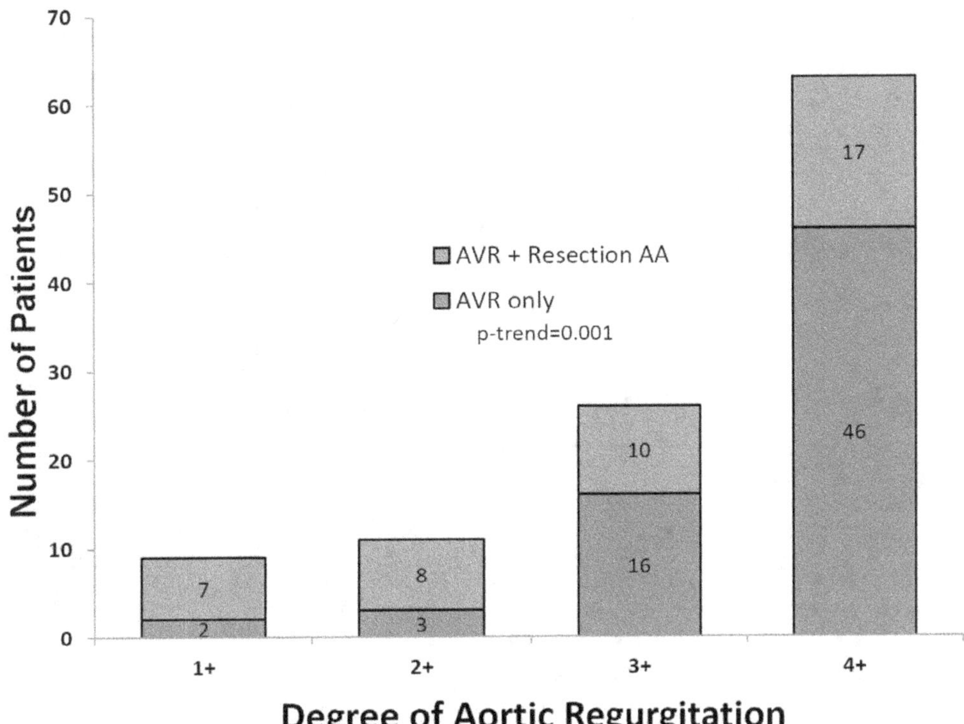

Figure 2. This bar graph shows the relation of the degree of aortic regurgitation, graded 1+ to 4+, involving a congenitally bicuspid aortic valve to the frequency of resection of the dilated ascending aorta. The orange indicates the patients who had resection of the ascending aorta in addition to aortic valve replacement. The patients with 1+ and 2+ aortic regurgitation had a higher frequency of ascending aorta resection than did the patients with grade 3+ or 4+ aortic regurgitation.

(either healed or active) or with aortic dissection (either acute or chronic). All patients were >20 years of age and most (86%) were men. The degree of AR ranged from mild to severe and the patients with mild AR had a significantly higher frequency of concomitant resection of the ascending aorta because of its large diameter than did the patients with more severe degrees of AR. A minority (52 of the 133) of the patients had the

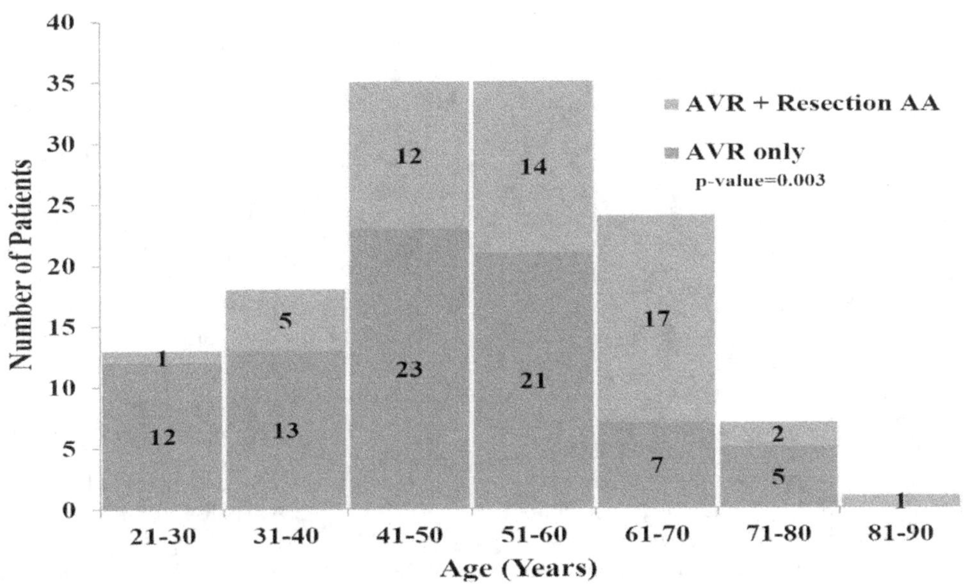

Figure 3. This bar graph shows the frequency of resection of ascending aorta according to age decade at the time of aortic valve replacement for pure aortic regurgitation involving a congenitally bicuspid aortic valve. The orange indicates the patients who had both valve and ascending aorta resected and the blue, the patients having only the aortic valve resected.

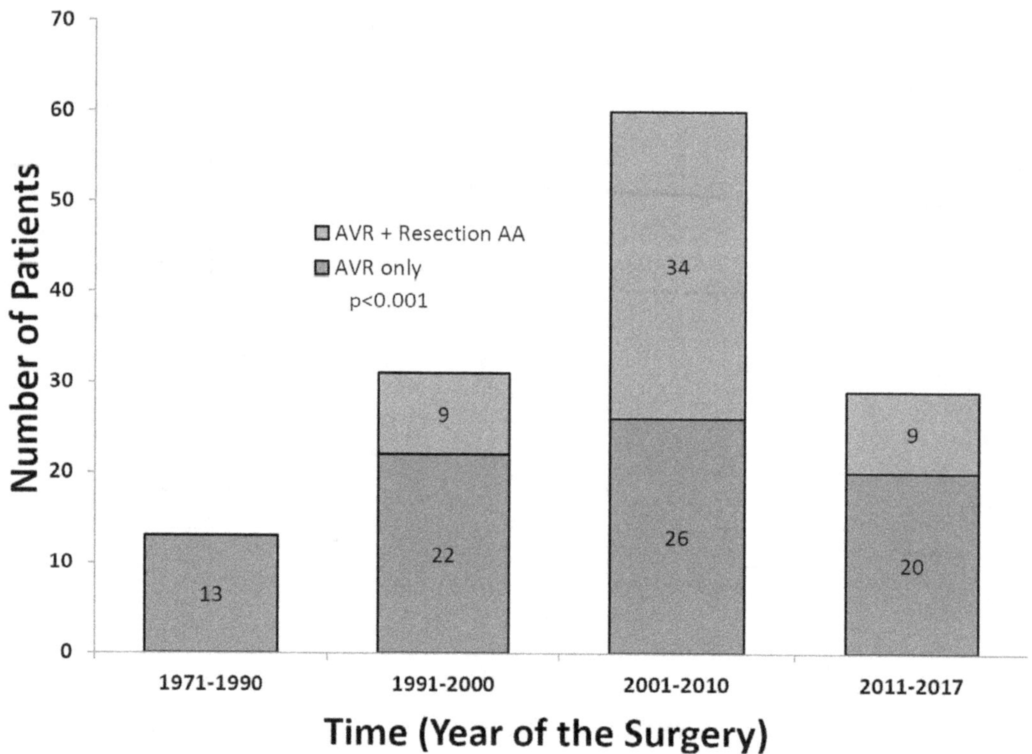

Figure 4. This bar graph shows the frequency of resection of ascending aorta by year decade at the time of aortic valve replacement for pure aortic regurgitation involving a congenitally bicuspid aortic valve. Among the 4 time periods the decade of 2001 through 2010 had the highest frequency of ascending aortic replacement.

ascending aorta resected at the time of AVR. Of them, 28 (54%) had a histologically normal or nearly normal aorta (grade 0 or 1+) and 24 (46%) had a histologically abnormal aorta (grade 2+ to 4+ loss of medial elastic fibers). In contrast, in an earlier study[14] of patients with aortic stenosis who had AVR and concomitant resection of the ascending aorta, 90% had no loss or only trace loss of aortic medial elastic fibers (grade 0 or 1+/4+) and only 10% had grade 2+ − 4+/4+ loss of medial elastic fibers.

The first report to point out that the congenitally BAV could be purely regurgitant (no element of stenosis) without superimposed IE or aortic dissection appeared in 1981 (36 years ago) by Roberts and colleagues[23] who described 13 patients aged 26 to 65 years (mean 43), all men, who also underwent AVR but without resection of the ascending aorta. The peak systolic left ventricular pressures in all 13 patients were equal to or lower than the peak systolic systemic arterial pressures. Subsequently, no report has appeared focusing exclusively on patients having AVR for pure AR involving a congenitally BAV unassociated with either IE or aortic dissection.

The BAV is frequent among patients with AR severe enough to warrant AVR. Olson et al[24] in 1984 examined 225 operatively excised aortic valves that were "either nonstenotic or only mildly stenotic." Some of the patients had "coexistent mitral and/or right-sided valvular disease." The cause of the AR among their 225 cases was "postinflammatory" (apparently rheumatic) in 103 cases (46%), "dilated aorta" in 48 (21%), BAV in 54 (24%), IE in 12 (5%), and miscellaneous in 8 (4%). Had the rheumatic cases not been included, the frequency of the BAV would have been higher. Of the 54 patients with BAV, the AR was attributed to superimposed IE in 9. Of the 21 cases with IE, 9 had a BAV and 12 had a tricuspid aortic valve. Of the 12 with a tricuspid aortic valve the valve was judged to be functionally normal before the IE appeared. Aortic dissection occurred in 3 of their 54 cases with a BAV and in none of their 171 cases with a tricuspid aortic valve. Roberts and colleagues[25] in 2006 described 268 patients who underwent AVR for pure AR: in 123 (46%) the AR resulted from disease of the aortic valve and in 146 (54%), from disease of the ascending aorta. (In the latter group, the aortic valve cusps were normal or only mildly thickened on their margins, mainly their central portions.) Of the 122 with disease of the aortic valve, 59 (48%) (49 men) had a congenitally BAV, 22 of whom had a dilated ascending aorta and it was resected. Of the 146 patients in whom the pure AR resulted from disease of the aorta (none had a BAV): aortic dissection was the cause in 28, the Marfan syndrome or its forme fruste variety in 15, syphilis in 12, and the cause was unclear in 91 (34%).

Among patients having AVR because of a malfunctioning BAV, pure AR is found far less commonly than the stenotic BAV. During the period April 1993 through April 2018 we examined 1,279 operatively excised BAVs, 87%

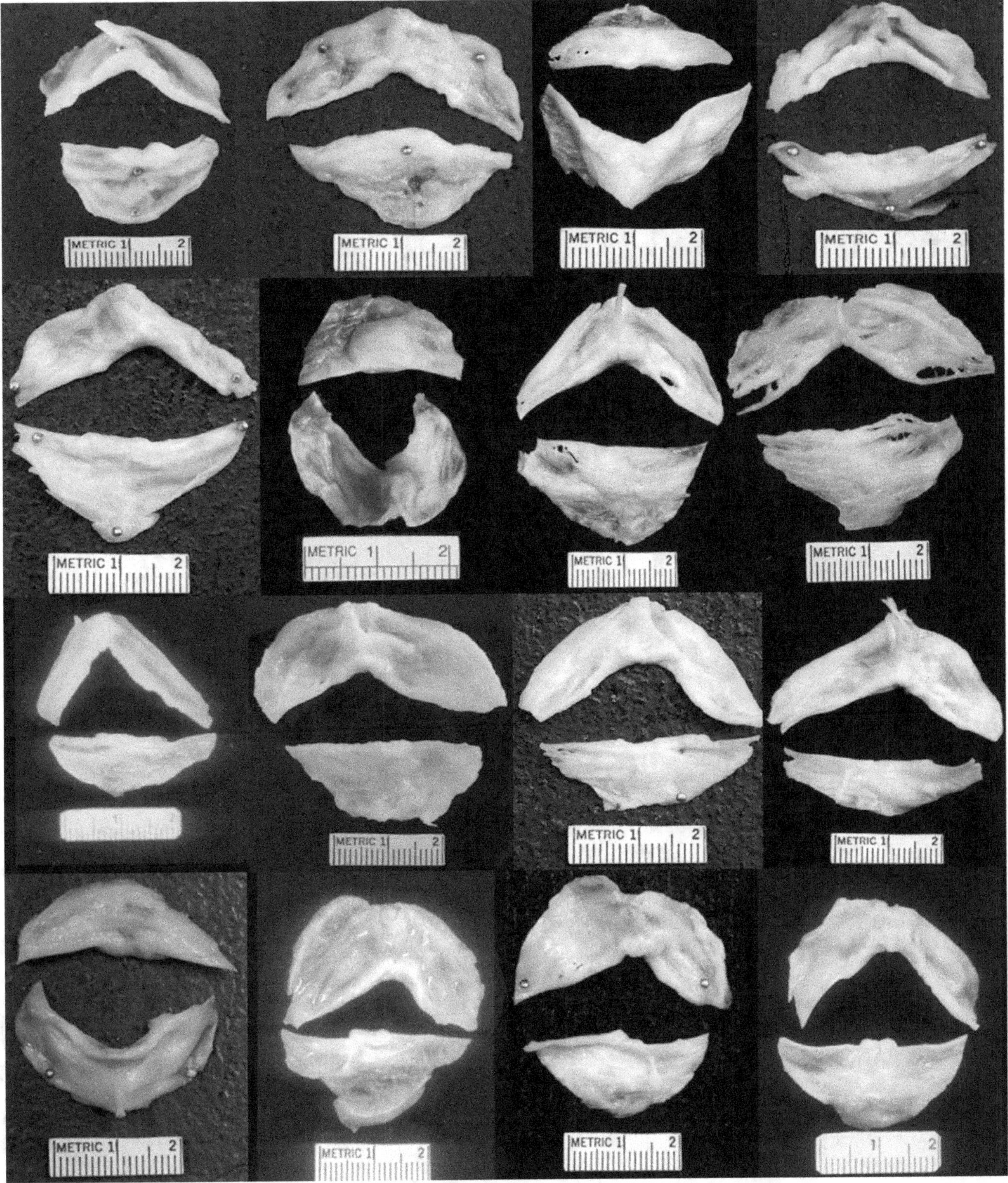

Figure 5. Shown here are photographs of congenitally bicuspid regurgitant aortic valves in 16 patients. The views are from the aortic aspect. The top row (*left to right*) are patients aged 21, 27, 36, and 36. In row 2 (*left to right*) the patients are aged 37, 40, 40, 45, and 47. In row 3 (*left to right*) the patients are aged 48, 48, 49, and 49. In the bottom row (*left to right*) the patients are aged 51, 54, 55, and 56. Raphes are present in these valves. None of these 16 patients had resection of any portion of ascending aorta.

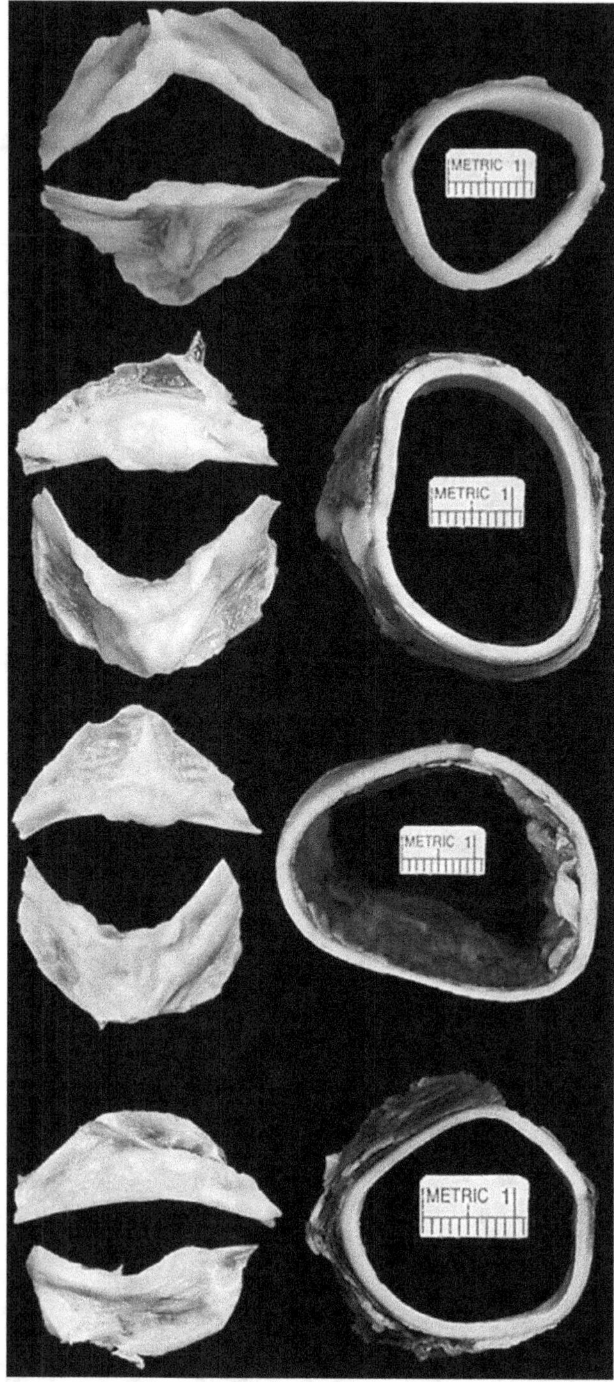

Figure 6. Shown here are the aortic valves and the intact ascending aorta in 4 patients with pure aortic regurgitation and a dilated ascending aorta. The *top panel* shows the aortic valve and aorta from a 38-year-old man; *top middle*, from a 48-year-old man; *bottom middle*, from a 57-year-old man, and *bottom panel*, from a 61-year-old man.

of which were stenotic (with or without some regurgitation) and 13% were purely regurgitant, indicating that during this time period stenotic valves were excised at a rate 6.6 times higher than that of purely regurgitant aortic valves. These numbers do not include the congenitally malformed unicuspid unicommissural aortic valves (usually called "bicuspid" by surgeons). If the unicuspid valves

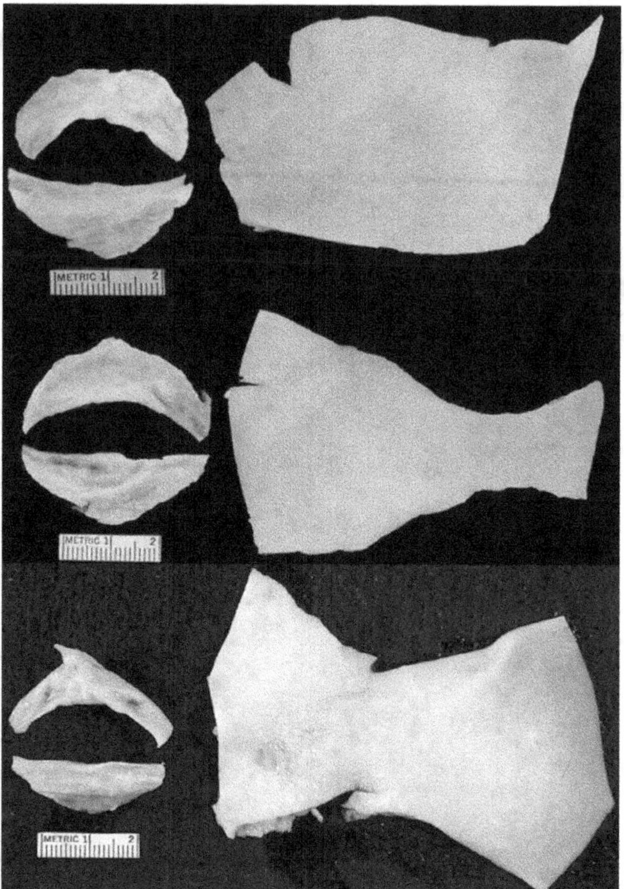

Figure 7. Shown here are bicuspid aortic valves and portions of ascending aorta removed in 3 patients with pure aortic regurgitation. The valve and aorta in the *top view* is from a 45-year-old man; in the *middle view*, from a 50-year-old man; and *bottom view*, from a 52-year-old man.

were included the frequency of the congenitally malformed stenotic valves, would be 7.4 times more frequent than the purely regurgitant bicuspid aortic valves. Sadee and colleagues[26] in 1992 reported 148 patients who had operative excision of a congenitally BAV: 14 (9%) had pure AR and 134 (91%) had aortic stenosis. There was no mention of either IE or aortic dissection and no purely regurgitant valves were illustrated. Sabet and associates[27] in 1999 reported 552 patients who had AVR and a congenitally BAV was resected: in 462 (85%) the BAV was stenotic; in 73 (13%), purely regurgitant, and in 7 the valve had functioned normally (although 2 of the 7 had IE). Of the 552 patients, 16 (3%) had IE, including 10 (14%) of the patients with pure AR. Eleven stenotic valves but no purely regurgitant valves were illustrated. The frequency of aortic dissection was not mentioned.

A purely regurgitant BAV is far less common among patients with BAV studied at autopsy than after operative resection. Roberts[1] in 1970, among 85 autopsied patients with BAV, found that 61 (82%) had aortic stenosis (with or without AR); 11 (13%) had pure AR (secondary to IE in 8 and unassociated with IE in 3), and 13 (15%) had a normally functioning aortic valve (an incidental autopsy finding). Thus, only 3 (4%) had pure AR involving a BAV unaffected by IE and unassociated with aortic dissection. Fenoglio and associates[3] in 1977, studied at necropsy 152 patients (aged 20 to 89 years) who had a congenitally BAV: only 5 (3%) had pure AR but "the majority...had perforated aortic valve cusps" indicating that most of these 5 patients almost certainly had had IE that healed.[28] Of their 152 patients, 60 (40%) had IE, 23 (15%) had aortic stenosis, and the remainder apparently had a normally functioning congenitally BAV. Thus, the complications of the BAV in their 152 autopsy cases stand at an unusual variance from most studies of patients with a BAV. Roberts and colleagues[10] in 2012 studied at necropsy 218 patients > 20 years of age with BAVs and none of the patients had ever undergone a cardiac operation or percutaneous transluminal aortic valve implantation. In other words, this was a true natural history study. Of the 218 patients, 142 (65%) had aortic stenosis (with or without AR) (11 of whom had superimposed IE); only 2 (1%) had pure AR not secondary to IE, and 74 (34%) had a normally functioning aortic valve that was the site of IE in 20. The IE produced severe AR in 15 (75%) of those 20 patients. Thus, in this large natural history study, only 2 patients (1%) had pure AR unrelated to IE or aortic dissection.

Limited data have been reported previously on the weights of operatively excised purely regurgitant aortic valves. In the present study the operatively excised purely regurgitant BAVs ranged in weight from 0.42 to 2.9 g (mean 1.27); the mean weights were significantly larger in the men than in the women (mean 1.32 g vs mean 1.05 g). (The weight of normal 3-cuspid aortic valves in adults ranges from 0.40 to 0.60 g [29]). The weight of normally functioning congenitally BAVs in adults has not been determined. The purely regurgitant tricuspid aortic valves in patients in whom aortic regurgitation resulted from disease of the aorta rather than from disease of the valve ranged from 0.4 to 0.7 g. In the present study, the weights of the purely regurgitant BAVs did not increase with age or with the degree of AR. The purely regurgitant aortic valves weigh considerably less than the stenotic aortic valves irrespective of the number of aortic valve cusps.[28–32] The purely regurgitant aortic valves are, with a few exceptions, devoid of calcific deposits whereas virtually all stenotic aortic valves in adults contain calcific deposits. It is the calcium that makes the stenotic valves weight so much more than the purely regurgitant aortic valves.

Disclosures

None of the authors have any relationships with industry relevant to the contents of this manuscript to disclose.

1. Roberts WC. The congenitally bicuspid aortic valve. A study of 85 autopsy cases. *Am J Cardiol* 1970;26:72–83.
2. Roberts WC. The structure of the aortic valve in clinically-isolated aortic stenosis: An autopsy study of 162 patients over 15 years of age. *Circulation* 1970;42:91–97.
3. Fenoglio JJ Jr, McAllister HA Jr, DeCastro CM, Davia JE, Cheitlin MD. Congenital bicuspid aortic valve after age 20. *Am J Cardiol* 1977;39:164–169.
4. Arnett EN, Roberts WC. Pathology of active infective endocarditis: A necropsy analysis of 192 patients. *Thorac Cardiovasc Surg* 1982;30:327–335.
5. Roberts WC, Ko JM. Frequency by decades of unicuspid, bicuspid, and tricuspid aortic valves in adults having isolated aortic valve replacement for aortic stenosis, with or without associated aortic regurgitation. *Circulation* 2005;111:920–925.
6. Lewin MB, Otto CM. The bicuspid aortic valve: adverse outcomes from infancy to old age. *Circulation* 2005;111:832–834.
7. Tzemos N, Therrien J, Yip J, Thanassoulis G, Tremblay S, Jamorski MT, Webb GD, Siu SC. Outcomes in adults with bicuspid aortic valves. *JAMA* 2008;300:1317–1325.
8. Michelena HI, Desjardins VA, Avierinos JF, Russo A, Nkomo VT, Sundt TM, Pellikka PA, Tajik AJ, Enriquez-Sarano M. Natural history of asymptomatic patients with normally functioning or minimally dysfunctional bicuspid aortic valve in the community. *Circulation* 2008;117:2776–2784.
9. Tribouilloy C, Rusinaru D, Sorel C, Thuny F, Casalta JP, Riberi A, Jeu A, Gouriet F, Collart F, Caus T, Raoult D, Habib G. Clinical characteristics and outcome of infective endocarditis in adults with bicuspid aortic valves: a multicentre observational study. *Heart* 2010;96:1723–1729.
10. Roberts WC, Vowels TJ, Ko JM. Natural history of adults with congenitally malformed aortic valves (unicuspid or bicuspid). *Medicine* 2012;91:287–308.
11. Pachulski RT, Weinberg AL, Chan KL. Aortic aneurysm in patients with functionally normal or minimally stenotic bicuspid aortic valve. *Am J Cardiol* 1991;67:781–782.
12. Hahn RT, Roman MJ, Mogtader AH, Devereux RB. Association of aortic dilation with regurgitant, stenotic and functionally normal bicuspid aortic valves. *J Am Coll Cardiol* 1992;19:283–288.
13. Bonow RO. Bicuspid aortic valves and dilated aortas: a critical review of the ACC/AHA practice guidelines recommendations. *Am J Cardiol* 2008;102:111–1114.
14. Roberts WC, Vowels TJ, Ko JM, Filardo G, Hebeler RF Jr, Henry AC, Matter GJ, Hamman BL. Comparison of the structure of the aortic valve and ascending aorta in adults having aortic valve replacement for aortic stenosis versus for pure aortic regurgitation and resection of the ascending aorta for aneurysm. *Circulation* 2011;123:896–903.
15. Michelena HI, Khanna AD, Mahoney D, Margaryan E, Topilsky Y, Suri RM, Eidem B, Edwards WD, Sundt TM 3rd, Enriquez-Sarano M. Incidence of aortic complications in patients with bicuspid aortic valves. *JAMA* 2011;306:1104–1112.
16. Roberts WC. Prophylactic replacement of a dilated ascending aorta at the time of aortic valve replacement of a dysfunctioning congenitally unicuspid or bicuspid aortic valve. *Am J Cardiol* 2011;108:1371–1372.
17. Michelena HI, Prakash SK, Della Corte A, Bissell MM, Anavekar N, Mathieu P, Bossé Y, Limongelli G, Bossone E, Benson DW, Lancellotti P, Isselbacher EM, Enriquez-Sarano M, Sundt TM 3rd, Pibarot P, Evangelista A, Milewicz DM, Body SC. BAVCon Investigators. Bicuspid aortic valve: identifying knowledge gaps and rising to the challenge from the International Bicuspid Aortic Valve Consortium (BAVCon). *Circulation* 2014;129:2691–2704.
18. Abbott ME. Coarctation of the aorta of the adult type. *Am Heart J* 1928;3:381–421.
19. Glancy DL, Morrow AG, Simon AL, Roberts WC. Juxtaductal aortic coarctation: Analysis of 84 patients studied hemodynamically, angiographically and morphologically after age 1 year. *Am J Cardiol* 1983;51:537–551.
20. Roberts WC. Major anomalies of coronary arterial origin seen in adulthood. *Am Heart J* 1986;11:941–963.
21. Roberts CS, Roberts WC. Dissection of the aorta associated with congenital malformation of the aortic valve. *J Am Coll Cardiol* 1991;17:712–716.
22. Roberts WC, Morrow AG, McIntosh CL, Jones M, Epstein SE. Congenitally bicuspid aortic valve causing severe, pure aortic regurgitation without superimposed infective endocarditis: Analysis of 13 patients requiring aortic valve replacement. *Am J Cardiol* 1981;47:206–209.
23. Vowels TJ, Gonzalez-Stawinski GV, Ko JM, Trachiotis GD, Roberts BJ, Roberts CS, Roberts WC. Anomalous cord from the raphe of a

congenitally bicuspid aortic valve to the aortic wall producing either acute or chronic aortic regurgitation. *J Am Coll Cardiol* 2014;63:153–157.

24. Olson LJ, Subramanian R, Edwards WD. Surgical pathology of pure aortic insufficiency: a study of 225 cases. *Mayo Clin Proc* 1984;59:835–841.

25. Roberts WC, Ko JM, Moore TR, Jones WH III. Causes of pure aortic regurgitation in patients having isolated aortic valve replacement at a single US tertiary hospital (1993-2005). *Circulation* 2006;114:422–429.

26. Sadee AS, Becker AE, Verheul RA, Beuma B, Hoedemaker G. Aortic valve regurgitation and the congenitally bicuspid aortic valve: a clinic-pathological correlation. *Br Heart J* 1992;67:439–441.

27. Sabat HY, Edwards WD, Tazelaar HD, Daly RC. Congenitally bicuspid aorta valves: a surgical pathology study of 542 cases (1992 through 1996) a literature review of 2, 715 additional cases. *Mayo Clinic Proc* 1999;74:14–26.

28. Roberts WC, Buchbinder NA. Healed left-sided infective endocarditis: a clinicopathologic study of 59 patients. *Am J Cardiol* 1977;40:876–888.

29. Silver MA, Roberts WC. Detailed anatomy of the normally functioning aortic valve in hearts of normal and increased weight. *Am J Cardiol* 1985;55:454–461.

30. Roberts WC, Ko JM. Frequency by decades of unicuspid, bicuspid, and tricuspid aortic valves in adults having isolated aortic valve replacement for aortic stenosis, with or without associated aortic regurgitation. *Circulation* 2005;111:920–925.

31. Roberts WC, Ko JM. Relation of weights of operatively excised stenotic aortic valves to preoperative transvalvular peak systolic pressure gradients and to calculated aortic valve areas. *J Am Coll Cardiol* 2004;44:1847–1855.

32. Roberts WC, Ko JM, Filardo G. Comparison of heavier versus lighter operatively excised stenotic aortic valves in adults with aortic stenosis and implications for percutaneous aortic valve implantation without replacement. *Am J Cardiol* 2009;104:393–405.

Orthotopic Heart Transplantation for Ankylosing Spondylitis Masquerading as Nonischemic Cardiomyopathy

Samarthkumar J. Thakkar, MD[a], Paul A. Grayburn, MD[a,b], Shelley Anne Hall, MD[a,b], and William C. Roberts, MD[a,b,c,*]

Described herein is a 48-year-old man who underwent orthotopic heart transplantation because of severe heart failure considered clinically due to idiopathic dilated cardiomyopathy, but examination of the operatively excised native heart disclosed classic features of ankylosing spondylitis. Orthotopic heart transplantation for this condition has not been reported previously.   © 2019 Elsevier Inc. All rights reserved. (Am J Cardiol 2019;123:1732−1735)

We recently studied the heart of a patient who had undergone orthotopic heart transplantation (OHT) for presumed idiopathic dilated cardiomyopathy and examination of the operatively excised heart disclosed it to have classic morphologic features of ankylosing spondylitis.[1,2] The patient clinically had aortic regurgitation, complete heart block, and periodic low back pain. Search of PubMed failed to disclose any report of OHT for ankylosing spondylitis. A description of this patient is the purpose of this report.

Case Description

A 48-year-old male roofer, who was born in March 1970, had been well until May 2011 (age 41) when he developed the sudden onset of dyspnea and was hospitalized. His systolic blood pressure was about 200 mm Hg, his coronary arteries were free of obstructive lesions, and his left ventricular ejection fraction was about 15%. He was started on valsartan, carvedilol, isosorbide dinitrate, and amlodipine, but despite these medicines, he had frequent episodes of acute heart failure. During one episode in March 2015, he was found to have abnormal kidney function and an atrophic left kidney (cause unknown) that was excised. The main artery to the right kidney was found to be stenotic and a stent was inserted. At that time, he developed complete heart block and a dual chamber pacemaker was inserted. In July 2016, he was started on peritoneal dialysis and 2 months later, hemodialysis. In July 2017, cardiac resynchronization therapy defibrillator was inserted.

In April 2018, he developed cardiogenic shock and pulmonary edema and was transferred to Baylor University Medical Center at Dallas. On arrival, his blood pressure was 160/80 mm Hg. A precordial murmur was not heard but his respirations were extremely rapid. The electrocardiogram (Figure 1) showed atrial-sensed ventricular-paced rhythm and total 12-lead QRS voltage of 152 mm (10-mm standard).[3] The echocardiogram (Figure 2) showed the left ventricular chamber to be severely dilated, the ejection fraction to be about 20%, and severe aortic regurgitation to be present. At cardiac catheterization, the cardiac index was 1.5 L/min/m^2. Certain laboratory findings are listed in Table 1.

He underwent combined heart and kidney transplant in May 2018. The native heart weighed 675 g (Figures 3 and 4). The left ventricular cavity was considerably dilated longitudinally: the distance from the base of the right aortic valve cusp to the apex was 9.5 cm. The anterior mitral leaflet was severely thickened by dense fibrous tissue, and the posterior mitral leaflet was normal. The bases of each aortic cusp were thickened by similar fibrous tissue which extended cephalad onto the aorta in the areas of the commissures. The epicardial coronary arteries were free of atherosclerotic plaques.

Discussion

Described herein is a 48-year-old man who underwent OHT because of severe heart failure attributed clinically to idiopathic dilated cardiomyopathy. Study of his explanted native heart, however, disclosed classic (specific) morphologic findings of ankylosing spondylitis,[1,2] distinctive and different from other cardiac conditions (Figure 5). Before OHT, echocardiogram disclosed severe aortic regurgitation. Although the degree of aortic regurgitation in our patient was severe by echocardiogram, a precordial murmur was not detected while in severe heart failure, probably the result of his rapid respiratory rate and his obesity (body mass index 33 kg/m^2). A precordial murmur had been present earlier when he was not in heart failure. His pulse pressure when hospitalized at our institution was 80 mm Hg.

Aortic regurgitation appears to occur in about 20% of patients with ankylosing spondylitis[4] and it usually appears after the appearance of the orthopedic consequences, although the reverse occurs, as in the present patient, on occasion. The severe thickening of the anterior mitral leaflet in ankylosing spondylitis in the

[a]Baylor Scott and White Heart and Vascular Institute, Baylor University Medical Center, Dallas, Texas; [b]Department of Internal Medicine (Division of Cardiology), Baylor University Medical Center, Dallas, Texas; and [c]Department of Pathology, Baylor University Medical Center, Dallas, Texas. Manuscript received November 1, 2018; revised manuscript received February 11, 2019; revised manuscript received and accepted February 11, 2019.

See page 1734 for disclosure information.

*Corresponding author: Tel: (214) 820-7911; fax: (214) 820-7533.

E-mail address: william.roberts1@BSWHealth.org (W.C. Roberts).

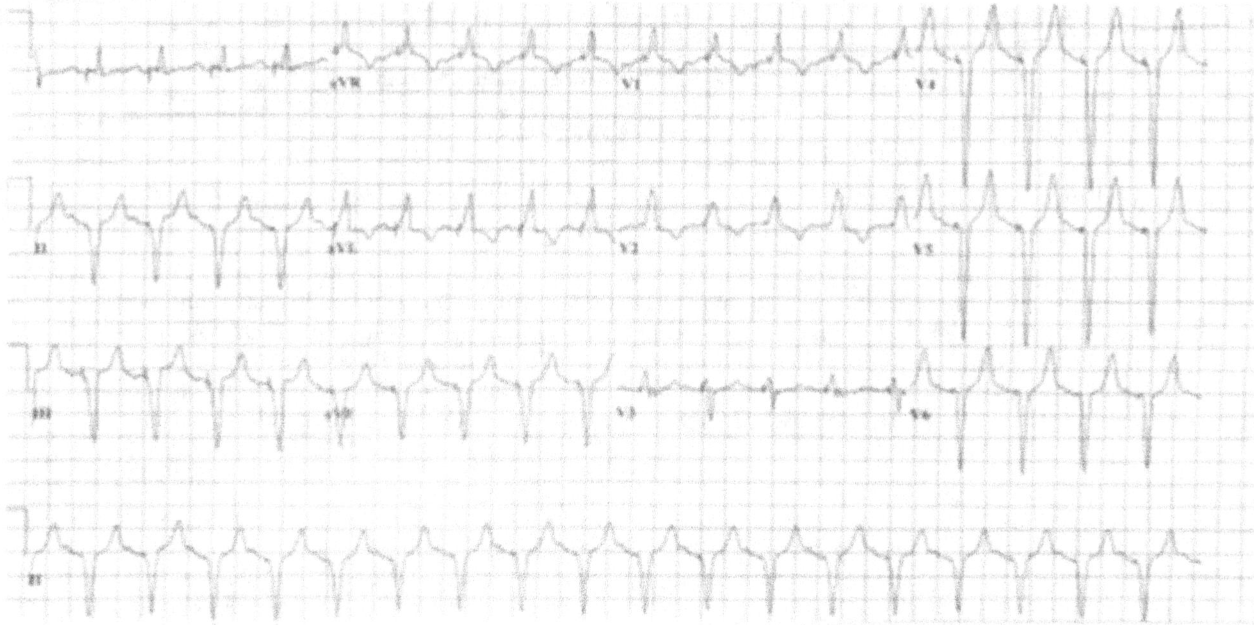

Figure 1. Electrocardiogram, recorded at the time of presentation, showing atrial-sensed ventricular-paced rhythm, biventricular pacemaker, and the total 12-lead QRS voltage of 152 mm.

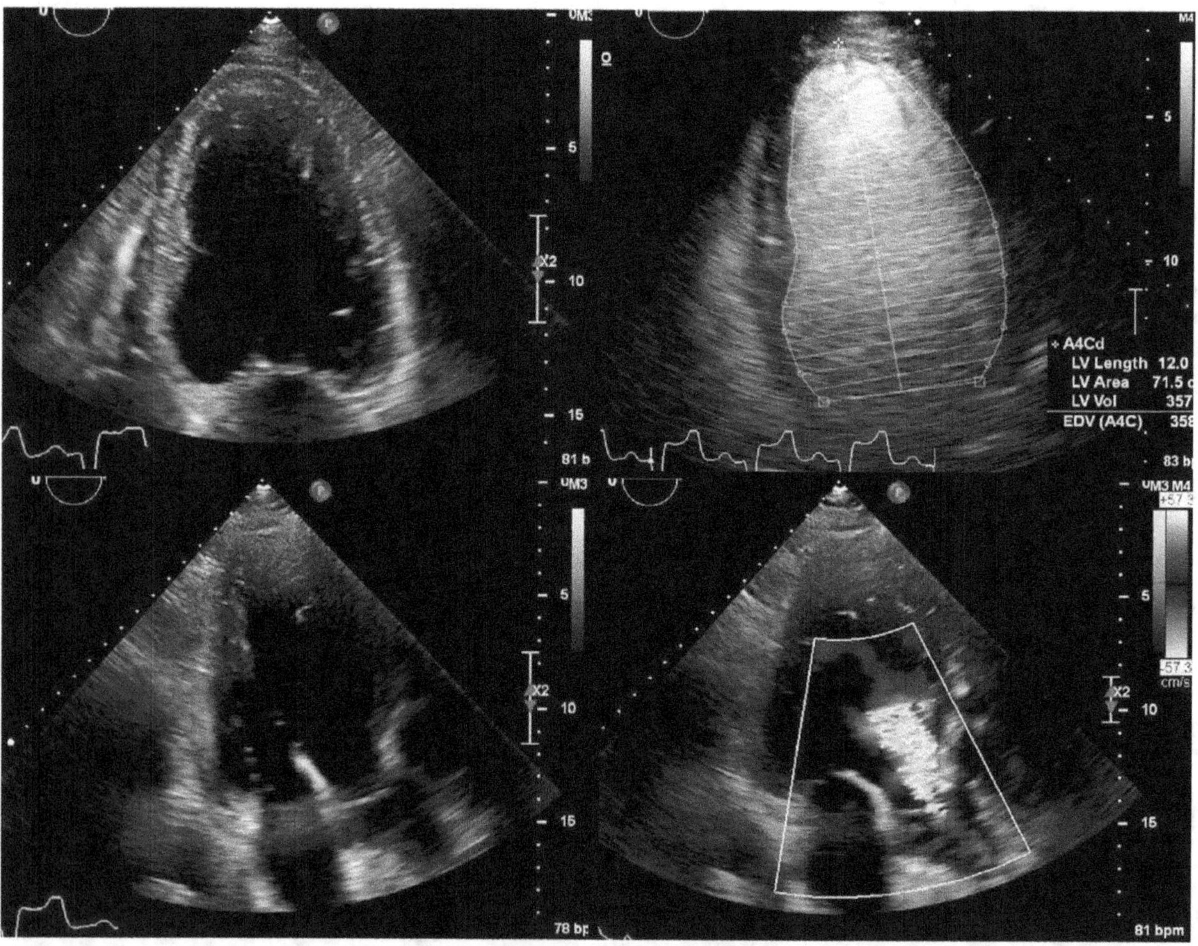

Figure 2. *Top left*: Apical 4-chamber view showing severely dilated, elongated left ventricle (LV) with normal right ventricular (RV) size and systolic function. An ICD lead is seen in the RV (arrow). *Top right*: Apical 4-chamber end-diastolic frame with ultrasound contrast. LV end-diastolic volume was 358 ml with LVEF 19% by biplane Simpson's method. *Bottom left*: Apical long-axis view showing severely thickened, restricted anterior mitral leaflet (yellow arrow). The posterior leaflet (white arrow) was of normal thickness and motion. *Bottom right*: Apical long-axis view with color Doppler imaging showing severe aortic regurgitation (AR).

Table 1
Pertinent admission laboratory findings in the patient described

B-type natriuretic peptide (pg/ml)	1895
Creatinine (mg/dl)	18
Blood urea nitrogen (mg/dl)	77
Estimated GFR (ml/min/1.73 m^2)	3
Sodium (meq/L)	136
Potassium (meq/L)	5.2
Calcium (mg/dl)	8.7
Magnesium (mg/dl)	2.2
Phosphorous (mg/dl)	2.0
Total cholesterol (mg/dl)	219
Low density lipoprotein cholesterol (mg/dl)	151
High density lipoprotein cholesterol (mg/dl)	35
Triglyceride (mg/dl)	241
Hemoglobin A1c (%)	5.8
Rheumatic factor ([IU]/ml)*	8
ANA*	Negative
HLA-B 27*	Negative
C-reactive protein (mg/dl)*	0.5

GFR = glomerular filtration rate.

* Test performed 6 months after the orthotopic heart transplant.

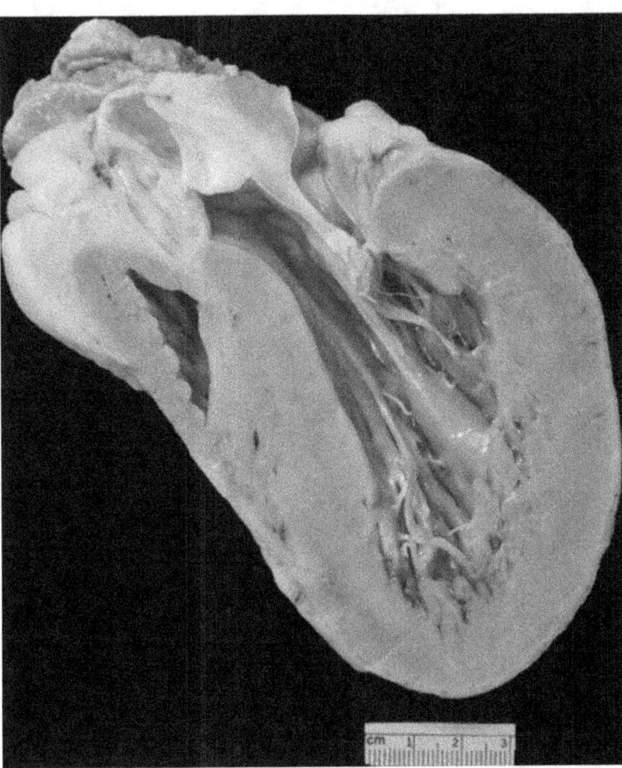

Figure 3. Shown here is the heart of a 48-year-old man showing a dilated ventricular cavity with thickened left ventricular walls, enlarged papillary muscles, and thickened anterior mitral leaflet. The posterior mitral leaflet is normal (not thickened).

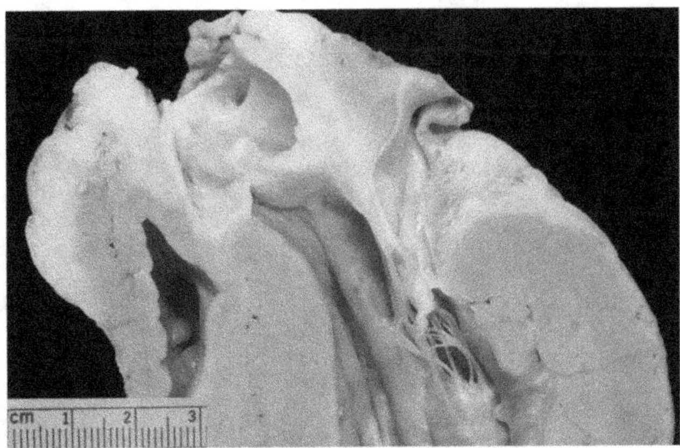

Figure 4. Shown here is a closer view of the mitral and aortic valve showing the remarkably thickened anterior mitral leaflet which is extending into the base of the posterior aortic valve cusp. The posterior mitral leaflet is normal.

absence of thickening of the posterior mitral leaflet as shown in the present patient is diagnostic (Figure 5). Although all 8 patients (all men) with ankylosing spondylitis studied by Buckley and Roberts[1] at necropsy had extremely severe aortic regurgitation, only one of the 187 patients with ankylosing spondylitis studied clinically by Klingberg et al[4] had "severe" aortic regurgitation; 24 others had "mild", and 9 had "moderate" aortic regurgitation.

Interview of the patient and his wife 3 months after the OHT revealed that the patient indeed had had low back pain periodically for years, but he attributed it to his kidney disease rather than to the arthritic problem. Thus, the cardiac features of ankylosing spondylitis in this patient probably appeared after the clinical onset of his orthopedic back problem. Lateral chest radiograph, however, did not show changes of ankylosing spondylitis.

The dense fibrous tissue — characteristic of ankylosing spondylitis — was present in the membranous ventricular septum just above the location of the atrioventricular node and its presence in that location appears to be the cause of the patient's complete heart block diagnosed initially about 2 years before the OHT.

We were unable to find a previous publication of a patient with ankylosing spondylitis having an OHT.

Disclosures

The authors have no conflicts of interest to disclose.

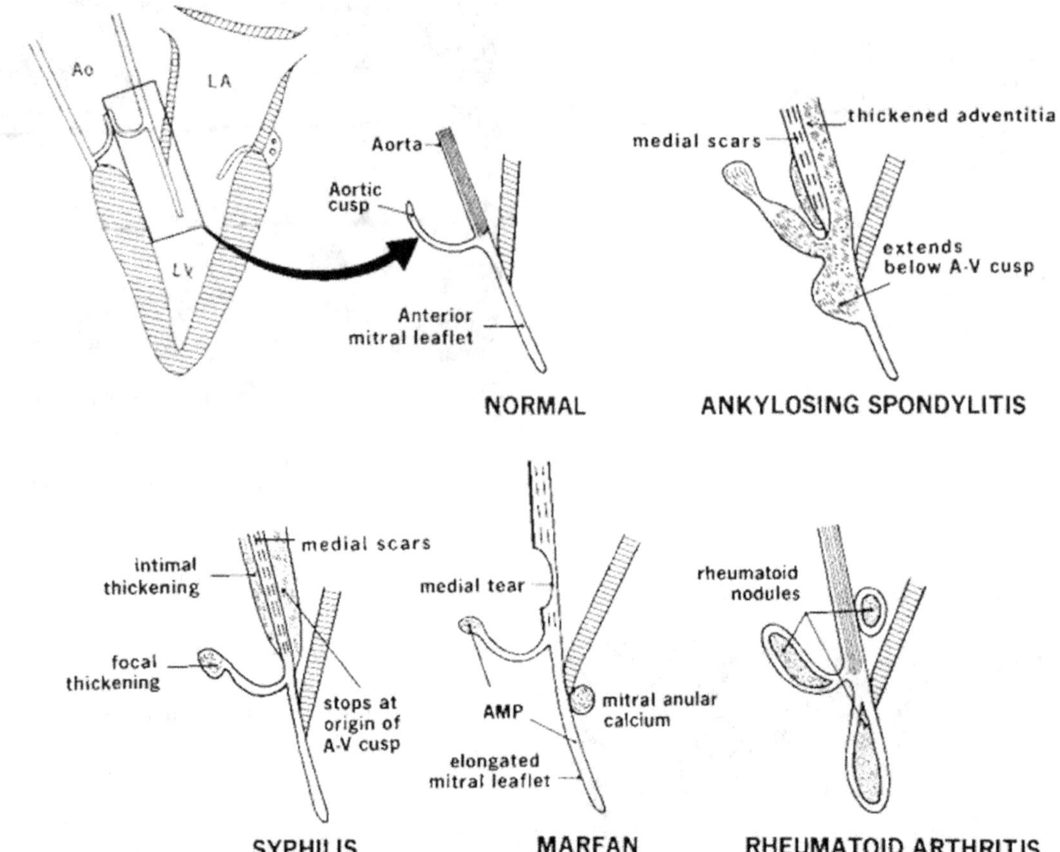

Figure 5. Diagram showing the distinctive morphologic features of 4 different cardiac conditions including *ankylosing spondylitis*. In *cardiovascular syphilis*, the aortic wall behind the sinuses of Valsalva is spared and the adventitial scar tissue does not extend below the aortic valve or involve mitral valve or ventricular septum. Only the distal margins of the aortic valve cusps are thickened in syphilis, not the proximal portions which are always involved in ankylosing spondylitis. In *rheumatoid arthritis*, the distinctive nodules similar to subcutaneous nodules, may infiltrate pericardium, myocardium and mural and valvular endocardium. If the valvular tissue is involved, regurgitation usually of only mild degree results. In the *Marfan syndrome*, aortic regurgitation is a consequence of disease of aortic wall, not of aortic valve; the aorta is thinner, and usually contains intimal-medial tears. The ascending aorta is diffusely involved, and dilatation of the aortic root causes the aortic regurgitation, which is usually severe. The mitral and rarely the aortic valve cusps may be redundant in patients with the Marfan syndrome.

Abbreviations: Ao = aorta; A-V = atrioventricular; LA = left atrium; LV = left ventricle.

Reproduced with permission from the authors and the publisher.[1]

1. Bulkley BH, Roberts WC. Ankylosing spondylitis and aortic regurgitation. Description of the characteristic cardiovascular lesion from study of eight necropsy patients. *Circulation* 1973;48:1014–1027.
2. Roberts WC, Hollingsworth JF, Bulkley BH, Jaffe RB, Epstein SE, Stinson EB. Combined mitral and aortic regurgitation in ankylosing spondylitis. Angiographic and anatomic features. *Am J Med* 1974;56:237–243.
3. Roberts WC, Filardo G, Ko JM. Comparison of total 12-lead QRS voltage in a variety of cardiac conditions and its usefulness in predicting increased cardiac mass. *Am J Cardiol* 2013;112:904–909.
4. Klingberg E, Sveälv BG, Täng MS, Bech-Hanssen O, Forsblad-D'Elia H, Bergfeldt L. Aortic regurgitation is common in ankylosing spondylitis: Time for routine echocardiography evaluation? *Am J Med* 2015;128:1244–1250.